Neuroanatomy Basics:
A Clinical Guide

Neuroanatomy Basics: A Clinical Guide

Mohammad Hassan A. Noureldine, MD
Neurosurgery Resident
Department of Neurosurgery
Lecturer, Neuroanatomy
Gilbert and Rose-Marie Chagoury School of Medicine
Lebanese American University
Byblos, Lebanon
Neuroimaging, MS Student
Faculty of Medical Sciences
Lebanese University
Beirut, Lebanon

ELSEVIER

ELSEVIER

7th Circle, Zahran Plaza, 7th Floor, PO Box 140825, Amman, 11814, Jordan

Neuroanatomy Basics: A Clinical Guide, by Mohammad Hassan A. Noureldine

Copyright © 2017 Elsevier.

ISBN: 978-0-7020-7542-1
e-ISBN: 978-0-7020-7543-8

Notices

Knowledge and best practice in this field are constantly changing. As new research and experience broaden our understanding, changes in research methods, professional practices, or medical treatment may become necessary.

Practitioners and researchers must always rely on their own experience and knowledge in evaluating and using any information, methods, compounds, or experiments described herein. In using such information or methods they should be mindful of their own safety and the safety of others, including parties for whom they have a professional responsibility.

With respect to any drug or pharmaceutical products identified, readers are advised to check the most current information provided (i) on procedures featured or (ii) by the manufacturer of each product to be administered, to verify the recommended dose or formula, the method and duration of administration, and contraindications. It is the responsibility of practitioners, relying on their own experience and knowledge of their patients, to make diagnoses, to determine dosages and the best treatment for each individual patient, and to take all appropriate safety precautions.

To the fullest extent of the law, neither the Publisher nor the authors, contributors, or editors, assume any liability for any injury and/or damage to persons or property as a matter of product liability, negligence or otherwise, or from any use or operation of any methods, products, instructions, or ideas contained in the material herein.

Although all advertising material is expected to conform to ethical (medical) standards, inclusion in this publication does not constitute a guarantee or endorsement of the quality or value of such product or of the claims made of it by its manufacturer.

Content Strategist: Rasheed Roussan
Sr Project Manager—Education Solutions: Shabina Nasim
Content Development Specialist: Amani Bazzari
Project Manager: Nayagi Athmanathan
Cover Designer: Milind Majgaonkar

Printed in India

Dedication

To Fatima and Ahmad . . .
My beloved parents who have always been the inspiration
to every achievement.

To Ali, Wared, Hussein, Mariam, and the youngest,
Nour Al Zahraa . . .
My siblings, the best you could ever get!

Mohammad Hassan

Contributors

Abeer J. Hani, MD
Assistant Professor of Pediatrics and Neurology
Gilbert and Rose-Marie Chagoury School of
Medicine
Lebanese American University
Byblos, Lebanon

Ahmad Sweid, MD
Neurosurgery Resident
Department of Neurosurgery
Gilbert and Rose-Marie Chagoury School of
Medicine
Lebanese American University
Byblos, Lebanon

Ali A. Haydar, MD
Gilbert and Rose-Marie Chagoury School of
Medicine
Lebanese American University
Byblos, Lebanon

Amanah Abraham, MS
Researcher in Medical Sciences
Tulane Medical Center
Tulane University
New Orleans, LA, USA

George Jallo, MD
Professor of Neurosurgery, Pediatrics and Oncology
Director, Institute for Brain Protection Sciences
Chief, Division of Pediatric Neurosurgery
Johns Hopkins All Children's Hospital
St. Petersburg, Florida, USA

Jade Nehmé, MD
Ear, Nose and Throat (ENT) Surgeon
Department of Otorhinolaryngology, Head and
Neck Surgery
Lebanese University
Beirut, Lebanon

Michel Kmeid, MD
Ear, Nose and Throat (ENT) Resident
Department of Otorhinolaryngology, Head and
Neck Surgery
Lebanese University
Beirut, Lebanon

Mohammad Hassan A. Noureldine, MD
Neurosurgery Resident
Department of Neurosurgery
Lecturer, Neuroanatomy
Gilbert and Rose-Marie Chagoury School of
Medicine
Lebanese American University
Byblos, Lebanon
Neuroimaging, MS Student
Faculty of Medical Sciences
Lebanese University
Beirut, Lebanon

Mohammad Shehade, MD
Neurosurgeon
Instructor, Neuroanatomy
Gilbert and Rose-Marie Chagoury School of
Medicine
Lebanese American University
Byblos, Lebanon

Nabil Moukarzel, MD
Chief, Department of Otorhinolaryngology,
Head and Neck Surgery
Lebanese University
Beirut, Lebanon
Adjunct Assistant Professor
Gilbert and Rose-Marie Chagoury School of
Medicine
Lebanese American University
Byblos, Lebanon

Naji Riachi, MD
Associate Professor of Neurology
Head, Division of Neurology and
EEG Laboratories
Gilbert and Rose-Marie Chagoury School of
Medicine
Lebanese American University
Byblos, Lebanon

Nour Estaitieh, MD
Neurologist
Department of Neurology
Rafic Hariri University Hospital
Beirut, Lebanon

Rajiv Iyer, MD
Neurosurgery Resident
Department of Neurosurgery
The Johns Hopkins University School of Medicine
Baltimore, MD, USA

Rechdi Ahdab, MD, PhD
Associate Professor of Neurology
Gilbert and Rose-Marie Chagoury School of
Medicine
Lebanese American University
Byblos, Lebanon

Samar S. Ayache, MD, PhD
Associate Professor of Clinical Neurophysiology
Faculty of Medicine, Paris-Est University
Department of Clinical Neurophysiology
Henri Mondor Hospital
Creteil, France
Adjunct Associate Professor of Neurology
Gilbert and Rose-Marie Chagoury School of
Medicine
Lebanese American University
Byblos, Lebanon

Reviewers

Abeer J. Hani, MD
Assistant Professor of Pediatrics and Neurology
Gilbert and Rose-Marie Chagoury School of
Medicine
Lebanese American University
Byblos, Lebanon

George Jallo, MD
Professor of Neurosurgery,
Pediatrics and Oncology
Director, Institute for Brain
Protection Sciences
Chief, Division of Pediatric Neurosurgery
Johns Hopkins All Children's Hospital
St. Petersburg, Florida, USA

Ibrahim Saikali, MD, FRCSC
Associate Professor of Neurosurgery
Program Director, Department of Neurosurgery
Gilbert and Rose-Marie Chagoury School of
Medicine
Lebanese American University
Byblos, Lebanon

Naji Riachi, MD
Associate Professor of Neurology
Head, Division of Neurology and
EEG Laboratories
Gilbert and Rose-Marie Chagoury School of
Medicine
Lebanese American University
Byblos, Lebanon

Pallab K. Ganguly, MBBS, MD, FACA
Professor and Chairman of Anatomy
College of Medicine
Alfaisal University
Kingdom of Saudi Arabia

Rechdi Ahdab, MD, PhD
Associate Professor of Neurology
Gilbert and Rose-Marie Chagoury School of
Medicine
Lebanese American University
Byblos, Lebanon

Samar S. Ayache, MD, PhD
Associate Professor of Clinical Neurophysiology
Faculty of Medicine, Paris-Est University
Department of Clinical Neurophysiology
Henri Mondor Hospital
Creteil, France
Adjunct Associate Professor of Neurology
Gilbert and Rose-Marie Chagoury School of
Medicine
Lebanese American University
Byblos, Lebanon

Waleed M. Renno
Professor of Anatomy
Department of Anatomy
Faculty of Medicine
Health Science Center
Kuwait University
Kuwait

Youssef G. Comair, MD, FRCSC
Professor of Neurosurgery
Clemenceau Medical Center
Beirut, Lebanon
Adjunct Professor of Neurosurgery
Baylor College of Medicine
Houston, Texas, USA

Foreword

Learning neuroanatomy has been traditionally one of the most challenging parts of a medical curriculum, particularly for the students who had little exposure to the fundamentals of neuroscience during their high school and college years. Traditional medical school curricula have a 2-year preclinical preparation where neuroanatomy teaching could be spread along several months and absorbed slowly by the students; neuroanatomy is reviewed again when the student is confronted by the elements of neurology and neurosurgery. Modern curricula that are system or organ based require that all of the neuroscience, from embryology to neurology and psychiatry, be taught in one module. This module is likely the most taxing of the entire medical years. Students initially attracted to the study of the nervous system become discouraged and disenchanted with the disciplines of neurology and neurosurgery. This situation was acutely experienced at the Lebanese American University (LAU) Gilbert and Rose-Marie Chagoury School of Medicine; many gifted students found the neuroscience module unattractive and unrewarding. Chief among their complaints was the neuroanatomy part that was difficult to absorb. The task of the teaching faculty was equally problematic; reducing the neuroanatomy material was perceived as inappropriate and could not procure the students with the necessary preparation needed for their career. In order to comply with the content of the neuroscience module, students adopted as a learning tool the texts that were simplistic and reduced neuroanatomy to cartoons, much to the chagrin of their mentors.

Mohammad Hassan A. Noureldine was one of the students struggling to balance the demands of the curriculum. He viewed all neuroanatomy texts as a 'bottom-down', somewhat anachronic and not keeping up with the self-learning expectations of the curriculum. He decided to create a text for the students by the students. Along the way, he found that mentors are still needed. Therefore, several contributors to the neuroanatomy teaching at LAU were requested to contribute by guiding the write-up and writing/reviewing chapters. This has resulted in the most balanced text that is amply and judiciously illustrated. I believe that one of the most important features of this book is the experiment that it has initiated, where a student is rethinking the process of medical education and becoming a true educator. With this, I believe it is a start of a 'mission accomplished'.

I acknowledge the exceptional contribution of a colleague and friend, Professor George Jallo, who has very kindly demonstrated his unique experience in the surgery of the brainstem by contributing a chapter and reviewing several others.

Youssef G. Comair, MD, FRCSC
Professor of Neurosurgery
Clemenceau Medical Center
Beirut, Lebanon
Adjunct Professor of Neurosurgery
Baylor College of Medicine
Houston, Texas, USA

Preface

This book serves as a guide for medical students and for other health care professionals studying basic neuroanatomy. Practitioners in all health care fields are encouraged to learn the basic anatomy of the different organ systems, since this establishes a base for a good understanding of the normal physiology, as well as pathologies of the human body. The nervous system is unique; the delicate and very well-organized structure obliges specific functions at different hierarchical levels.

Studying for the neuroanatomy course requires special considerations, some of which are as follows:

(1) Neuroanatomy is a relatively dry material where many structures are described anatomically but their clinical relevance is not elucidated yet.

(2) Unless students enrol in a neuroscience programme, there is minimal exposure to neuroanatomy in the undergraduate years of study. Thus, medical students literally 'suffer' while studying for neuroanatomy in the preclinical medical years as well as while preparing for standardized exams.

(3) The organ-based system of modules covering medical disciplines other than the neuroscience module in the first two medical years does not allow sufficient time to be allocated for studying neuroanatomy for the first time.

(4) Compared to the anatomy of other organ systems, neuroanatomy is a vast discipline and cannot be studied in one course and at one time. The decision of what to and what not to include in the course tailored to medical students remains a matter of debate.

This book primarily demonstrates the student perspective and is a fruit of the self-learning process that is very much encouraged in modern teaching curricula. Among the goals of medical education is graduating future physicians who are equally scholars, researchers, self-learners and health care leaders as much as excellent clinicians.

Although several neuroanatomy references are already published, this book has been prepared to fill the teaching gaps where other books failed. It is heavily illustrated, clinically oriented with clinical correlations pertaining to most of the described anatomical structures, and relatively short in terms of content, yet comprehensive in terms of what medical students should learn at their level.

It is important to note that feedback on the preparation of this book was sought from medical students as well as from experienced professors in the neuroscience field; the approach, style and extent of this book are a result of the successful implementation of thoughts from both parties, the student and the instructor.

Mohammad Hassan A. Noureldine, MD

Acknowledgement

I extend my sincerest thanks to the contributors of the first edition; their support was endless and went beyond the preparation of their corresponding chapters. I am greatly in debt to them and could not have completed this work without their contribution to the write-up and cross-review of the book contents, as well as their continuous advising through every phase of preparing this book.

Special thanks goes on to my family, especially mom and dad, who were very supportive and understanding when I broke the 'pleasant routine' of meeting up with family members at our home village on weekends during the preparation of this edition; they realized it was a sacrifice that was, with no doubt, worth it!

Most of all, many thanks to Elsevier staff who were closely following up on every detail since the first contact up until the day of publishing, especially Mr Rasheed Roussan, Senior Content Strategist; Ms Shabina Nasim, Senior Project Manager; Mr Shravan Kumar and Ms Amani Bazzari, Content Development Specialists; Ms Nayagi Athmanathan, Project Manager; and Mr Milind Majgaonkar, Cover Designer.

Mohammad Hassan A. Noureldine, MD

Contents

CHAPTER 1

Microstructural Organization – Cellular Level

Mohammad Hassan A. Noureldine

CASE STUDY

Presentation and Physical Examination: A 27-year-old previously healthy female presented to the neurology unit complaining of right leg instability causing her to fall several times during the past week. She also reported changes in sensation over the left side of her body. Two days prior to presentation, her symptoms significantly worsened after spending an hour in sauna and she developed intolerable tremors and fatigue, which disappeared in the next morning. Previous history revealed right-eye vision problems dating back to 10 months prior to consultation where she had a sudden partial loss of vision accompanied by pain. Although her vision had improved, she noticed that colours seem to be 'washed out' when looking with the right eye compared to the left. On examination, the patient was anxious. Right upper quadrant vision was impaired, whereas funduscopic examination and the remaining cranial nerves (CNs) were normal. Sensory exam showed decreased touch, pinprick and pain sensations over the left face and body and decreased vibration sensations over the distal lower extremities bilaterally. Motor power was decreased in the right leg without apparent spasticity. Ankle and knee-deep tendon reflexes were increased on both sides (3+). Babinski sign was present bilaterally. Tandem gait was impaired. Dysdiadochokinesia was noted on the right hand.

Diagnosis, Management and Follow-Up: Brain magnetic resonance imaging (MRI) showed multifocal hyperintense lesions on T2 sequence suggesting demyelination (Fig. 1.1). Lesions affected the white matter and were mostly located around the lateral ventricles and in the corpus callosum. Lumbar puncture was performed, and cerebrospinal fluid analysis revealed the presence of oligoclonal bands and high immunoglobulin G (IgG) index. Visual evoked potential revealed conduction abnormalities in the right optic nerve.

A preliminary diagnosis of **multiple sclerosis (MS)** was evoked, and the patient was treated with high doses of intravenous methylprednisone. Symptoms improved over the following week. Subsequent follow-up led to the diagnosis of the relapsing–remitting subtype of MS, and the patient was started on a disease-modifying agent (DMA).

Try to guess the pathophysiology, clinical features, management and prognosis of MS after studying this chapter!

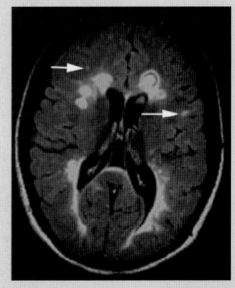

FIGURE 1.1 MRI of brain lesions of a patient with multiple sclerosis. The large lesions appear as nodes and rings. The arrows point to small lesions.
Source: *Brody T, PhD. Endpoints in immune diseases. Clinical trials: study design, endpoints and biomarkers, drug safety, and FDA and ICH guidelines. p. 355–67, Chapter 19.*

BRIEF INTRODUCTION

The complex function of the human nervous system necessitates the presence of finely tuned structures and highly organized patterns of specialized cells.

- The cellular components of the central nervous system (CNS) comprise a wide spectrum of cell types.
- Nerve fibres carry specific messages between different regions of the nervous system and from the nervous system to peripheral organs in the form of electrical impulses.
- Accurate processing of electrical impulses occurs at microstructures acting as checkpoints that allow or prevent signal transmission.
- The blood–brain and blood–cerebrospinal fluid (CSF) barriers ensure complete separation of the nervous system from the peripheral milieu.

This chapter aims at introducing the microstructural anatomy of the nervous system and correlates it to some of the pathological processes that occur at the cellular level.

THE NEURON: BASIC CONCEPTS

Neurons are specialized, excitable cells that function by processing and transmitting information through electrical and chemical impulses.

Morphology (Fig. 1.2)
Typically, a neuron cell consists of three components: (1) **cell body** or **soma**, (2) **dendrites**, i.e. highly branched thin extensions of the soma and (3) **axon**, i.e. an extension of the soma arising at a site called the axon hillock and travelling distances that may reach as long as 1 m.

Nissl Substance (Fig. 1.3)
- Specific to neuronal cells
- Has a granular structure
- Composed of stacks of **rough endoplasmic reticulum** interfering with free polysomes in rosettes
- Located in the soma and dendrites but not the axons
- Neuronal proteins are synthesized in the Nissl substance, many of which travel along the axon towards the **terminal bouton** (synaptic endings)

Axonal Transport (Fig. 1.4)
Mechanisms of axonal transport are essential to maintain the health as well as the function of neuronal cells.

- **Anterograde transport** refers to the movement of organelles and molecules (secretory and cytoskeletal proteins) from the soma to the axonal terminals.
  - Newly synthesized vesicles containing **neurotransmitter precursors**, among other elements that are essential for neurotransmission, are

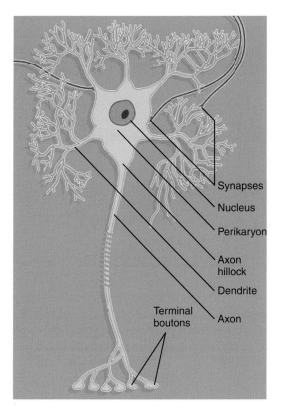

FIGURE 1.2   The neuron consists of a large cell body containing the nucleus surrounded by cytoplasm, known as the perikaryon. Processes of two types extend from the cell body, namely a single axon and one or more dendrites. Dendrites are highly branched tapering processes which either end in specialized sensory receptors (as in primary sensory neurons) or form synapses with neighbouring neurons from which they receive stimuli. In general, dendrites function as the major sites of information input into the neuron. Each neuron has a single axon arising from a cone-shaped portion of the cell body called the axon hillock. The axon is a cylindrical process up to 1 m in length, terminating on other neurons or effector organs by way of a variable number of small branches, which end in small swellings called terminal boutons.
Source: *Young B, BSc Med Sci (Hons), PhD, MB BChir, MRCP, FRCPA. Nervous tissues. Wheater's functional histology. p. 122–42, Chapter 7.*

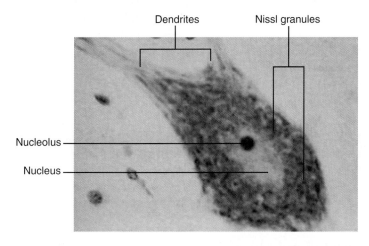

FIGURE 1.3   A spinal motor neuron cell body. Cresyl violet (a basophilic dye) stain shows prominent Nissl granules.
Source: *Crossman AR, PhD DSc. Cells of the nervous system. Neuroanatomy: an illustrated colour text. p. 32–5, Chapter 2.*

rapidly transported **(fast anterograde, 100–400 mm/day)** to the terminal bouton.

■ **Cytosolic and cytoskeletal elements** are relatively slow **(slow anterograde, 1–8 mm/day).**

■ **Kinesins** direct the anterograde movement and microtubules carry the molecules/organelles.

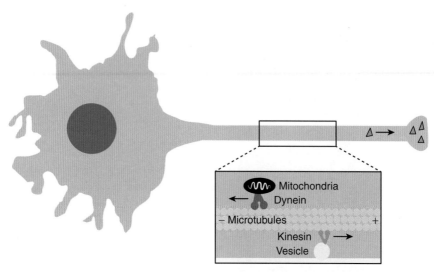

FIGURE 1.4   Basic mechanisms of axonal transport. In healthy neurons, anterograde axonal transport (towards the nerve terminal) is performed by the microtubule plus-end-directed motor kinesin, whereas the minus-end-directed motor dynein is responsible for retrograde transport (towards the cell body). In general, newly synthesized proteins and synaptic vesicles are transported in the anterograde direction, recycling organelles such as endosomes and lysosomes in the retrograde direction and mitochondria in both directions. Source: *Lamberts JT. Spreading of α-synuclein in the face of axonal transport deficits in Parkinson's disease: a speculative synthesis. Neurobiol Dis 77:276–83.*

- **Retrograde transport** is similar to the fast anterograde transport but occurs in the opposite direction (from the terminal bouton to the soma).
  - Carries nerve growth factors, endocytic vesicles and degradation products back to the cell
  - Occurs at a relatively **slow speed (100–200 mm/day)**
  - Is directed by the action of **dyneins**

CLINICAL INSIGHT

- **Neurotropic viruses**: Neurotropic viruses such as rabies, polio, tetanus and herpes simplex are carried to the soma by retrograde transport.

Classification

Neurons can be classified on the basis of their
- **Structure**: bipolar, unipolar or pseudo-unipolar and multipolar (Fig. 1.5)
- **Direction of message (or impulse) transmission**: afferent, interneuron and efferent
- **Function**: action (excitatory, inhibitory), production of neurotransmitters (glutamatergic, GABAergic, cholinergic, dopaminergic, etc.) and electro-physiology (pattern of firing)

Bipolar neuron

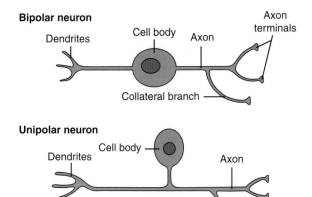

Unipolar neuron

Multipolar neuron

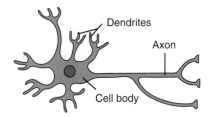

FIGURE 1.5   Types of neurons. There are many different types of neuron, which are shaped according to their function. Bipolar cells are commonly interneurons, whereas unipolar cells tend to be sensory neurons and multipolar cells are often motor neurons. Source: *Lowe JS, BMedSci, BMBS, DM, FRCPath. Nervous tissue. Stevens & Lowe's human histology. p. 84–104, Chapter 6.*

ADDITIONAL CLINICAL INSIGHTS

Pathologies Associated with Histologic Pigments/Inclusions

See Fig. 1.6 and Table 1.1.

CENTRAL NERVOUS SYSTEM

The cerebral and cerebellar microstructures consist of distinct layers where billions of different cell types synapse and interact in a highly organized manner; this interaction would ultimately lead to a well-defined function.

Cerebral Cellular Components (Fig. 1.7)

The structure and function of cerebral cells can be roughly summarized as follows:

Neurons

- The **neocortex** is the largest part of the human cerebral cortex consisting of **six distinctive layers**. Higher brain functions such as spatial and sensory perception, language and thinking are processed in the neocortex. Of the cells found in the neocortical layers, we describe:
  - **Cortical association neurons**, also known as **interneurons**, convey impulses from one neuron to another.

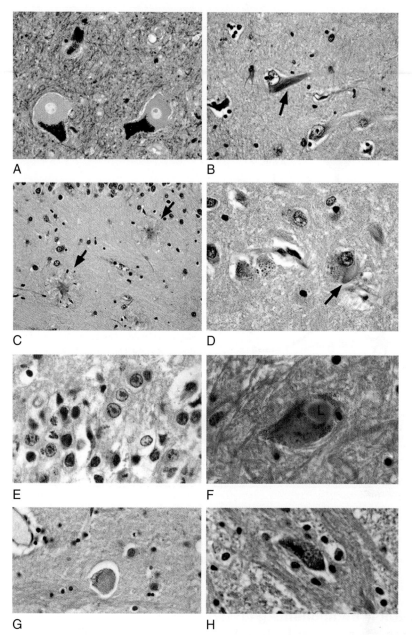

FIGURE 1.6   (A) Lipofuscin granules; (B) neurofibrillary tangles; (C) senile plaques; (D) Hirano bodies; (E) Cowdry type A inclusions; (F) Lewy body (L); (G) Pick bodies; (H) Negri body.

Source: *(A) Bolon B. Nervous system. Haschek and Rousseaux's handbook of toxicologic pathology. p. 2005–93, Chapter 52. (B–D) Brat DJ. Overview of central nervous system anatomy and histology. Neuropathology 1:1–39. (E) Beckham JD. Viral encephalitis and meningitis. Bradley's neurology in clinical practice. p. 1121–46.e4, Chapter 78. (F) Ironside JW. Central and peripheral nervous systems. Underwood's pathology: a clinical approach. p. 674–720, Chapter 26. (G) Ellison D. MD, PhD, MA, MSc, BChir, MRCP(UK), FRC-Path, FRCPCH. Dementias. Neuropathology 31:609–58. (H) Perkin GD. BA, MB, FRCP. Infections. Atlas of clinical neurology. p. 312–42, Chapter 12.*

Table 1.1 List of selected pathologies and the associated typical pigments, deposits and/or inclusions detected on histopathologic specimens

Pathologic Process(es)	Pigments/Inclusions	Localization	Comments
Ageing	Lipofuscin granules	Cytoplasmic	Yellow-brown lipid lysosomal degradation products
Alzheimer disease	Neurofibrillary tangles	Cytoplasmic	Insoluble aggregates of hyperphosphorylated tau, a microtubule-associated protein
	Senile plaques	Extracellular	Deposits of β-amyloid (core) surrounded by neural degradation products
	Hirano bodies	Cytoplasmic	Rod-shaped, eosinophilic aggregates of actin filaments found in the hippocampus
Herpes encephalitis	Cowdry type-A inclusions	Nuclear	Eosinophilic aggregates of nucleic acids and proteins
Parkinson disease and Lewy body dementia	Lewy bodies	Cytoplasmic	Spherical, eosinophilic aggregates of α-synuclein filaments and ubiquitin
Pick disease (frontotemporal dementia)	Pick bodies	Cytoplasmic	Spherical aggregates of straight tau filaments
Rabies	Negri bodies	Cytoplasmic	Eosinophilic aggregates of ribonuclear proteins produced by rabies virus; these aggregates are mostly found in the hippocampus and cerebellum

α, alpha; β, beta.

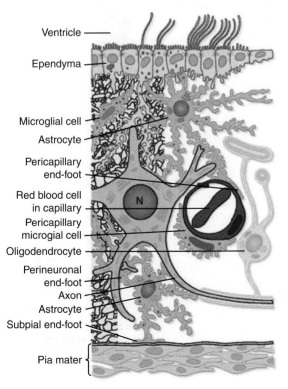

Ventricle
Ependyma
Microglial cell
Astrocyte
Pericapillary end-foot
Red blood cell in capillary
Pericapillary microgial cell
Oligodendrocyte
Perineuronal end-foot
Axon
Astrocyte
Subpial end-foot
Pia mater
N

FIGURE 1.7 Cellular elements of the CNS. Two astrocytes are shown ending on a neuron's soma and dendrites. They also contact the pial surface or capillaries, or both. An oligodendrocyte provides the myelin sheaths for axons. Also shown are microglia and ependymal cells. N, neuron.
Source: *Redrawn from Williams PL, Warwick R. Functional neuroanatomy of man. Edinburgh: Churchill Livingstone; 1975.*

- Large pyramidal cells of Betz, the largest cells in the CNS, are motor neurons with very long axons extending through the corticospinal tract to the anterior horn of the spinal cord. Their cell bodies are located in the fifth layer of the neocortex.

CLINICAL INSIGHT

- **Amyotrophic lateral sclerosis**
  - Betz cells, in addition to other pyramidal cells in the primary motor cortex and the anterior horn cells of the spinal cord, undergo degeneration in a debilitating motor neuron disease called amyotrophic lateral sclerosis.

- Retinal ganglion cells
  - Are located in the **ganglion cell layer** of the retina.
  - Receive visual information from the photoreceptors (rods and cons).
  - Relay electrical impulses to brain visual centres by their long axons that converge to form the **optic nerves**.
- Olfactory receptor/sensory neurons
  - Are highly sensitive ciliated cells located at the **roof of the nose**.
  - Are **bipolar** in shape, with dendrites extending to the nasal cavity.
  - Their unmyelinated axons pass through the **cribriform plate** and form the **olfactory nerve** that reaches the olfactory bulb.

Neuroglia

Neuroglia are non-neuronal cells of the nervous system with variable supportive and protective functions. They essentially consist of:
- Oligodendrocytes
  - Are large glial cells found only in the CNS.
  - Produce **myelin**, a modified plasma membrane composed of a mixture of proteins and phospholipids, which wraps around axons in a **spiral sheath-like** structure.
    - **Myelination** occurs rapidly from infancy through childhood and is responsible for the appearance of many developmental milestones such as crawling and walking.
    - Myelin functions as an insulator, leading to a **saltatory** rather than continuous electrical conduction over nerve fibres. Action potentials 'jump' between nonmyelinated spaces known as **nodes of Ranvier**. This significantly increases the speed of conduction of action potentials.
  - Have extensive processes that may extend and myelinate as many as **20–30 neuronal axons** simultaneously.
  - Are subdivided into two types:
    - **Interfascicular oligodendrocytes:** Arranged in rows between nerve fibres and fascicles of the CNS white matter.
    - **Perineuronal oligodendrocytes:** Found next to somata of grey matter neurons.

CLINICAL INSIGHT

- **Oligodendrocyte injury**
  - In immunocompromised patients, the John Cunningham (JC) virus infects oligo-dendrocytes leading to **progressive multifocal leukoencephalopathy**.
  - Oligodendrocytes, and eventually myelin sheaths and neuronal axons, are damaged in demyelinating diseases such as **MS**.

- **Microglia**
  - Are the **smallest** of all neuroglia.
  - Their embryologic origin is **mesoderm** in contrast to other neuroglia, which originate from ectoderm.
  - Are generated from monocytes and considered as the **CNS phagocytes**.
  - Are activated by degenerative or infectious processes of the CNS.
- **Astrocytes**
  - Are **star-shaped** cells with multiple foot processes extending from the soma in a radial fashion and surrounding synapses, neurons and capillaries; these processes form the external and internal limiting membranes of the CNS.
  - Can be identified by A_2B_5 **monoclonal antibodies** and are **glial fibrillary acidic protein (GFAP)** and **glutamine synthetase** positive.
  - Are divided into two types:
    - **Fibrous astrocytes:** Mostly located in the white matter of the CNS, surrounding myelinated nerve fibres.
    - **Protoplasmic astrocytes:** Mostly located in the grey matter of the CNS, surrounding neurons and proximal ends of unmyelinated fibres.
  - Proliferate and occupy areas of neuronal injury; they are involved in **gliosis**, i.e. scarring of CNS tissue.
  - Modulate synaptic transmission through uptake and storage of neurotransmitters such as gamma-aminobutyric acid (GABA), glutamate and serotonin, among others.
- **Ependymal cells**
  - Form the epithelial lining of ventricles, central canal of the spinal cord and choroid plexuses.
  - Produce the **CSF**.
  - Are covered by cilia that beat in a uniform pattern leading to unidirectional flow of CSF; this facilitates the washout of metabolic wastes and the neuronal uptake of nutrients and neurotransmitters.
  - Are connected by **loose desmosomes** between cells surrounding CNS cavities, allowing CSF to diffuse to CNS tissue; and by **tight junctions** between cells lining choroid plexuses, preventing blood constituents from leaking to CSF.
  - **Tanycytes**
    - Are **modified, nonciliated ependymal cells** found in the lining of the floor of the third ventricle.

- Possess **long processes** with large end-feet that contact distant capillaries and neurons.
- Facilitate transport of hormones and neurotransmitters, e.g. transport along the hypothalamic–pituitary axis.

Cerebellar Cellular Components (Fig. 1.8)

Cerebellar cells are organized in **highly distinctive layers and nuclei**. Neuroglia of the cerebellum are essentially the same as those of the cerebrum.

Molecular Layer

- Is the outermost synaptic layer.
- Contains **dendritic extensions of the Purkinje cells,** which reside in the layer just below it.

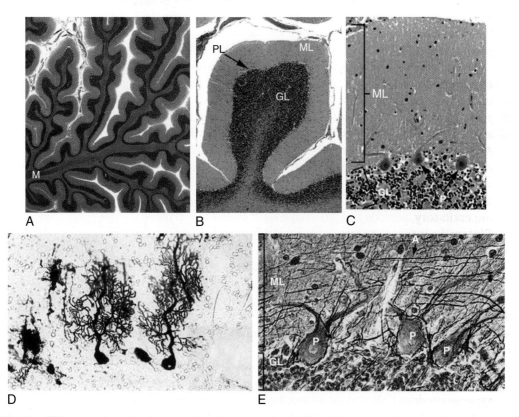

FIGURE 1.8   (A) The cerebellar cortex forms a series of deeply convoluted folds or folia supported by a branching central white matter (M); (B) the cortex is seen to consist of three layers. The outer molecular layer (ML) contains relatively few neurons and large numbers of unmyelinated fibres. The inner granular cell layer (GL) is extremely cellular. Between the two, there is a single layer of huge neurons called Purkinje cells (PL); (C) Purkinje cells (P). They have very large cell bodies, a relatively fine axon extending down through the granular cell layer (GL) and an extensively branching dendritic system which arborizes in the molecular layer (ML); (D) the extraordinary dendritic system of Purkinje cells; (E) the deep granular cell layer of the cortex contains numerous small neurons, the nonmyelinated axons of which pass outwards to the molecular layer where they bifurcate to run parallel to the surface to synapse with the dendrites of Purkinje cells. The axons (A) are stained black and their cell bodies in the granular cell layer GL are counter-stained with neutral red. Source: *Young B, BSc Med Sci (Hons), PhD, MB BChir, MRCP, FRCPA. Central nervous system. Wheater's functional histology. p. 384–401, Chapter 20.*

- **Parallel fibres** run perpendicular to and synapse with the Purkinje dendritic extensions.
- **Basket and stellate cells**
  - Are **inhibitory interneurons**.
  - Form GABAergic synapses onto the dendritic extensions and the initial axonal segments of Purkinje cells.

Purkinje Layer

The **Purkinje layer** is also known as the intermediate discharge layer, where Purkinje somata reside.

- **Purkinje cells**
  - Are large **GABAergic neurons** stacked in a narrow zone.
  - Have extensive dendrites reaching the molecular layer.
  - Have axonal inhibitory projections onto the deep cerebellar nuclei and the vestibular nuclei located in the brainstem.
  - Purkinje axonal projections are the **only motor coordination outputs** from the cerebellum.

Granular Layer

The **granular layer**, i.e. the innermost receptive layer, is relatively thick and densely packed with granule cells.

- **Granule cells**
  - Are very numerous and account for more than two-thirds of the total number of brain cells.
  - Their axons extend vertically to the molecular layer and split into two branches in a T-shaped manner to give rise to **parallel fibres**.
  - Are **excitatory** cells in nature.
  - **Glutamine** is their neurotransmitter.
- **Golgi and brush cells**
  - Are unipolar **interneurons**.
  - Synapse on the granule cells dendrites and inhibit them.

Cerebellar White Matter

The **cerebellar white matter** is essentially similar to the cerebral white matter in that it constitutes nerve fibres and tracts crossing from one area to another.

- **Mossy fibres**
  - Originate from the **spinal cord and pontine nuclei**.
  - Synapse on dendrites of deep cerebellar nuclei cells, granule cells and vestibular nuclei.
  - Have an **excitatory** effect.
- **Glomeruli**
  - Contain **mossy fibre enlargements** called **rosettes** at their centres.
  - Are microstructures, where granule and Golgi cell dendrites interact with mossy fibres.
- **Climbing fibres**
  - Carry **excitatory** inputs from the contralateral **inferior olivary nucleus**, which is located in the medulla oblongata, to Purkinje cells and deep cerebellar nuclei (to a lesser extent).

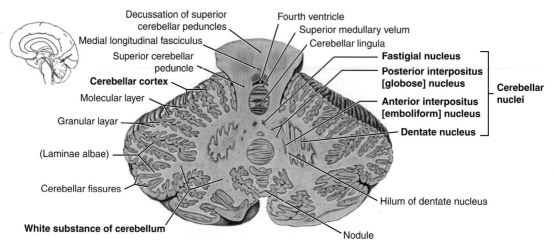

Decussation of superior cerebellar peduncles
Fourth ventricle
Superior medullary velum
Medial longitudinal fasciculus
Cerebellar lingula
Superior cerebellar peduncle
Fastigial nucleus
Cerebellar cortex
Posterior interpositus [globose] nucleus
Molecular layer
Anterior interpositus [emboliform] nucleus
Granular layar
Dentate nucleus
Cerebellar nuclei
(Laminae albae)
Cerebellar fissures
Hilum of dentate nucleus
White substance of cerebellum
Nodule

FIGURE 1.9   Cerebellum with cerebellar nuclei; posterior view. The cerebellum is composed of the white substance of cerebellum (medullary centre) with embedded cerebellar nuclei and the surrounding cerebellar cortex. The oblique section reveals all four cerebellar nuclei in both hemispheres. The dentate nucleus is U-shaped and jagged. Medial to the dentate nucleus lies the anterior interpositus nucleus (emboliform nucleus) and even further medial the posterior interpositus nucleus (globose nucleus), both collectively named interpositus nucleus. Both nuclei share functional similarities and connect with the paravermal and vermal zone of the cerebellum. Located in the medulla of the vermis are the right and left fastigial nucleus, which have close functional connections with the cortex of the flocculonodular lobe.

Source: *Paulsen F. Brain and spinal cord. Sobotta atlas of human anatomy. vol. 3, p. 211–342, Chapter 12.*

Deep Cerebellar Nuclei (Fig. 1.9)

The **deep cerebellar nuclei** constitute distinct collections of neurons embedded in the white matter, around the centre of the cerebellum.

- Each cerebellar hemisphere houses a set of **four nuclei.**
- From lateral to medial and largest to smallest, they are the **dentate, emboliform** and **globose** – collectively known as the **interpositus nucleus** – and **fastigial**.
- Almost all of the cerebellar outputs originate from these nuclei.
- Within each nucleus, most of the **cells are large sized** and use **glutamate.**
- Sparse **smaller cells** are **GABAergic** and project onto the inferior olivary nucleus to counteract the excitatory effect carried on by the climbing fibres.
- Purkinje cell axons synapse on and inhibit the cells of the deep nuclei.

Spinal Cord Cellular Components (Fig. 1.10)

Although it is mainly considered as a highway for tracts crossing from the peripheral body into the brain and vice versa, the spinal cord contains many cell types whose function is to ensure proper relay of neuronal impulses. Distinctive cell types include the following.

Alpha Motor Neurons

Alpha motor neurons, also known as **anterior horn cells,** are located in the anterior (ventral) grey column of the spinal cord.

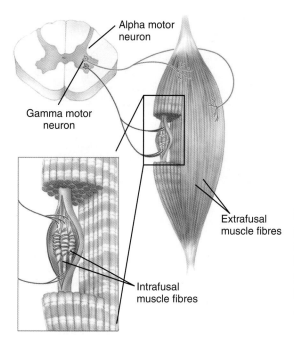

Alpha motor neuron

Gamma motor neuron

Extrafusal muscle fibres

Intrafusal muscle fibres

FIGURE 1.10 The parallel organization of the alpha and gamma lower motor neurons. The alpha motor neuron innervates extrafusal skeletal muscle; the gamma motor neuron innervates the intrafusal muscle fibres to ensure proper sensory feedback from the muscle spindle.
Source: *From Bear MF, Connors BW, Paradiso MA: Neuroscience, Exploring the Brain, 2nd ed. Baltimore, Lippincott Williams & Wilkins, 2001.*

- Are **lower motor neurons**, innervating **extrafusal muscle fibres** and leading to muscle contraction.
- Receive inputs from three main sources: (1) upper motor neurons, (2) interneurons, such as Renshaw cells and (3) sensory neurons

Renshaw Cells
- Are **inhibitory interneurons**.
- Are closely associated with alpha motor neurons and modulate the activity of these cells.

Gamma Motor Neurons
Gamma motor neurons are located in the anterior grey column of the spinal cord.
- Are **lower motor neurons**, innervating **intrafusal muscle fibres** located inside the muscle spindles *(see chapter 5)*.
- Are coactivated along with the alpha motor neurons.
- Keep the muscle spindles tense by detecting changes in muscle stretch during contraction.

PERIPHERAL NERVOUS SYSTEM

Cells
Nerve fibres, rather than cells, account for the largest portion of the peripheral nervous system (PNS). Cells of the PNS are either present in ganglia – clusters of neuron cells outside the CNS – or disseminated along the nerve fibres for supportive or protective functions, and thus considered as the neuroglia of the PNS.

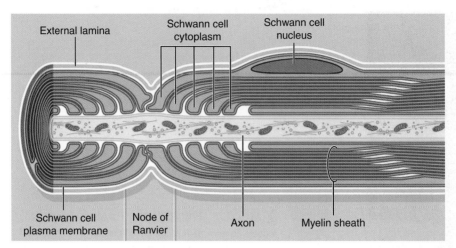

External lamina | Schwann cell cytoplasm | Schwann cell nucleus

Schwann cell plasma membrane | Node of Ranvier | Axon | Myelin sheath

FIGURE 1.11 Schwann cells. Note the manner in which cytoplasmic processes of adjacent Schwann cells interdigitate at the node; also note the continuation of the Schwann cell basement membrane (external lamina) across the node. The myelin sheath prevents the nerve action potential from being propagated continuously along the axon, and the action potential travels by jumping from node to node. This mode of conduction, known as saltatory conduction, greatly enhances the conduction velocity of axons. The internodal length is related to the diameter of the axon and may be up to 1.5 mm in the largest fibre.
Source: *Young B, BSc Med Sci (Hons), PhD, MB BChir, MRCP, FRCPA. Nervous tissues. Wheater's functional histology. p. 122–42, Chapter 7.*

Schwann Cells (Fig. 1.11)

- Are **oligodendrocyte analogues** and have important functions in the PNS.
- Are divided into two subtypes: myelinating and nonmyelinating cells.
  - **Myelinating** cells produce and maintain myelin sheaths around axons; a Schwann cell myelinates **only one axon**, in contrast to an oligodendrocyte that can myelinate around 20–30 axons simultaneously.
  - **Nonmyelinating** as well as myelinating cells encircle nerve axons providing structural, nurturing and protective support.
- Are considered as essential components of the axonal **regeneration** and **re-innervation** process after injuries; they form tunnels that guide sprouting axons towards their targets.

CLINICAL INSIGHT

- **Schwann cell injury**
  - Damage to Schwann cells significantly contributes to the pathophysiology of inherited, acquired and infectious peripheral nerve diseases such as Charcot–Marie–Tooth disease, Guillain–Barre syndrome and leprosy neuropathy.

Satellite Cells (Fig. 1.12)

- Have a very similar role to that of astrocytes in the CNS.
- Form unilayered and multilayered sheaths – connected by gap junctions – that cover the somata of nerve cells located in the autonomic (sympathetic, parasympathetic) and sensory ganglia.

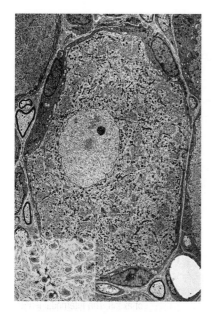

FIGURE 1.12   Satellite cells (Sa) surrounding a single dorsal root ganglion. The inset at the lower left is a light micrograph of part of a dorsal root ganglion, in which the nuclei (arrows) can be seen in flattened satellite cells surrounding individual, much larger, dorsal root ganglion cells (arrowheads).

Source: *Pannese E. Electron micrograph. Neurocytology: fine structure of neurons, nerve processes, and neuroglial cells, New York: Thieme Medical Publishers; 1994. Inset courtesy Dr. Nathaniel T. McMullen, University of Arizona College of Medicine.*

- ▨ Provide a structural support, protective barrier and homeostatic environment to nerve cells inside the ganglia.
- ▨ Are **GFAP, S-100 proteins** and **glutamine synthetase** positive.

CLINICAL INSIGHT

- ■ **Neuropathic pain**: Satellite glial cells are implicated in the development and persistence of neuropathic pain after nerve injury due to secretion of cytokines.

Olfactory Ensheathing Cells [Fig. 1.13]

- ▨ Wrap around the nonmyelinated axons of olfactory cells and provide support and protection to these cells.
- ▨ Are also found in the outer layers of the olfactory bulb inside the CNS.
- ▨ Are similar in function to the nonmyelinated type of Schwann cells.

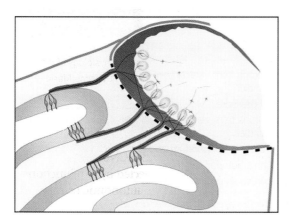

FIGURE 1.13   Anatomy of the primary olfactory nervous system. Primary olfactory neurons (purple) are located in the neuroepithelium (blue) in the nasal cavity. The neurons project axons through the lamina propria (green) to the glomeruli (dark yellow) in the olfactory bulb. As soon as the axons enter the lamina propria, they form fascicles and get enwrapped by olfactory ensheathing glia (OEG) (red). OEG guide them through the cribriform plate (black-dotted line) into the olfactory nerve layer.

Source: *Franssen EHP. Olfactory ensheathing glia: their contribution to primary olfactory nervous system regeneration and their regenerative potential following transplantation into the injured spinal cord. Brain Res Rev 56(1):236–58.*

- Phagocyte debris from dead axons and cells, secrete neurotrophic factors and guide the **regeneration** of severed olfactory axons.
- Are **GFAP, S-100 proteins, p75, nestin** and **vimentin** positive.

Enteric Glial Cells

- Are mostly found within the enteric nervous system, more specifically the **ganglia of the submucosal and myenteric plexuses** but some are also found in the mucosal lamina propria and circular muscles.
- Are involved in a wide spectrum of functions related to the gastrointestinal tract such as motility, protection and mucosal secretion.
- Are activated by synaptic stimulation and may have a role in synaptic transmission.

Classification of Nerve Fibres (Fig. 1.14)

- **Conduction velocity** is the most important variable in the classification of nerve fibres.
- Factors affecting the conduction velocity are fibre **diameter** and **myelination**. As a rule, conduction velocities are highest in large myelinated fibres and lowest in small unmyelinated fibres.
- Nerve fibre diameter and conduction velocity may range from **0.5 to 20 µm** and **0.5 to 120 m/s**, respectively.
- Table 1.2 summarizes the different types of nerve fibres on the basis of both the **sensory classification** and the **motor and sensory classification**.

Table 1.2 Sensory classification and motor and sensory classification of nerve fibres

Type of Fibre	Diameter	Conduction Velocity	Myelin	Function
Sensory Classification				
Ia	++++	++++	Present	Muscle spindle afferents and proprioception (joint position)
Ib	++++	++++	Present	Golgi tendon organ afferents and proprioception
II	+++	+++	Present	Secondary afferents of muscle spindles, touch, pressure and vibration
III	++	+++	Present	Touch, pressure, temperature and fast pain
IV	+	+	Absent	Temperature, slow pain and olfaction
Motor and Sensory Classification				
Aα	++++	++++	Present	α Motoneurons from ventral horn of spinal cord to extrafusal muscle spindles
Aβ	+++	+++	Present	Touch and pressure
Aγ	+++	+++	Present	γ Motoneurons from ventral horn of spinal cord to intrafusal muscle spindles
Aδ	++	+++	Present	Touch, pressure, temperature and fast pain
B	++	+++	Present	Preganglionic autonomic fibres
C	+	+	Absent	Postganglionic autonomic fibres, slow pain and olfaction

Aα, A-alpha; Aβ, A-beta; Aγ, A-gamma; Aδ, A-delta; ++++, large diameter/fast velocity; +++, medium diameter/medium velocity; ++, small diameter; +, smallest diameter/slowest velocity.

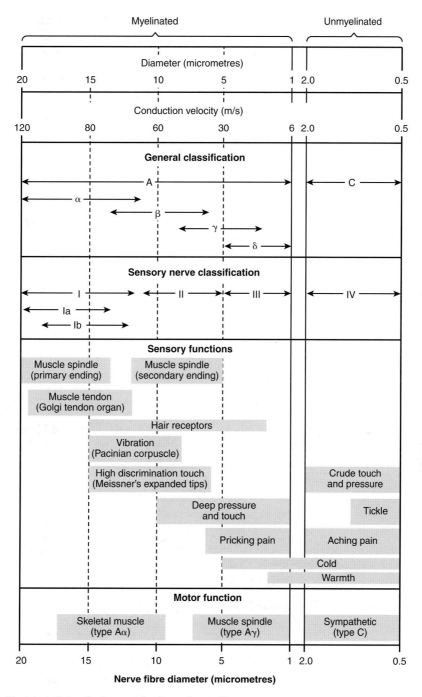

FIGURE 1.14 Physiological classifications and functions of nerve fibres.

Source: *Hall JE, PhD. Sensory receptors, neuronal circuits for processing information. Guyton and Hall textbook of medical physiology. p. 595–606, Chapter 47.*

CLINICAL INSIGHT

■ **Microstructural changes in nervous system injury**

In response to injury, one or more of the following mechanisms take place in the nervous system:

■ **Chromatolysis (Fig. 1.15)**
- The process of degradation of Nissl substance and ultimately apoptosis of the soma; occurs post exposure to any significant injury such as ischaemia, infection, axotomy or toxins

■ **Wallerian (anterograde) degeneration (Fig. 1.16)**
- Refers to degeneration of the **distal segment** of a transected nerve axon, degradation of myelin and invasion of the dead area by Schwann cells and macrophages to clear the debris if it is a PNS injury
- Slowly and less effectively, the clearance of debris in the CNS is performed by microglia transforming into phagocytic cells
- Unlike Schwann cells, oligodendrocytes have no role in CNS injuries
- In the CNS, astrocytes proliferate to fill the dead area in a process known as gliosis, which is similar to the proliferation of fibrocytes in fibrosis

■ **Regeneration (Fig. 1.17)**
- A repair process of injured parts of the nervous system
- Occurs more significantly in the PNS compared to the CNS
- The presence of endoneurium investing axons of nerve cells in the PNS is a key factor in the process of regeneration
- The live, proximal axonal tip sprouts and grows at a rate ranging between **1** and **5 mm/day** by the help of Schwann cells that direct the growth inside the **endoneurial tube**

■ Peripheral nerve injuries are classified into three types (Fig. 1.18):

■ **Neuropraxia**
- Mildest form, leading to **blockage of action potential conduction** and temporary loss of nerve function
- Repetitive or prolonged insult to the nerve causes ischaemia and myelin sheath damage; the nerve itself is not injured
- Wallerian degeneration does not occur
- Full recovery is completed within 2 months

■ **Axonotmesis**
- Results from a **nerve contusion**
- Myelin sheaths and axons are injured, whereas nerve coverings (endoneurium, perineurium and epineurium) are undamaged
- Wallerian degeneration occurs in the distal axonal segment
- Nerve regeneration is initiated post injury and may lead to complete recovery if the distance to the effector organ is relatively short

■ **Neurotmesis**
- Most severe type with **worst prognosis**
- Axons, myelin sheaths and nerve coverings are damaged and Wallerian degeneration ensues
- Partial recovery may occur either spontaneously or by the help of surgery

Denervation atrophy and flaccid paralysis of muscles result from loss of neuronal innervation due to any severe and permanent nerve damage (Fig. 1.16)

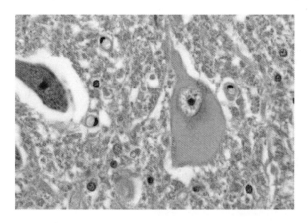

FIGURE 1.15   Neuronal chromatolysis. This neuron shows central chromatolysis. The neuron is swollen with no visible Nissl substance. The nucleus is large, centrally placed with an open chromatin pattern.
Source: *Stevens A, MB BS, FRCPath. Nervous system and muscle. Core pathology. p. 453–94, Chapter 21.*

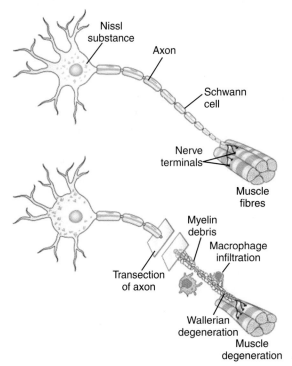

FIGURE 1.16   Wallerian degeneration. After axotomy, axon and myelin sheath distal to transection begin to degenerate. Within a few days, macrophages are recruited into injury site and digest debris. Changes also occur proximal to site of injury. A degree of Wallerian degeneration takes place up to the first encountered node of Ranvier. If regeneration does not take place, target tissue is not re-innervated, and degeneration of target organ eventually occurs.
Source: *Tsao B. Trauma of the nervous system: peripheral nerve trauma. Bradley's neurology in clinical practice. p. 903–19.e2, Chapter 64.*

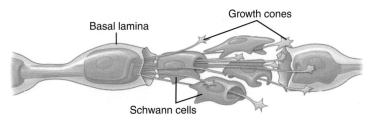

FIGURE 1.17   After transection of a single axon, multiple axons will 'sprout' from the proximal nerve stump forming a regenerating unit, whereas Wallerian degeneration will occur distal to the injury.
Source: *Tung TH. Nerve reconstructive techniques in the hand. Hand and upper extremity reconstruction. p. 233–43, Chapter 17.*

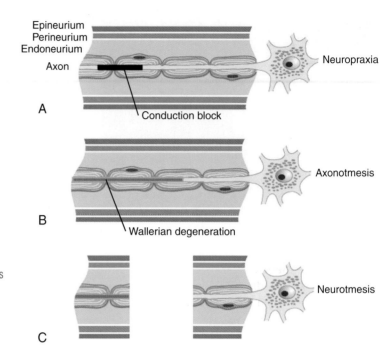

FIGURE 1.18 Classification of nerve injury. (A) Neuropraxia: physiologic conduction block; (B) axonotmesis leading to Wallerian degeneration of axon distal to the site of injury. Note, all three neural supporting structures are intact; (C) neurotmesis: axonotmesis with injury to one or more neural supporting structures.
Source: *Patel D. Brachial plexopathy. Pain management. p. 529–40, Chapter 59.*

Ganglia

A **ganglion** is a collection of nerve cell bodies located outside the CNS. It functions as a **relay station** for information that is communicated between the PNS and CNS. Ganglia are classified into three categories:

- **Dorsal (posterior) root ganglia**, also known as **spinal ganglia** (Fig. 1.19)
  - Reside in the intervertebral foramina and house the **somata of the afferent sensory nerves**, which relay sensory stimuli from body organs to the spinal cord
  - Interestingly, an action potential can bypass the somata of sensory nerves residing in spinal ganglia; the **pseudo-unipolar** shape of these cells may explain this unusual nervous electrical activity

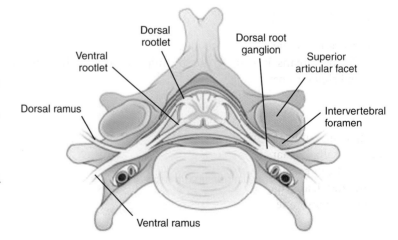

FIGURE 1.19 Each spinal nerve has a dorsal (sensory) and a ventral (motor) root. Dorsal roots are branches from dorsal root ganglia cells; ventral roots are motor axons from cells in the ventral horn.
Source: *From Bradley WG et al., editors. Neurology in clinical practice, 5th ed., Philadelphia: Butterworth-Heinemann; 2008.*

CLINICAL INSIGHT

- **Shingles (Fig. 1.20)**
  - Is a recurrent infection due to reactivation of the **varicella zoster virus**, the causative agent of chickenpox
  - The virus remains **dormant** in the dorsal root or trigeminal ganglia, but replicates when the immune system is compromised (i.e. immunosuppressive therapy and stress)
  - After replication in the neuronal somata, the virus travels down the sensory axons and causes inflammation of the nerves and blistering over the corresponding dermatome (skin area innervated by sensory nerve)
  - Chronic pain, also known as **postherpetic neuralgia**, may occur after shingles and may persist for months or years

- **Autonomic ganglia** are classified into the following:
  - **Sympathetic ganglia,** which are organized in bilateral symmetrical chains extending from the cervical to sacral regions. These ganglia are located in close proximity to the spinal cord, and thus referred to as paravertebral and prevertebral ganglia
  - **Parasympathetic ganglia,** which unlike the sympathetic ganglia, are located near or inside the organs that they innervate
- **CN ganglia**
  - Are found along the path of some cranial nerves
  - Some are sensory, such as those of CNs V (trigeminal), VII (facial), VIII (vestibulocochlear), IX (glossopharyngeal) and X (vagus)
  - Others are parasympathetic, such as those of CNs III (oculomotor), VII, IX and X

ADDITIONAL CLINICAL INSIGHTS

Tumours of the Nervous System

See Figs 1.21 and 1.22.

CROSSTALK AT THE CELLULAR LEVEL

Communication between different components of the nervous system and their effective organs is carried out by microstructures that ensure a well-controlled signal transmission.

Synapse

A **synapse** is a unit of communication between two neurons. It consists of a small gap called synaptic cleft between the pre- and postsynaptic cell membranes and can conduct electrical and chemical signals.

- In **chemical synapses**, neurotransmitters are released from the presynaptic membrane upon the arrival of an electrical stimulus, cross the

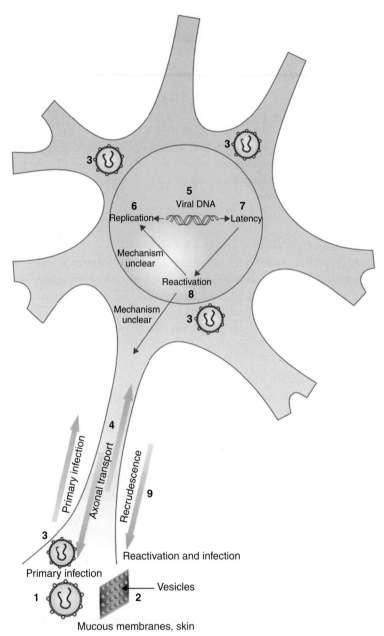

FIGURE 1.20 Herpes virus cycle in the human host. During primary infection, the virus (1) attaches to nerve endings at the peripheral mucocutaneous region. Replication at the periphery is associated with typical vesicles (2). With or without replication, the viral capsid (3) is transported through axonal transport (4) into the neuronal cell body. Viral DNA (5) enters the nucleus of the neuron where it can take two directions: a full replication cycle (6) or go into latency (7). Reactivation (8) is associated with transport of virus into the axon and recrudescence (9) at the periphery. The mechanism of reactivation in vivo is yet unknown and it is unclear whether it is associated with a full replication cycle, and hence lytic infection.

Source: *Steiner I, Prof. The neurotropic herpes viruses: herpes simplex and varicella-zoster. The Lancet Neurology 6(11):1015–28.*

Meningiomas

- derived from arachnoid cap cells and represent the second most common primary intracranial brain tumour after astrocytomas (15%)
- are not invasive; they indent the brain; may produce hyperostosis
- pathology: concentric whorls and calcified psammoma bodies
- location: parasagittal and convexity
- gender: females > men
- associated with neurofibromatosis-2 (NF-2)

Germinomas

- germ cell tumours that are commonly seen in the pineal region (>50%)
- overlie the tectum of the midbrain
- cause obstructive hydrocephalus due to aqueductal stenosis
- the common cause of Parinaud syndrome

Astrocytomas

- represent 20% of the gliomas
- histologically benign
- diffusely infiltrale the hemispheric white matter
- most common glioma found in the posterior fossa of children

Brain abscesses

- may result from sinusitis, mastoiditis, hematogenous spread
- location: frontal and temporal lobes, cerebellum
- organisms: streptococci, staphylococci and pneumococci
- result in cerebral oedema and herniation

Ependymomas

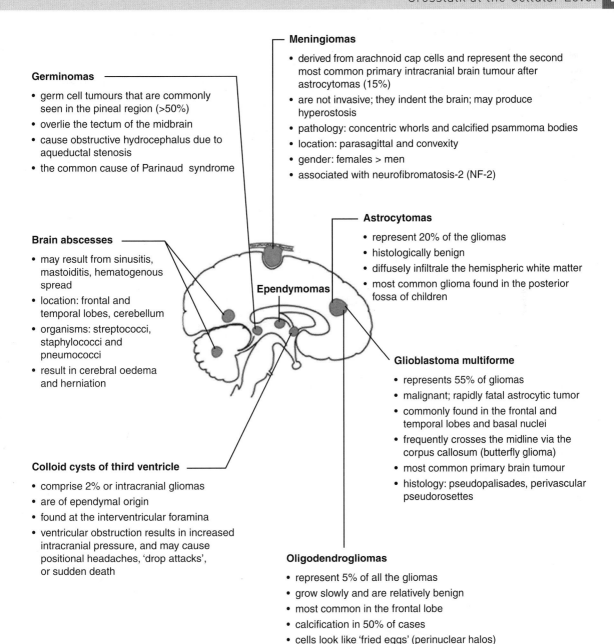

Glioblastoma multiforme

- represents 55% of gliomas
- malignant; rapidly fatal astrocytic tumor
- commonly found in the frontal and temporal lobes and basal nuclei
- frequently crosses the midline via the corpus callosum (butterfly glioma)
- most common primary brain tumour
- histology: pseudopalisades, perivascular pseudorosettes

Colloid cysts of third ventricle

- comprise 2% or intracranial gliomas
- are of ependymal origin
- found at the interventricular foramina
- ventricular obstruction results in increased intracranial pressure, and may cause positional headaches, 'drop attacks', or sudden death

Oligodendrogliomas

- represent 5% of all the gliomas
- grow slowly and are relatively benign
- most common in the frontal lobe
- calcification in 50% of cases
- cells look like 'fried eggs' (perinuclear halos)

FIGURE 1.21   Supratentorial tumours of the central and peripheral nervous systems. In adults, 70% of tumours are supratentorial. Source: *High-yield neuroanatomy, 4th ed.; Fig. 1.3.*

Choroid plexus papillomas

- histologically benign
- represent 2% of the gliomas
- one of the most common brain tumours in patients < 2 years of age
- occur in decreasing frequency: fourth, lateral and third ventricle
- CSF overproduction may cause hydrocephalus

Cerebellar astrocytomas

- benign tumours of childhood with good prognosis
- most common paediatric intracranial tumour
- contain pilocytic astrocytes and Rosenthal fibres

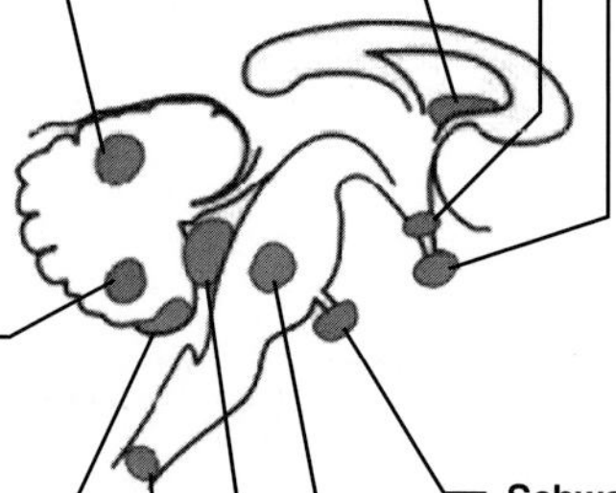

Medulloblastomas

- represent 7% of primary brain tumours
- represent a primitive neuroectodermal tumour (PNET)
- second most common posterior fossa tumour in children
- responsible for the posterior vermis syndrome
- can metastasize via the CSF tracts
- highly radiosensitive

Hemangioblastomas

- characterized by abundant capillary blood vessels and foamy cells; most often found in the cerebellum
- when found in the cerebellum and retina, may represent a part of the von Hippel–Lindau syndrome
- 2% of primary intracranial tumours; 10% of posterior fossa tumours

Intraspinal tumours

- Schwannomas 30%
- Meningiomas 25%
- Gliomas 20%
- Sarcomas 12%
- Ependymomas represent 60% of intramedullary gliomas

Craniopharyngiomas

- represent 3% of primary brain tumours
- derived from epithelial remnants of Rathke's pouch
- location: suprasellar and inferior to the optic chiasma
- cause bitemporal hemianopia and hypopituitarism
- calcification is common

Pituitary adenomas (PA)

- most common tumours of the pituitary gland
- prolactinoma is the most common PA
- derived from the stomodeum (Rathke's pouch)
- represent 8% of primary brain tumours
- may cause hypopituitarism, visual field defects (bitemporal hemianopia and cranial nerve palsies CNN III, IV, V-1 and V-2, and postganglionic sympathetic fibres to the dilator muscle of the iris)

Schwannomas (acoustic neuromas)

- consist of Schwann cells and arise from the vestibular division of CN VIII
- compromise approx. 8% of intracranial neoplasms
- pathology: Antoni A and B tissue and Verocay bodies
- bilateral acoustic neuromas are diagnostic of NF-2

Brainstem glioma

- usually a benign pilocytic astrocytoma
- usually causes cranial nerve palsies
- may cause the 'locked-in' syndrome

Ependymomas

- represent 5% of the gliomas
- histology: benign, ependymal tubules, perivascular pseudorosettes
- 40% are supratentorial; 60% are infratentorial (posterior fossa)
- third most common posterior fossa tumour in children and adolescents

FIGURE 1.22 Infratentorial (posterior fossa) and intraspinal tumours of the central and peripheral nervous systems. In children, 70% of tumours are infratentorial.

Source: *High-yield neuroanatomy, 4th ed.; Fig. 1.4.*

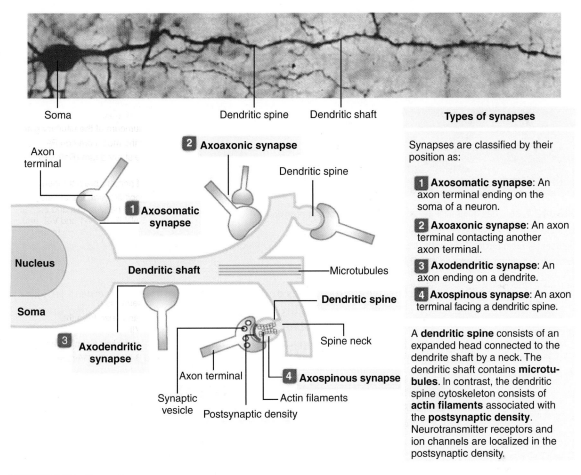

Soma   Dendritic spine   Dendritic shaft

Types of synapses

Synapses are classified by their position as:

Axon terminal

2 Axoaxonic synapse

Dendritic spine

1 Axosomatic synapse

Nucleus

Dendritic shaft ——— Microtubules

Soma

3 Axodendritic synapse

Dendritic spine

Spine neck

Axon terminal   **4 Axospinous synapse**

Synaptic vesicle   Actin filaments

Postsynaptic density

1 Axosomatic synapse: An axon terminal ending on the soma of a neuron.

2 Axoaxonic synapse: An axon terminal contacting another axon terminal.

3 Axodendritic synapse: An axon ending on a dendrite.

4 Axospinous synapse: An axon terminal facing a dendritic spine.

A **dendritic spine** consists of an expanded head connected to the dendrite shaft by a neck. The dendritic shaft contains **microtubules**. In contrast, the dendritic spine cytoskeleton consists of **actin filaments** associated with the **postsynaptic density**. Neurotransmitter receptors and ion channels are localized in the postsynaptic density.

FIGURE 1.23 Types of synapses.

Source: *Kierszenbaum AL, MD, PhD. Nervous tissue. Histology and cell biology: an introduction to pathology. p. 227–58, Chapter 8.*

synaptic cleft and activate receptors on the postsynaptic membrane that ultimately generates or inhibits the passage of an electrical signal.

- **Electrical synapses** do not utilize neurotransmitters but rather allow the electrical signal to cross rapidly from pre- to postsynaptic membranes through gap junctions.

Neurotransmission can be bidirectional in electrical synapses, whereas only unidirectional transmission is possible in chemical synapses. The different types of synapses are summarized in Fig. 1.23.

Neuromuscular Junction (Fig. 1.24)

Somehow similar in structure to a chemical synapse, a **neuromuscular junction (NMJ)** allows unidirectional transmission of an action potential from a motor neuron to a muscle fibre.

- Upon arrival of an action potential, the presynaptic axonal terminal (terminal bouton) releases acetylcholine (ACh) into the synaptic

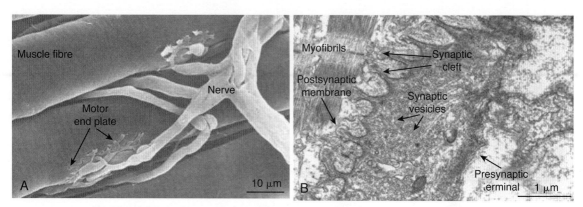

FIGURE 1.24   Neuromuscular junction. (A) scanning electron micrograph of an α-motoneuron innervating several muscle fibres in its motor unit; (B) transmission electron micrograph.
Source: *(A) From Bloom W, Fawcett DW. A textbook of histology, 10th ed., Philadelphia: WB Saunders; 1975 (B) Courtesy Dr. Clara Franzini-Armstrong, University of Pennsylvania, Philadelphia.*

cleft, where it diffuses and binds to nicotinic ACh receptors (nAChR) clustered on the highly folded muscle fibre membrane, also known as the **motor endplate**.

◼ **Dystrophin** and **rapsyn** are essential structural proteins that stabilize the cytoskeleton and nAChR at the motor endplate.

CLINICAL INSIGHT

◼ **Myasthenia gravis**
  ▪ Is a disease of the NMJ manifesting as **muscle fatigue and weakness after usual activity;** weakness significantly **improves after rest**
  ▪ Patients produce **antibodies that target nAChR** at the postsynaptic NMJ
  ▪ Is associated with **thymomas** in 10% of cases, which require surgical removal
  ▪ Electromyographic studies reveal **action potential decrements** on repetitive nerve stimulation and 'jitter' on single fibre studies; these findings help in confirming the diagnosis
  ▪ Medical treatment includes **acetylcholinesterase inhibitors** such as **pyridostigmine**, steroids and immunosuppressants; intravenous immunoglobulins and plasmapheresis are usually indicated in the treatment of myasthenic crisis, a life-threatening condition where weakness involves the respiratory muscles

◼ **Lambert Eaton syndrome**
  ▪ Is another disease of the NMJ, which manifests as **muscle weakness**; such weakness mainly involves proximal muscles of the arms and legs, and typically **improves after exercise**
  ▪ Is due to autoimmune production of **antibodies against presynaptic voltage-gated calcium channels**
  ▪ Is a **paraneoplastic** syndrome in 60% of cases and highly associated with **small cell lung cancer**
  ▪ Electromyographic studies reveal a large **increment of motor compound action potentials after voluntary muscular contraction**; in addition, typical action potential decrement occurs following repetitive nerve stimulation

- Management plan includes treatment of the underlying malignancy, if present
- Medical treatment includes **acetylcholinesterase inhibitors (pyridostigmine)** and an ACh-releasing agent called **3,4-diaminopyridine**; in severe and refractory cases, plasmapheresis and IVIG provide temporary improvement
- **Duchenne muscular dystrophy**
  - Is an **X-linked recessive** muscular disorder caused by a mutation in the gene coding for the **dystrophin** protein
  - Has early signs and symptoms, including weakness and atrophy of **proximal leg and pelvis muscles**; these start to appear in infancy and progress to involve other muscles
  - Is associated with paradoxical enlargement of muscles, known as **pseudo-hypertrophy**, which occurs due to replacement of muscle mass by fat and fibrotic tissue
  - Has a very bad prognosis; most of the patients are **wheelchair-bound by age 12** and pass away by age 25

Neuroglandular Junction

A **neuroglandular junction** permits the passage of neural stimuli to a secretory gland. A notable example is the junction between a preganglionic sympathetic neuronal axon and a chromaffin cell of the adrenal medulla.

- The electrical signal causes the release of ACh that crosses the synaptic cleft and binds to nAChR on the postsynaptic membrane.
- After effective stimulation, adrenaline and other hormones such as noradrenaline and enkephalins are secreted into the blood circulation.

Neurotransmitters (Table 1.3)

Table 1.3 List of the most important neurotransmitters, their secretion sites in the nervous system and the associated clinical correlations

Category	Neurotransmitter	Location of Secretion in the Nervous System	Clinical Insights	Comments
Acetylcholine	Acetylcholine	<ul><li>ANS, PNS and NMJ (parasympathetic nerve fibres, preganglionic sympathetic fibres, postganglionic sympathetic fibres to sweat glands and blood vessels in skeletal muscles)</li><li>Brainstem and spinal cord (somatic and visceral nuclei)</li><li>Forebrain (basal nucleus of Meynert)</li><li>Striatum (interneurons in caudate and putamen)</li></ul>	<ul><li>Deficiency: Contributes to the pathophysiology of Alzheimer disease – due to degeneration of the basal nucleus of Meynert</li><li>Antibodies against nicotinic ACh receptors: Myasthenia gravis – due to inability of ACh to activate the receptors</li></ul>	<ul><li>Important role in neuromodulation and plasticity, attention and arousal, learning and motivation</li><li>Binds to and activates nicotinic (in muscles, ANS and CNS) and muscarinic (in PNS and CNS) receptors</li></ul>

Continued

Table 1.3 List of the most important neurotransmitters, their secretion sites in the nervous system and the associated clinical correlations—cont'd

Category	Neurotransmitter	Location of Secretion in the Nervous System	Clinical Insights	Comments
Catechol-amine	Norepinephrine	■ ANS (postganglionic sympathetic fibres) ■ Pons (locus ceruleus) ■ Medulla (solitary nucleus)	■ Increased: Mania, anxiety and panic attacks ■ Decreased: Depression	■ Important role in memory, arousal and attention ■ Binds to and activates α and β adrenergic receptors

	Dopamine	■ Midbrain (substantia nigra and ventral tegmental area)
		■ Hypothalamus (arcuate nucleus, periventricular nucleus and posterior hypothalamus)
		■ Zona incerta
		■ Retina (amacrine neurons)
		■ PNS (local effect)
			■ Increased: Schizophrenia
			■ Decreased: Parkinson disease, ADHD and restless legs syndrome
				■ Important role in motor control and executive functions, reward system (pleasure, learning, approach behaviour), motivation and reinforcement
				■ Controls the release of certain hormones (inhibit prolactin release from pituitary)
				■ Activity through two receptors:
				  ■ D1: excitatory postsynaptic receptors that are activated by psychostimulants
				  ■ D2: inhibitory pre- and postsynaptic receptors that are blocked by antipsychotic drugs

Amino acids: Excitatory	Glutamate	■ Neocortex (projecting to thalamus, subthalamus and striatum)
		■ Cerebellar granule cells
		■ Corticobulbar and corticospinal tracts
		■ Large primary afferent fibres entering the spinal cord and brainstem
			■ Neurodegenerative brain diseases by long-term excitotoxicity:
			  ■ Huntington disease
			  ■ Hyperalgesia
			  ■ Autism
			  ■ Rasmussen encephalitis
			  ■ Epilepsy
			  ■ Ischaemic stroke
				■ Chief excitatory neurotransmitter of the brain
				■ Precursor for GABA
				■ Important role in learning, memory formation, modulation of synaptic plasticity, long-term potentiation, and neural communication
				■ Binds to and activates two types of receptors:
				  ■ Ionotropic (NMDA, Kainate, and AMPA)
				  ■ Metabotropic (mGluR)

	Aspartate	■ Climbing fibres projecting to the cerebellum from the inferior olivary nucleus	___	■ Major excitatory neurotransmitter of the brain ■ Binds to and activates NMDA receptors, but weaker than glutamate

Table 1.3 List of the most important neurotransmitters, their secretion sites in the nervous system and the associated clinical correlations—cont'd

Category	Neurotransmitter	Location of Secretion in the Nervous System	Clinical Insights	Comments

Amino acids: Inhibitory	Gamma-aminobutyric acid	▪ Several cortical projections with subsets of GABAergic neurons (Globus pallidus to thalamus; Striatum to substantia nigra and Globus pallidus; Striatum to thalamus and subthalamic nucleus; Substantia nigra to thalamus)
		 ▪ Cerebellar cells (Purkinje, Golgi, stellate and basket) exerting their actions
			▪ Disrupted inhibitory function:
			   ▫ Epilepsy
			   ▫ Anxiety disorder
			   ▫ Stiff-person syndrome
			   ▫ Schizophrenia
			   ▫ Huntington disease
				▪ Chief inhibitory neurotransmitter of the mature brain
				 ▪ Major excitatory neurotransmitter in the developing brain, i.e. before the maturation of glutamatergic synapses
				 ▪ Binds to and inhibits pre- and postsynaptic membranes by two types of receptors:
				   ▫ GABA$_A$ ligand-activated chloride channels
				   ▫ GABA$_B$ metabotropic receptors

	Glycine	▪ Brainstem ▪ Spinal cord ▪ Retina	▪ Spasticity ▪ Hyperekplexia	▪ Major inhibitory neurotransmitter of the brainstem and spinal cord ▪ Excitatory effect in the forebrain by acting as a co-agonist with glutamate binding to NMDA receptors
Amino acids: Other	Nitric oxide	▪ Neocortex ▪ Striatum ▪ Hypothalamus (supra-optic nucleus) ▪ Hippocampus ▪ Olfactory nerve and bulb ▪ Cerebellum ▪ ENS	—	▪ Role in learning and memory through long-term potentiation ▪ Nonadrenergic, noncholinergic with short half-life and its action is not limited to synapses, thus can affect nonsynapsed local neurons
Peptides: Endogenous Opiates	Endorphins	▪ Hypothalamus (arcuate nucleus projecting to nucleus accumbens and other limbic system regions)	▪ Depersonalization disorder	▪ Classified as α-, β-, γ-, α-neo-, and β-neo-endorphins ▪ Bind to and activate μ-receptors ▪ Chief subtype in brain is the extremely potent β-endorphin ▪ Function by blocking transmission and increasing resistance to pain signals ▪ Produce analgesia, euphoria, physical dependence, miosis, and respiratory depression

Continued

Table 1.3 List of the most important neurotransmitters, their secretion sites in the nervous system and the associated clinical correlations—cont'd

Category	Neurotransmitter	Location of Secretion in the Nervous System	Clinical Insights	Comments
	Enkephalins	▪ Brain (Globus pallidus mainly, but also cortex, thalamus, olfactory bulb, amygdala) ▪ Brainstem (medulla, pons, periaqueductal grey of midbrain) ▪ Spinal cord (substantia gelatinosa)	___	▪ Bind to and activate δ- and μ-receptors ▪ Produce similar effects as endorphins, but less potent
	Dynorphins	▪ Brain (hypothalamus, striatum, claustrum, hippocampus) ▪ Brainstem (medulla, pons, periaqueductal grey of midbrain) ▪ Spinal cord (substantia gelatinosa)	___	▪ Bind to and activate κ-receptors ▪ Produce spinal analgesia, miosis, and sedation ▪ Inhibit ADH release
Peptides: Nonopioids	Somatostatin/ Somatotropin-release-inhibiting factor	▪ Hypothalamus (ventro-medial nucleus projecting to median eminence, then carried to anterior pituitary through the hypothalamic–hypophysial portal system, arcuate nucleus) ▪ Hippocampus ▪ Striatum ▪ Medulla (solitary nucleus)	▪ Decreased: Alzheimer disease ▪ Increased: Huntington disease	▪ Functions by inhibiting the release of growth hormone, thyroid-stimulating hormone, and prolactin
	Substance P	▪ Substantia nigra mainly and striatonigral tract ▪ Brain (hypothalamus, amygdala); spinal cord (substantia gelatinosa) ▪ Dorsal root ganglion cells	▪ Decreased: Huntington disease ▪ Role in mood disorders, anxiety disorder, major depressive disorder, and movement disorders	▪ First responder in pain transmission (released from sensory nerve terminals during inflammation) ▪ Role in emotion regulation ▪ Binds to and activates neurokinin 1 receptor

Indolamine	Serotonin/5-HT	▪ Brainstem (raphe nucleus)	▪ Decreased:
			  ▪ Insomnia
			  ▪ Depression
			  ▪ Obsessive-compulsive disorder
			  ▪ Increased risk of sudden infant death syndrome
			▪ Increased: Mania
				▪ Important role in regulating mood, sleep, appetite, memory and learning
				▪ Selective serotonin reuptake inhibitors are antidepressant drugs that increase serotonin levels in the brain

Notes: *ACh, acetylcholine; ADHD, attention deficit hyperactivity disorder; AMPA, α-amino-3-hydroxy-5-methyl-4-isoxazolepropionic acid; ANS, autonomic nervous system; CNS, central nervous system; ENS, enteric nervous system; GABA, gamma-aminobutyric acid; mGluR, metabotropic glutamine receptor; NMDA, N-methyl-D-aspartate; NMJ, neuromuscular junction; PNS, peripheral nervous system; α, alpha; β, beta; γ, gamma; δ, delta; μ, mu; κ, kappa; 5-HT, 5-Hydroxytryptamine.*

Cutaneous Receptors: Classification and Function (Figs 1.14 and 1.25)

Cutaneous receptors constitute essential components of the somatosensory nervous system. Each receptor responds to one or more sensory modalities. Table 1.4 lists the different types of cutaneous receptors and summarizes the associated sensory modalities and nerve fibres types (see Table 1.2 for more details on classification of nerve fibres).

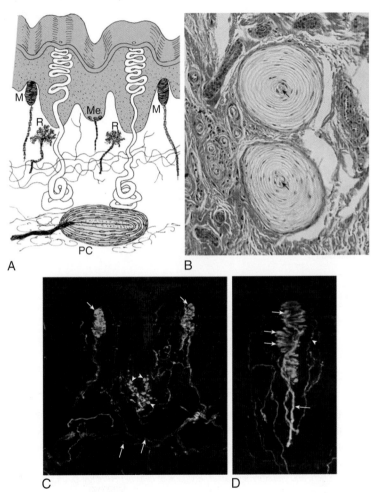

FIGURE 1.25 Some of the sensory endings found in glabrous skin. (A) Schematic overview. M, Meissner corpuscle; Me, Merkel cell; PC, Pacinian corpuscle; R, Ruffini ending. (B) Two Pacinian corpuscles, sectioned transversely. Multiple thin layers of each capsule surround a central mechanosensitive ending (arrows). (C) Section of biopsied skin from a fingertip, stained to show epidermis (blue fluorescence), myelin (red fluorescence) and nerve fibres (green fluorescence). Myelinated and unmyelinated axons course horizontally in a dermal plexus (thick arrows), giving off branches that end in Meissner corpuscles (thin arrows) and as Merkel endings (arrowheads). (D) Meissner corpuscle, stained as in C. A myelinated axon (thick arrow) enters the corpuscle, loses its myelin and winds back and forth (thin arrows) between the stacked Schwann cells. Other unmyelinated fibres (arrowhead) head off into the epidermis to form free nerve endings.

Source: *(A) Vanderah TW, PhD. Sensory receptors and the peripheral nervous system. Nolte's the human brain. p. 207–32, Chapter 9. (B) courtesy Dr. Nathaniel T. McMullen, University of Arizona College of Medicine. (C) and (D) courtesy Dr. Maria Nolano, Salvatore Maugeri Foundation, Terme, Italy.)*

Table 1.4 List of the different types of cutaneous receptors

Cutaneous Receptors	Type of Endings	Type of Fibres	Sensory Modality	Conduction Velocity/Rate of Adaptation (Fig. 1.26)
Thermoreceptors	Unspecialized free nerve endings	Aδ (warm) and C (cold)	Temperature	Fast (Aδ) and slow (C) conduction velocity
Nociceptors	Unspecialized free nerve endings	Aδ and C	Pain	Fast (Aδ) and slow (C) conduction velocity
Hair follicle receptors	Specialized free nerve endings (root hair plexus)	Aβ	Touch	Rapid adaptation
Meissner corpuscles	Encapsulated	Aβ	Touch	Rapid adaptation
Pacinian corpuscles	Oval lamellar (onion-like) capsules	Aβ	Vibration	Rapid adaptation
Merkel disks	Large myelinated free endings	Aβ	Touch	Slow adaptation
Ruffini corpuscles	Elongated capsules	Aβ	Pressure	Slow adaptation

Notes: *β, beta; δ, delta.*

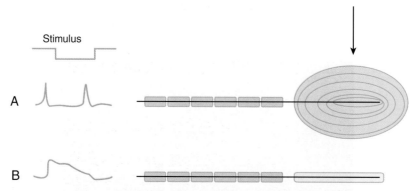

FIGURE 1.26   Rapidly adapting (RA) versus slowly adapting (SA) mechanoreceptors. (A) RA mechanoreceptors quickly adapt to a sustained stimulus. Thus, generator potentials primarily fire at stimulus onset and offset, and they provide information regarding changes in sensory stimuli. (B) SA mechanoreceptors are slowly adapting and fire throughout the duration of stimulation. They provide information regarding sustained stimulation.

Source: *Rowin J. Proprioception, touch, and vibratory sensation. Textbook of clinical neurology. p. 343–61, Chapter 19.*

BLOOD–CENTRAL NERVOUS SYSTEM BARRIERS
(Fig. 1.27)

Blood–brain and blood–CSF barriers are dynamic tissues with significant physiologic functions as much as anatomical barriers that ensure almost complete separation of the delicate CNS tissues from the blood milieu.

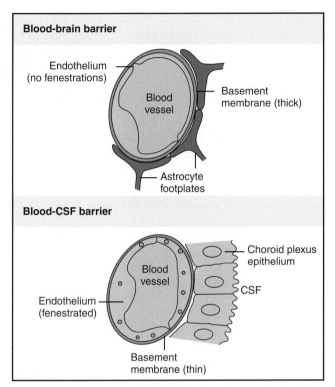

FIGURE 1.27 Structures of the blood–brain and blood–cerebrospinal fluid (CSF) barriers.
Source: *Goering RV, BA MSc PhD. Central nervous system infections. Mims' medical microbiology. p. 311–27, Chapter 24.*

Blood–Brain Barrier (BBB)

The **BBB** is a functional physical barrier, whereby the highly specialized, brain-specific, **nonfenestrated, overlapping endothelial cells** are interconnected by **tight junctions** and implement **permanently active transport systems** that allow nutrients but no other blood-borne molecules to cross to the brain tissues. Tight junctions are formed by a well-structured combination of trans-membrane and plasma accessory proteins that closely interact with an actin-based cytoskeleton. These junctions form a tight seal that prevents paracellular diffusion of water and solutes (including drugs). In addition, a **thick, continuous basement membrane** and **footplates of nearby astrocytes** establish structural support and further restrict the permeability.

Blood–CSF Barrier (BCSFB)

The **BCSFB** is located at the **choroid plexuses**. Unlike the BBB that is mostly located at the endothelium, a layer of **modified cuboidal epithelial cells** forms the BCSFB. Thus, **apical tight junctions** firmly connect these epithelial cells and prevent paracellular diffusion of water and solutes and retrograde passive flow of CSF. Although the main function of the choroid epithelium is to secrete CSF, epithelial cells utilize **active transport systems** that carry nutrients and essential solutes to the brain side and remove metabolic wastes and toxins out of the CNS.

CLINICAL INSIGHT

- **Cerebral oedema**
    - Results from excessive accumulation of water in and around cerebral cells
    - Fluids accumulate due to **disruption of the BBB and/or BCSFB** from traumatic or nontraumatic causes
    - Symptoms progress depending on the aetiology, rate of development and severity of oedema; these may include headache, confusion, psychosis, ataxia, seizures and coma, among others
    - Classified into four types, the characteristics of which are summarized in Table 1.5

Table 1.5 Types of cerebral oedema (Fig. 1.28)

Oedema Type	Aetiology	Pathophysiology
Cytotoxic	Ischaemia Drug-induced; Severe hypothermia; Reye syndrome	▪ Disrupted cellular metabolism leads to cerebral cell swelling due to intracellular retention of sodium and calcium
Vasogenic	Brain cancer; Malignant hypertension; Quick ascent to high-altitudes (HACE)	▪ Breakdown of endothelial tight-junctions allowing plasma proteins and water to cross capillary walls into the brain extracellular space ▪ Cancer: Secretion of VEGF and other molecules that weaken or destroy cerebral capillaries ▪ Malignant hypertension: Elevated hydrostatic pressure leads to forcible transudation of plasma into the extracellular space ▪ HACE: Cerebral endothelial cell dysfunction that is induced by hypoxia
Interstitial	Obstructive hydrocephalus (see chapter 3)	▪ Transependymal flow of CSF from brain ventricles into the extracellular space ▪ Cerebral capillaries are not involved and plasma proteins are not elevated in the brain extracellular compartment
Osmotic	SIADH; Hyponatremia due to any cause; Hemodialysis	▪ Rapid and significant decrease in plasma osmolality leads to shift of water from plasma into the brain extracellular space

Notes: CSF, cerebrospinal fluid; HACE, high-altitude cerebral oedema; SIADH, syndrome of inappropriate antidiuretic hormone secretion; VEGF, vascular endothelial growth factor.

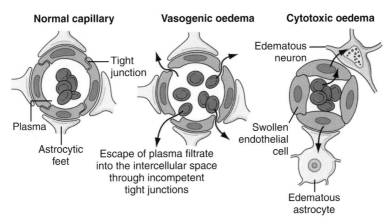

FIGURE 1.28   Normal appearance of a cerebral capillary contrasted with the changes that occur in vasogenic or cytotoxic oedema. Under normal conditions, the intercellular tight junctions are intact. In vasogenic oedema, the tight junctions are not competent, allowing leakage of plasma into the interstitial space. In cytotoxic oedema, there is a primary failure of adenosine triphosphate (ATP)-dependent sodium pump mechanism resulting in intracellular accumulation of sodium and secondarily water.
Source: *Morton R. Intracranial hypertension. Principles of neurological surgery. p. 311–23, Chapter 19.*

CASE STUDY DISCUSSION

MS is a chronic inflammatory, demyelinating disease whereby the immune system erroneously attacks myelin, myelinated axons and oligodendrocytes **at different times** and **in different regions** of the CNS. Neurologic sequelae from different episodes accumulate and ultimately lead to physical disability and cognitive dysfunction. A summary of the disease is depicted in Fig. 1.29.

Classification

A set of clinical criteria has been proposed to distinguish between different categories of MS. Thus, almost all patients will fall into one of the following categories (Fig. 1.30):

- **Relapsing–remitting**
  - The majority of patients (more than 80%) fall into this category
  - Repetitive pattern of exacerbations followed by remissions
  - Neurologic sequelae may persist in periods of remission
  - Newer relapses are more severe than the previous ones
- **Secondary progressive**
  - An advanced stage of the relapsing–remitting course
  - Remission periods become progressively shorter in duration until they disappear and the disease continuously evolves over time
- **Primary progressive**
  - Around 10% of MS patients have this disease subtype

- Neurologic symptoms have an insidious onset and progress slowly without early relapses or remissions
- There may be periods of levelling off of symptoms, i.e. plateaus in the disease course, but there is an overall trend of disease progression over time
- **Progressive relapsing**
  - A rare subtype affecting less than 5% of MS patients
  - Patients experience progressive onset of symptoms, which is later accompanied by intermittent flare-ups (relapses)

Clinical Features

Signs and symptoms may involve any part of the CNS. Some of the neurologic features are as follows:

- **Sensory**: Paraesthesia, tingling
- **Motor**: Muscle weakness, cramping, twitching
- **Autonomic**: Bladder and bowel incontinence, sexual dysfunction
- **Cerebellar**: Tremor, ataxia, dysarthria
- **Ophthalmologic**: Eye pain, visual disturbances, diplopia
- **Constitutional**: Fatigue, pain, dizziness, heat intolerance
- **Cognitive and psychiatric**: Dementia, depression, hypomania/mania, impairments in attention, judgment and concentration

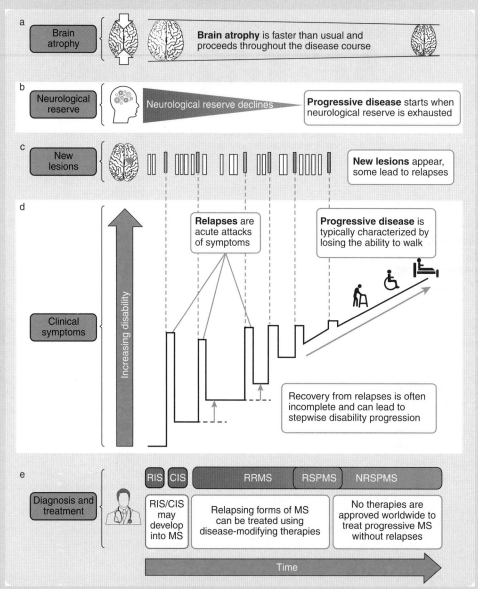

FIGURE 1.29 The damage caused by MS typically leads to relapses followed by progressive disease. (A) The brain of people with MS shrinks (atrophy) more rapidly than usual as a result of damage caused by the disease; (B) the brain can use its neurological reserve to compensate for damage by remodelling itself. However, when neurological reserve is used up, the clinical symptoms of the disease may progress; (C) MS causes lesions – acute areas of damage to the brain and spinal cord that accumulate over time. If a lesion noticeably disrupts nerve function, it leads to a relapse (an attack of clinical symptoms); (D) a typical MS disease course involves relapses, followed by progressive disease; (E) a person with MS may have a variety of diagnoses over time, but disease-modifying therapies are effective only in the early stages when relapses are still present. NRSPMS, nonrelapsing secondary progressive multiple sclerosis; RIS, radiologically isolated syndrome; RRMS, relapsing–remitting multiple sclerosis; RSPMS, relapsing secondary progressive multiple sclerosis.
Source: *Reproduced with permission from Oxford PharmaGenesis Ltd.*

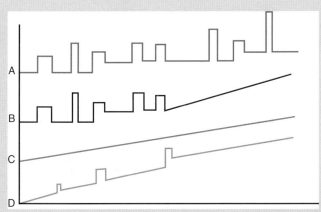

FIGURE 1.30   A diagrammatic representation of disability by time for different subtypes of MS:
(A) Relapsing–remitting MS; (B) secondary progressive MS; (C) primary progressive MS; (D) progressive
relapsing MS.
Source: Greenberg BM. Multiple sclerosis. Pharmacology and therapeutics: principles to practice.
p. 685–702, Chapter 46.

Pathophysiology

The hallmark of MS is **inflammation** and **demyelination** of
CNS nerve fibres with or without axonal damage. The proposed pathologic process may be summarized as follows:

- **Myelin-reactive T-cells** are activated in the periphery,
  cross the BBB and produce proinflammatory cytokines
  that augment the inflammatory process and recruit
  other inflammatory cells
- Once activated by myelin-reactive T-cells, **peripheral
  B-cells** produce antibodies against myelin
- The location of plaques, the demyelinating lesions
  formed by destruction of myelin and oligodendrocytes,
  dictate the specific neurologic symptoms of MS
  patients
- Although the nervous system succeeds at some
  point in remyelinating the affected areas, some
  lesions may be irreparable and thus replaced by
  gliosis tissue

Management

The management plan is best accomplished through a
multidisciplinary approach.

- Medical therapy is essential to relieve neurologic
  symptoms after an attack, prevent new attacks and
  delay disability as much as possible
  - **Acute attacks** are managed with **corticosteroids
    and/or plasmapheresis** depending on the severity
  - **Chronic treatment** comprises **immunomodulatory** and
    immunosuppressive therapy with DMA such as inter-
    ferons beta-1a and beta-1b, glateramer acetate, mito-
    xantrone, fingolimod and teriflunomide, among others
- **Behavioural therapy and physical rehabilitation** significantly improve the quality of life of MS patients

Prognosis

Prognosis depends on multiple factors including disease
course and severity of attacks.

- After disease onset, 30% of untreated patients will
  progress to physical disability within 20–25 years
- Worst prognosis is seen in male patients with primary
  progressive course
- The best long-term prognosis is significantly associated
  with early treatment with DMA and a clinically isolated
  syndrome (CIS)

CHAPTER 2

Embryology and Development of the Nervous System

Rechdi Ahdab

CASE STUDY

Presentation and Physical Examination: A 21-year-old man was brought by his family to the emergency department (ED) with confusion and disorientation after 10–15 min of continuous tonic–clonic movements. He is known to have intractable epilepsy since 11 months of age and has been on anti-epileptic medications since then. His seizures occurred three to four times a month, lasting less than 3 min. His family reported a consistently similar seizure pattern and described it as 'a moment of staring where he does not respond but gulps and picks up his cloth repeatedly'. Carbamazepine and phenytoin partially controlled his seizures until 11 years of age. At 12 years of age, the first secondarily generalized tonic–clonic seizure occurred and he was started on valproic acid. Several combinations and dose escalations of anti-epileptic medications did not effectively control his seizures. Upon admission, he was on valproic acid, levetiracetam and lamotrigine; regardless, his seizures still occurred at a rate of 2–3 episodes per week. His prenatal and postnatal histories were negative and early developmental milestones were not delayed. He barely completed secondary education, was not able to enrol in high school and could not obtain a driver's license or any employment due to his frequent seizures. His family history is negative for epilepsy. Neurological examination is normal with no focal deficits in the motor or sensory systems. Gait and coordination are normal as well.

Diagnosis, Management and Follow-Up: The scalp video electroencephalogram (EEG) showed ictal left temporoparietal discharges. The patient reported auras consisting of a combination of fear and déjà vu. The seizures were almost identical in symptomatology and progression; they started with staring, followed by swallowing, loss of responsiveness and incomprehensible speech and then progressed to right

arm dystonic posturing and postictal confusion. The seizures lasted between 5 and 7 min.

Brain magnetic resonance imaging (MRI) revealed multiple confluent nodules of heterotopic grey matter lining the lateral walls of the ventricles bilaterally, often protruding into the lumen (Fig. 2.1).

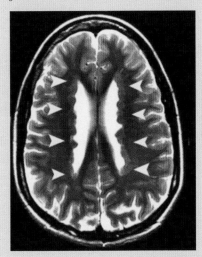

FIGURE 2.1 Bilateral periventricular nodular heterotopia. A T2-weighted axial magnetic resonance image from the patient demonstrates multiple confluent nodules of heterotopic grey matter lining the lateral walls of the ventricles bilaterally, often protruding into the lumen (white arrowheads).
Source: *Selvitelli MF. Sleep spindle alterations in patients with malformations of cortical development. Brain & Develop 31(2): 163–8.*

The patient was diagnosed with **bitemporal periventricular nodular heterotopias** (PNHs) causing intractable complex partial seizures. The culprit nodules were those on the left side, while the right nodules seemed to be silent, as depicted by the ictal left temporoparietal discharges.

Surgical management was recommended, and the patient underwent surgical resection of the left nodules. Over 2 years of follow-up, valproic acid and lamotrigine were discontinued and levetiracetam dose was decreased. No seizures occurred since the surgery.

BRIEF INTRODUCTION

Neuroembryology provides the key to understanding congenital malformations of the nervous system. Maturation of the nervous system progresses in a predictable sequence with precise timing. Even brief insults may have a profound impact on later development of the nervous system by interfering with processes essential to initiate the next stage of development.

The nervous system is among the earliest embryological structures to develop and the last to be completed. Before the formation of the nervous system, the embryo has already become differentiated into the three basic layers.

- **Ectoderm**, which gives rise to the epidermis and nervous system.
- **Mesoderm**, which forms the muscles, vessels and connective tissue.
- **Endoderm**, which forms the gastrointestinal tract, lungs and liver.

NEURULATION

During the **third week** of development, the **neural plate** develops as a thickening of the ectoderm between the buccopharyngeal membrane and primitive notch.

- The neural plate is **pear-shaped**.
- The **wider cranial** region will give rise to the **brain,** whereas the **narrower caudal** region will form the **spinal cord**.
- The neural plate will progressively transform into a **neural tube** in a process known as **neurulation**.
- The neural tube will eventually give rise to the **entire nervous system**.

Neurulation proceeds as follows (Fig. 2.2 and Table 2.1):

- The neural plate develops a **longitudinal groove** along its rostrocaudal axis.
- The neural groove deepens and becomes bound by **neural folds** on both sides.
- The neural folds come together and eventually fuse to form the **neural tube**.
  - Fusion starts at the midportion.
  - It then proceeds cranially and caudally in a continuous zipper-like fashion.
  - Fusion is more rapid cranially than caudally.
- The unclosed cephalic and caudal parts of the neural tube are called the anterior (cranial) and posterior (caudal) **neuropores**.

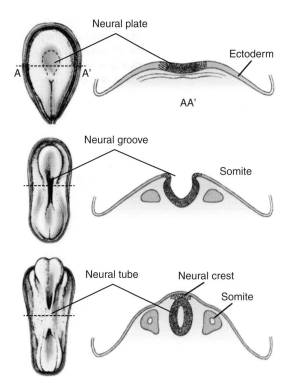

FIGURE 2.2 Primary neurulation: Schematic illustration of formation of the neural tube during the third and fourth weeks of gestation.
Source: *From Cowan WM. The development of the brain. Sci Am 1979;241:113.*

Table 2.1 Chronology of neurulation					
			Neural Groove Closure		
Embryonic Structure	**Neural Plate Formation**	**Neural Groove Formation**	**Middle Portion**	**Cranial End**	**Caudal End**
Chronology	Day 18	Day 20	Day 21	Day 26	Day 28

- The cranial neuropore closes at **around 24 days** and forms the **lamina terminalis**, an essential primordium of the **forebrain**.
- The last portion of the groove to fuse is the caudal end (**28 days**).
- Initially, the neural tube is a straight structure. Progressive growth of surrounding structures exerts an external physical force that causes bending at precise points: the **pontine** and **cervical flexures**.

CLINICAL INSIGHT

- **Neural Tube Defects**
  - Since the fusion process starts in the midportion of the neural tube, the caudal and cranial portions of the tube initially remain in contact with the amniotic fluid. **Neural tube defects** occur when the neural tube fails to close. These are the most common central nervous system (CNS) malformations. Its incidence can be reduced by supplementation of maternal diet with folic acid.

- An unclosed caudal neuropore causes **spina bifida**, in which the vertebral arch of the spinal column is either incompletely formed or absent (Fig. 2.3). The severity of spina bifida is variable, ranging from asymptomatic to severe neurological sequelae including lower extremity paralysis, loss of sensation and bowel/bladder dysfunction. Spina bifida can be broadly categorized into:
  - **Spina bifida occulta:**
    - Failure of vertebral elements to fuse posteriorly
    - Neural elements remain in the spinal canal
    - Mostly asymptomatic
  - **Spina bifida cystica:**
    - The posterior arch fails to form and is replaced by a cyst
    - When the cyst contains the dura and arachnoid, it is called meningocele
    - When the cyst contains neural elements, it is called myelomeningocele
  - An unclosed cranial neuropore causes a lethal condition called **anencephaly** (Fig. 2.4). In this condition, the lamina terminalis and its derivative (the forebrain) fail to develop. The lack of forebrain neuroectoderm results in failure of induction of the overlying mesoderm, and the cranium, meninges and scalp fail to close in the midline, exposing the remaining brain tissue to the surrounding amniotic fluid.

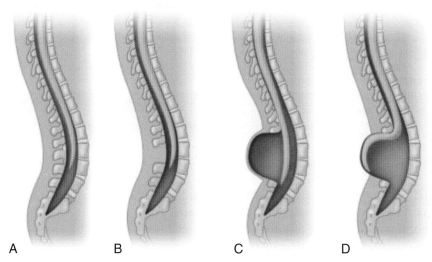

A   B   C   D

FIGURE 2.3 Schematic representation of the spectrum of spina bifida. (A) Intact neural tube; (B) spina bifida occulta; (C) meningocele; (D) myelomeningocele.

Source: *Reproduced with permission from Visual encyclopedia of ultrasound in obstetrics and gynecology. 2011. www.isuog.org.*

NEURAL CREST CELLS

While the neural tube is in the process of closing, it sinks below the surface.

- **Neuroectodermal cells** at the lateral margins of the neural plate do not become incorporated into the tube.
- They form a strip of cells between the neural tube and the overlying ectoderm known as the **neural crest cells** (Fig. 2.5).

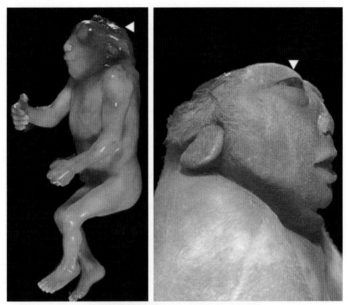

FIGURE 2.4   Anencephaly characterized by the absence of development of the fetal cranial vault.
Source: *Klatt EC, MD. The central nervous system. Robbins and Cotran atlas of pathology. p. 493–546.e7, Chapter 19.*

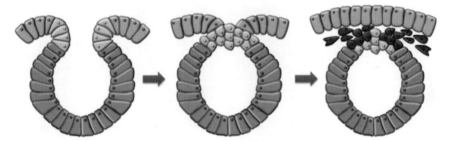

FIGURE 2.5   Neural crest cells: The lateral margins of the neural grooves (green) do not incorporate into the neural tube and form the neural crest cells (red).
Source: *Strobl-Mazzulla PH. Epithelial to mesenchymal transition: new and old insights from the classical neural crest model. Semin Cancer Biol 22(5–6):411–6.*

- These will later migrate extensively along **predetermined routes** and give rise to much of the **peripheral nervous system** in addition to other differentiated cell types.
- They terminally differentiate only after reaching their final destination.
- The major derivatives of the neural crest cells are as follows:
  - **Cells of the dorsal root ganglion**
  - **Sensory ganglia of the cranial nerve**
  - **Autonomic ganglia**
  - **Cells of the suprarenal medulla**
  - **Melanocytes**

In addition, the neural crest cells contribute to the development of the **outer layers of the eye** and **many of the skull bones**.

CLINICAL INSIGHT

■ **Syndromes of migration and differentiation**
  ■ Altered migration and/or abnormal differentiation of neural crest cells are the cause of several disease states.
    - **Hirschsprung disease:**
      - Ganglion cells derived from the neural crest migrate caudally with the vagal nerve fibres along the intestine.
      - These ganglion cells reach their final destination in the rectum by 12 weeks of gestational age.
      - Arrest of migration leads to an aganglionic segment with impaired motility (Fig. 2.6).
    - **Neurocutaneous melanosis:**
      - Patients with this disease have:
        - **Multiple large pigmented naevi** (Fig. 2.7A)
        - Excessive production of melanin in the leptomeninges (Fig. 2.7B)

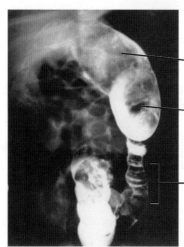

— Transverse colon

— Expanded segment of colon proximal to constriction (parasympathetic ganglia are normal)

— Constricted aganglionic segment of descending colon

FIGURE 2.6 Radiograph after a barium enema showing the aganglionic distal colon in Hirschsprung disease.
Source: *Schoenwolf GC, PhD. Development of the gastrointestinal tract. Larsen's human embryology. p. 341–74, Chapter 14.*

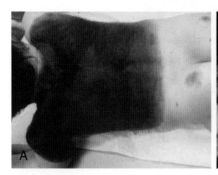
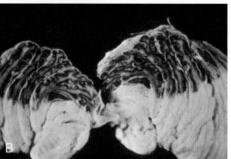

FIGURE 2.7 (A) Large, dark, hairy naevus covering most of the back of an infant with neurocutaneous melanosis; (B) leptomeningeal melanosis at autopsy in a patient with neurocutaneous melanosis.
Source: *Islam MP. Neurocutaneous syndromes. Bradley's neurology in clinical practice. p. 100, 1538–1562.e1.*

PRIMARY AND SECONDARY BRAIN VESICLES FORMATION

Once the neuropores close, the future **CNS** is organized in a way that resembles an **irregular cylinder** sealed at both ends.

- Neural tube stem cells generate the two major classes of cells that form the nervous system: **neurons** and **glia**.
- Most mitotic activity in the neuroepithelium occurs at the ventricular surface.
- Cell proliferation is most active in the:
  - **Spinal cord** and **brainstem** during the **early first trimester**.
  - **Forebrain** during the **late first** and **early second trimester**.

During the **fourth week** of development, cells at the cephalic end of the neural tube actively proliferate causing it to dilate and form the three primary brain vesicles (Fig. 2.8):

- **Forebrain** vesicle (**prosencephalon**)
- **Midbrain** vesicle (**mesencephalon**)
- **Hindbrain** vesicle (**rhombencephalon**)

The **caudal end** of the neural tube elongates and remains smaller in diameter; it will form the **spinal cord**. As development continues, the three primary vesicles form **five secondary brain vesicles (fifth week)**. These vesicles, from rostral to caudal, are as the following (Fig. 2.8):

- The prosencephalon, which divides into:
  - **Telencephalon**
  - **Diencephalon**
- The mesencephalon
- The rhombencephalon, which divides into:
  - **Metencephalon**
  - **Myelencephalon**

Each secondary vesicle develops into specific components of the adult nervous system (Fig. 2.8).

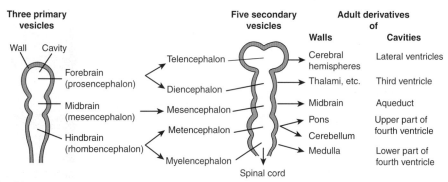

FIGURE 2.8 Primary and secondary brain vesicles and their main derivatives in the adult brain.

Source: *Moore KL, BA, MSc, PhD, DSc, FIAC, FRSM, FAAA. Nervous system. Before we are born. p. 251–75.e1, Chapter 16.*

DEVELOPMENT OF THE SPINAL CORD

The spinal cord derives from the caudal portion of the neural tube.

- In its earliest stage, the future spinal cord is formed of a single layer of pseudostratified epithelium centred by the neural tube. These cells are known as the **matrix cells** (or **neuroepithelium cells**).
- Repeated division of the matrix cells forms the **early neuroblasts**.
    - Neuroblasts are neuroepithelial cells committed to the **neuronal lineage**.
    - These cells have not yet achieved all functions of mature neurons and are often still migratory.
    - Neuroblasts are incapable of further division.

As the number of neuroblasts increases, the neural tube progressively increases in length and diameter. As development continues:

- Neuroblasts migrate **peripherally** to form the **mantle layer** (the future **grey matter**) (Fig. 2.9).
- Neuroblasts in the mantle layer give rise to **nerve fibres** that grow **peripherally** and form the **marginal zone** (Fig. 2.9).
- Nerve fibres in the marginal zone then become **myelinated**. As a result, this zone turns white in colour and is called the **white matter** of the spinal cord.

Matrix cells also give rise to **non-neural** components of the nervous system:

- **Astrocytes** (nerve fibre supporting cells)
- **Oligodendrocytes** (myelin producing cells)
- **Ependymal cells** (cells lining the central canal)

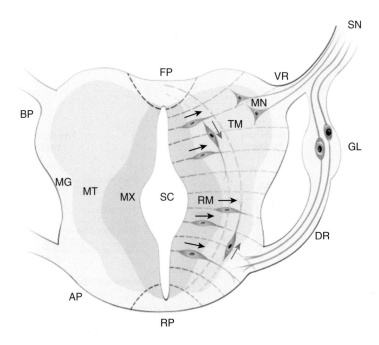

FIGURE 2.9 Transverse section of the spinal cord at 6 weeks of intrauterine life. AP, alar plate; BP, basal plate; DR, dorsal root; FP, foot plate; GL, dorsal root ganglion; MN, motoneurons; MG, marginal layer; MT, mantle layer; MX, matrix layer; RM, radially migrating neuroblasts; RP, roof plate; SC, spinal canal; SN, spinal nerve; TM, tangentially migrating neuroblasts; VR, ventral root.

Source: *(Adapted and modified from Nieuwenhuys et al.). Spinal cord anatomy and clinical syndromes. Diaz, Eric, MD; Morales, Humberto, MD. Published October 1, 2016. Volume 37, Issue 5. Pages 360–371.*

Matrix cells **do not form** the **microglial cells**. Along with blood vessels, these cells derive from the **mesenchyme** and **later migrate** into the nervous system.

Movement of maturing neuroblasts is **centrifugal**, radiating towards the surface of the spinal cord (Fig. 2.9).

- This process is governed by **glial cells** with **elongated radial processes** that guide the neuroblasts from the germinating matrix to their final destination.
- The same process guides neuroblast migration throughout the CNS.
- Once migration is accomplished, **radial glial cells** transform into astrocytes and ependymal cells.

As a result of continuous addition of neuroblasts to the mantle layer, **ventral** and **dorsal thickenings** form on both sides of the midline, the **basal** and **alar plates** respectively (Fig. 2.10).

- The **basal plate** is destined to contain most of the **motor neurons**.
- The **alar plate** contains **sensory neurons**.
- The two plates are separated by a longitudinal groove, the **sulcus limitans**.
- The midline portion of the neural tube remains thin and forms the **roof** and **floor plates**; these contain no neuroblasts and serve as **pathways for crossing fibres**.

As development proceeds, the spinal cord progressively achieves its mature appearance (Fig. 2.11).

- Progressive enlargement of the basal plate on both sides of the midline creates a deep longitudinal groove, the **ventral fissure**, which will later contain the **anterior spinal artery**.

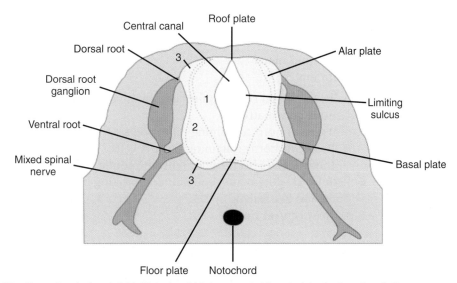

FIGURE 2.10 The early spinal cord divided into dorsal (alar) and ventral (basal) plates by the sulcus limitans.

Source: *Swanson LW. Basic plan of the nervous system. Fundamental neuroscience. p. 15–38, Chapter 2.*

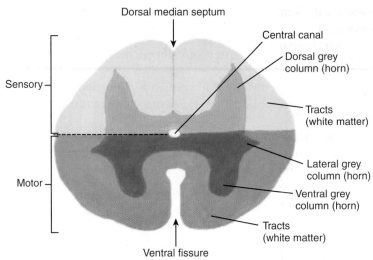

FIGURE 2.11 General organization of the mature spinal cord.
Source: *Hansen JT, PhD. Back. Netter's clinical anatomy. p. 49–86, Chapter 2.*

- The alar plates also enlarge and project medially. The median walls will eventually fuse and form the **dorsal median septum.**
- The **roof** and **floor plates** remain thin and contribute to the **ependyma.**
- As a result of the expansion of the basal and alar plates, the lumen of the neural tube becomes limited to a thin dorsiventral cleft that will eventually form the **central canal.**
- Accumulation of cells between alar and basal plates results in an **intermediate horn (lateral grey column)**, which contains **motor neurons of the autonomic nervous system.**

The **mesenchyme** surrounding the neural tube forms the:
- **Pia mater**
- **Arachnoid mater**
- **Dura mater**

Eventually, the spinal cord acquires its definitive form (Fig. 2.11).
- **Central grey matter:**
  - **Anterior** horn containing **motor** cells
  - **Posterior** horn containing **sensory** cells
  - **Intermediate** horn containing **autonomic** cells
- Peripheral white matter containing projecting fibres to and from the brain and brainstem
- **Narrow central canal**

DEVELOPMENT OF THE BRAINSTEM

Throughout the **brainstem**, the general organization of the spinal cord is maintained.
- **Anterior** thickening (**basal plates**) that gives rise to the **motor cranial nerve nuclei.**

- **Posterior** thickening (**alar plates**) that gives rise to the **sensory cranial nerve nuclei**.
- The **sulcus limitans** that marks the boundary between the anterior motor and posterior sensory areas.
- The **roof** and **floor plates** (and their lateral boundaries) that delineate the cavities of the neural tube, the **future ventricles** and the **interventricular communications**.

One exception is the **rostral myelencephalon** and **caudal metencephalon**, where the expanding fourth ventricle displaces the **alar plates** that come to lie **dorsolateral** to the **basal plates** (Fig. 2.12). Consequently, the **sensory** nuclei develop **dorsolateral** to the **motor** nuclei at this level. Cranial nerve **nuclei located near the sulcus limitans** are associated with **visceral functions**.

The **grey matter**, derived from the alar and basal plates, forms:
- **Segmental** nuclei, the **cranial** and **autonomic nuclei**
- **Suprasegmental** structures, which serve as relay or association centres. Their development is the result of extensive cellular migration and consists of:
  - **Discrete** structures such as the **red nucleus** and **substantia nigra**
  - **Diffuse** structures such as the **reticular formation**, which occupies the **ventral** aspect of the brainstem.

Myelencephalon

The **myelencephalon** will give rise to the **medulla oblongata**. The caudal part is cylindrical and closely resembles the spinal cord, whereas the rostral part is wide and flat. The **myelencephalic cavity** (**fourth ventricle**) remains in communication with the spinal canal caudally and the mesencephalic cavity

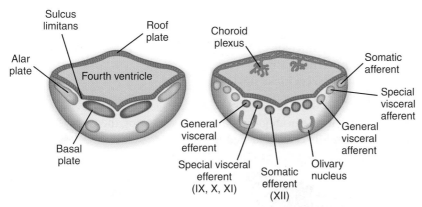

FIGURE 2.12 Cross-sections through the developing myelencephalon at early (left) and later (right) stages of embryonic development. Motor tracts (from the basal plate) are shown in green; sensory tracts (from the alar plate) are orange.

Source: *Adapted from Sadler T. Langman's medical embryology, 6th ed. Baltimore: Williams & Wilkins; 1990.*

rostrally via the **metencephalic cavity**. During the **4th–5th month** of development, local resorption of the roof plate forms:

- The paired **lateral** foramina (**Luschka**)
- A **median** foramen (**Magendi**)

At this stage, **cerebrospinal fluid (CSF)** is free to leave the ventricular system and enter the subarachnoid space. Eventually, CSF is reabsorbed via the **arachnoid granulations** into the venous system.

With further development:

- Neurons of the **basal plate** develop into the **motor nuclei** of **cranial nerves (CNs) IX, X, XI and XII** (Fig. 2.12).
- Neurons of the **alar plate** will form (Fig. 2.12):
  - **Sensory nuclei** of CNs V, VIII, IX and X
  - **Gracile** and **cuneate nuclei**
  - **Olivary nuclei**

As a result of the expanding fourth ventricle:

- The **roof plate** becomes stretched into a thin layer of **ependymal tissue**.
- The latter is covered by the **highly vascular pia mater** (derived from the mesenchyme).
- The two layers form the **tela choroidea**.
- Vascular tufts of the tela choroidea project into the cavity of the fourth ventricle to form the **choroid plexus** (Fig. 2.12).

Metencephalon

At a more rostral level, the **metencephalon** differentiates into two major structures:

1. **Pons** ventrally
2. **Cerebellum** dorsally

The **cavity of the metencephalon** forms the **superior part of the fourth ventricle**. Its **ventral** aspects will form the **pons** (Fig. 2.13). Neurons of the **basal plate** develop into the **motor nuclei** of CNs V, VI and VII. Neurons of the **alar plate** will form the:

- **Main sensory nucleus** of **V**
- **Sensory nucleus** of **VII**
- **Vestibular** and **cochlear nuclei**
- **Pontine nuclei**

Axons of the pontine nuclei grow transversely forming the transverse pontine fibres and the middle cerebellar peduncle.

The **cerebellum** arises from the **dorsal aspect** of the **metencephalon** (Fig. 2.14).

- The **alar plate** becomes thickened to form two lateral plates, the **rhombic lips**.
- The rhombic lips expand medially and eventually fuse in the midline producing a **thick lamina** that constitutes the rudiment of the cerebellum (**tuberculum cerebelli**).

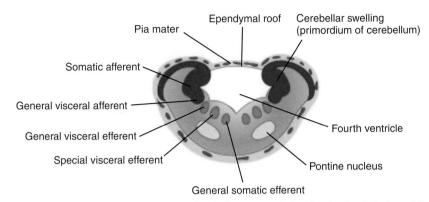

FIGURE 2.13 Cross-sections through the developing metencephalon showing the derivatives of the basal and alar plates.

Source: *Moore KL, BA, MSc, PhD, DSc (OSU), DSc (WU), FIAC, FRSM, FAAA. The developing human. p. 379–416.e1, Chapter 17.*

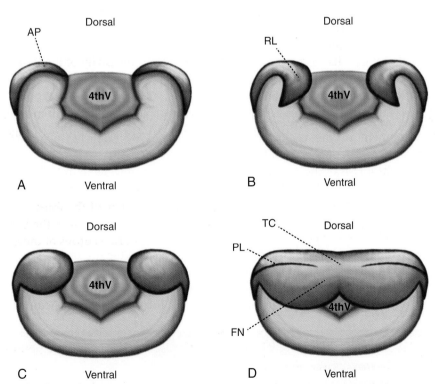

FIGURE 2.14 Development of the cerebellum. (A) Allar plate (AP) cell proliferation in the most rostral aspect of the metencephalon; (B) the AP hypertrophy at its medial aspect creates the rhombic lips (RL); (C) cerebellum originates entirely from rhombomere 1; (D) fusion of the RL at the midline creates the cerebellar primordium or tuberculum cerebelli (TC). PL, posterolateral fissure; FN, flocculonodular lobule.

Source: *Nuñez S, MD. Midline congenital malformations of the brain and skull. Neuroimag Clin North Am 21(3):429–82.*

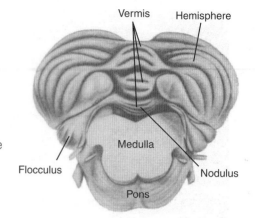

FIGURE 2.15 Late development of the cerebellum. By about 5 months, the cerebellum is composed of a midline (vermis) and two lateral (hemisphere) components. A series of deep fissures appear on its surface.
Source: *From Hochstetter F. Beiträge zur Entwicklungsgeschichte des menschlichen Gehirns. II. Teil, Vienna: Franz Deuticke; 1929.*

- At **12 weeks** of development, the cerebellum is formed of (Fig. 2.15):
  - A small **midline** portion, the **vermis**
  - Two **lateral** portions, the **cerebellar hemispheres**

The outer surface of the cerebellum is originally smooth but **deep fissures** soon appear (Fig. 2.15).

- These first appear during the **third month** of development in the vermis and floccular region.
- Continued **fissuration** subdivides the expanding cerebellum into further **lobes** and then into **lobules**.
- Fissures on the cerebellar hemispheres do not appear until the **fifth month**.

Development of the cerebellum is characterized by extensive neuroblast migration and axonal growth to and from the cerebellum.

- Neuroblasts of the **mantle zone** of the **alar plate** migrate to the **marginal zone** and form the **cerebellar hemispheres**. These cells have a long migratory period, which is not complete until after the **first year of life**.
- Others remain close to the ventricular surface and develop into **deep cerebellar nuclei**.
- Axons grow out into the mesencephalon to reach the forebrain and form much of the **superior cerebellar peduncles**.
- Conversely, axonal growth from the spinal cord, vestibular nuclei and olivary nuclei into the cerebellum form the **inferior cerebellar peduncle**.

CLINICAL INSIGHT

- **Dandy–Walker Syndrome**
  - **Dandy–Walker syndrome** is the result of failure of development of the **midline cerebellum** (Fig. 2.16). It is characterized by
    - Aplastic cerebellar vermis
    - Deficient or absent corpus callosum
    - Greatly dilated fourth ventricle often with a large posterior fossa cyst
    - Dilation of the aqueduct
    - Dilatation of the third and lateral ventricles

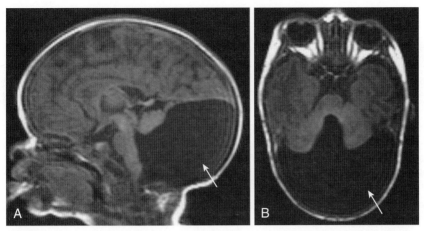

FIGURE 2.16 Magnetic resonance imaging (MRI) of a patient with Dandy–Walker syndrome showing a hypoplastic cerebellum and a large posterior fossa cyst in continuation with the fourth ventricle. Source: *Coban D, MD. Dandy-Walker malformation: a rare association with hypoparathyroidism. Pediatr Neurol 43(6):439–41.*

Mesencephalon

The mesencephalon is the middle portion of the future brain and is therefore called 'the **midbrain**'. In contrast to the prosencephalon and the rhombencephalon, the mesencephalon does not undergo further division during neuronal development. The mesencephalon gives rise to (Fig. 2.17):

- **Dorsal** midbrain, which is composed of:
  - The **tectum** that derives from the **alar** and **roof plates**
  - **Superior** and **inferior colliculi** that also derive from the **alar plates**
- **Ventral** midbrain, where neuroblasts of the **basal plate** differentiate into:
  - **CNs III** and **IV**
  - **Red nucleus**
  - **Substantia nigra**
  - **Reticular formation**
- The marginal zone within the ventral midbrain, which enlarges to form the basis pedunculi containing:
  - **Corticopontine** fibres
  - **Corticobulbar** fibres
  - **Corticospinal** tracts
- The cavity of the midbrain becomes much reduced to form the aqueduct of Sylvius.

DEVELOPMENT OF THE DIENCEPHALON

The **diencephalon** ('middle brain') develops from the median portion of the prosencephalon. Its general organization is fundamentally different from that of the spinal cord and brainstem. This is because the sulcus limitans ends in the region of the mammillary recess (ventral part of the diencephalon).

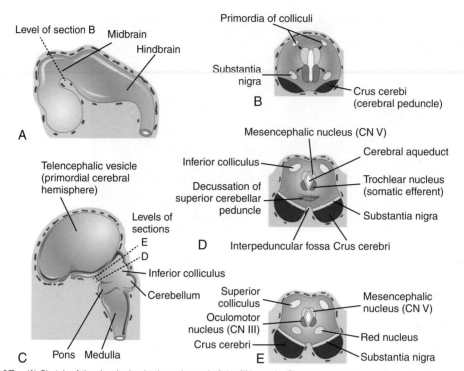

FIGURE 2.17   (A) Sketch of the developing brain at the end of the fifth week; (B) transverse section of the developing midbrain shows the early migration of cells from the basal and alar plates; (C) sketch of the developing brain at 11 weeks; (D and E) transverse sections of the developing midbrain at the level of the inferior and superior colliculi respectively.
Source: *Moore KL, BA, MSc, PhD, DSc (OSU), DSc (WU), FIAC, FRSM, FAAA. Nervous system. The developing human. p. 379–416.e1, Chapter 17.*

Therefore, neural tissue at this level is an extension of the alar plate. Its function is either **sensory** or **associative**. The two main components of the diencephalon are the **thalamus** and **hypothalamus**.

Initially, the diencephalon consists of:
  ▪ **Roof plate** formed of a single layer of **ependymal cells**
  ▪ **Alar plates**
  ▪ **Third ventricle**

The **roof plate's ependymal cells** combined with the covering **mesenchyme** form the **choroid plexus** of the **third ventricle**. The roof plate also gives rise to:
  ▪ **Pineal gland:**
    ▪ Initially arises as a caudal midline thickening immediately anterior to the midbrain.
    ▪ The thickening evaginates towards **week 7**.
    ▪ The evagination eventually forms a solid organ.
    ▪ The mature pineal gland secretes **melatonin**, a sleep modulator.
  ▪ **Epithalamus:**
    ▪ Develops on both sides of the midline near the pineal gland.
    ▪ It will eventually form the **habenular nuclei**.

- The habenular nuclei are linked by the **habenular commissure**.
- The habenular nuclei are involved in multiple functions including pain processing, sleep–wake cycle, stress response and reward processing, among others.

The cavity of the diencephalon is formed by the third ventricle (Fig. 2.18). The alar plate forming the lateral wall of the third ventricle thickens and gives rise to:

- **Thalamus:**
  - Progressively enlarges and bulges into the lateral wall of the diencephalic cavity.
  - Ultimately differentiates into:
    - A large number of **thalamic nuclei**
    - The **medial** and **lateral geniculate bodies** that develop posteriorly as solid buds; these are important relays in the auditory and visual pathways
- **Hypothalamus:**
  - An **autonomic** centre
  - Differentiates into a large number of nuclei that serve as regulation centres of visceral functions, sleep, digestion, body temperature and emotional behaviour
  - One pair of nuclei becomes conspicuous on the **ventral aspect** of the diencephalon, the **mammillary bodies** (part of the limbic system)
  - The thalamus and hypothalamus are separated by the **hypothalamic sulcus**
- **Pallidum,** which is the only striated intercerebral structure having a diencephalic origin

The **floor** of the diencephalon gives rise to:

- **Optic vesicles** and **stalk** that ultimately form the retina and optic nerve
- Funnel-shaped **infundibulum**
- **Stalk** and **pars nervosa** of the **hypophysis** (pituitary gland)

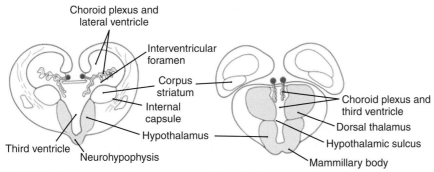

FIGURE 2.18   Developing diencephalon at 8 (left) and 9 (right) weeks of gestation.
Source: *Mihailoff GA. The diencephalon. Fundamental neuroscience for basic and clinical applications. p. 198–210.e1, Chapter 15.*

DEVELOPMENT OF THE TELENCEPHALON

The **telencephalon** is the most rostral part of the brain. At **30 days** of development, it consists of (Fig. 2.19):

- **Two lateral diverticula**, the **cerebral hemispheres**, which are composed of two major structures:
    - **Pallium** or vault (the future cortex)
    - **Floor** (the future striated bodies)
- A median structure, the lamina terminalis (located at the anterior end of the third ventricle)
- Two lateral ventricles, which communicate with the cavity of the diencephalon via the foramina of Monroe

The separation of the brain into two hemispheres is completed by the **end of week 5**. The cerebral hemispheres are initially oval shaped, but **ventral bending** then occurs to create the **operculum** and eventually the **lateral (Sylvian) fissure** (Fig. 2.20). Later on, the **mesenchyme** between the hemispheres will condense to form the **falx cerebri**.

CLINICAL INSIGHT

- **Holoprosencephaly**
    - **Holoprosencephaly** results from **failure of cleavage of the forebrain** that usually occurs around the **33rd week** of gestation. In the most severe form (**lobar** form), the **interhemispheric fissure** and **corpus callosum** are **completely absent** (Fig. 2.21). Milder forms (**semilobar** forms) are associated with some hemispheric separation posteriorly. Holoprosencephaly is often seen as part of **trisomy 13**, but it has also been mapped to several other chromosomes.

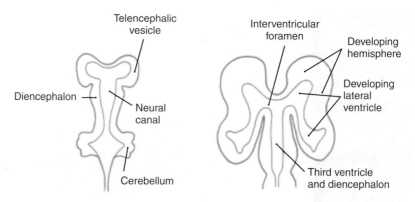

FIGURE 2.19 Development of the telencephalon.
Source: *Haines DE. The telencephalon. Fundamental neuroscience for basic and clinical applications. p. 211–24.e1, Chapter 16.*

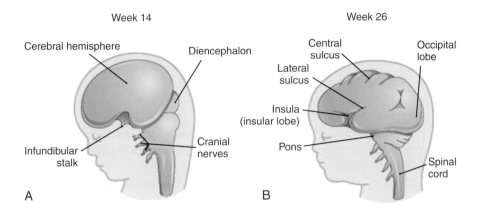

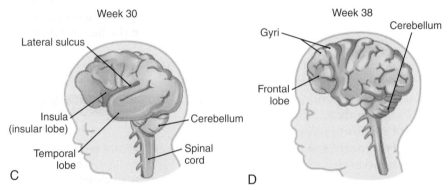

FIGURE 2.20 Development of the cerebral hemispheres. At week 14, the surface of the telencephalon is still smooth. Thereafter, sulci and gyri develop. The insula becomes buried within the Sylvian fissure as a result of the expansion of the frontal, parietal and temporal lobes.
Source: *Paulsen F. Brain and spinal cord. Sobotta Atlas Hum Anat 3(12):211–342.*

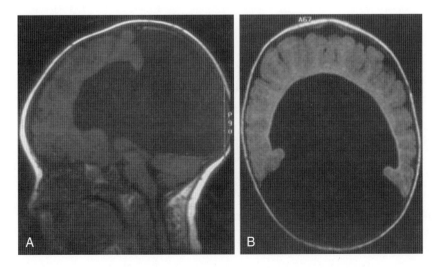

FIGURE 2.21 Alobar holoprosencephaly shows a pancake of brain anteriorly (A), with the single, midline ventricle leading into a large, dorsal cyst (B). The corpus callosum is absent.
Source: Courtesy of Joseph Pinter, MD, Children's Hospital and Regional Medical Center, Seattle, WA.

All neurons of the cerebral cortex are generated remotely in the neuroepithelium of the **subventricular zone**.

- Once formed, neuroblasts:
  - Migrate to their final destination in the cortex
  - Establish synaptic connections with neighbouring neurons
  - Send their axons to their targets
- Migration follows very specific pathways.
- It is guided by specialized fetal astrocytes with long radial processes that extend from the ventricular zone to the surface of the brain (radial glial fibres) (Fig. 2.22).
- Starting at **6 weeks** of gestation, forebrain neuroblasts migrate in waves.
- Each successive wave moves past the preceding wave to add a more superficial layer.
- Eventually, migrating neuroblasts form the **six-layered neocortex**.
- By the 16th week of gestation, the majority of neuroblasts have reached their destination and most of the remaining immature cells of the periventricular germinal matrix yet to migrate will become glioblasts.

As development proceeds, the hemispheres greatly expand and progressively cover the diencephalon and midbrain (Fig. 2.20). Between the **fifth week** and **2 months** of gestation, cortical expansion proceeds in the following order:

- **Anteriorly** to form the **frontal lobe**
- **Laterally** to form the **parietal lobe**
- **Posteriorly** and **inferiorly** to form the **occipital** and **temporal lobes** respectively

Conversely, the cortex covering the **lentiform nucleus** (future insula) remains fixed. It becomes **buried within the lateral fissure** because of the continuous growth of the adjacent frontal, parietal and temporal lobes (Fig. 2.20).

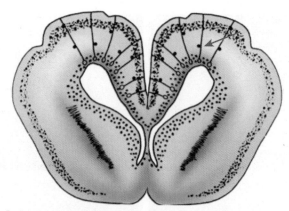

FIGURE 2.22   Radial glial cells (arrow) form long radial processes that extend from the ventricular zone to the surface of the brain. These cells guide the migrating cells to their final destination.
Source: *From Sarnat HB. Cerebral dysgenesis. New York: Oxford University Press; 1992. p. 263.*

CLINICAL INSIGHT

■ **Disorders of migration and lamination**

■ Many brain malformations are the direct or indirect consequence of faulty neuroblast migration. The most severe migratory defects occur in early gestation (**8th–15th weeks**), whereas insults during the **third trimester** cause more subtle or focal abnormalities of cerebral architecture that typically manifest as **epilepsy**.

■ Most disturbances of neuroblast migration are the result of arrested migration before they reach their final destination. These are mostly genetic disorders that fall into three categories depending on where the migratory arrest occurred.

- **PNH** is a condition where neuroblasts never migrated from the **periventricular region (Fig. 2.23A)**

- **Subcortical laminar heterotopia (double cortex or band heterotopia)** results when neuroblasts begin migration but undergo arrest in the **subcortical white matter** before reaching the cortical plate (Fig. 2.23B)

- In other conditions, neuroblasts reach the cortical plate but **lack correct lamination**. These include:

- **Lissencephaly**, which refers to a smooth cerebral cortex without convolutions (Fig. 2.23C)

- **Pachygyria**, which refers to abnormally large and poorly formed gyri

- **Polymicrogyria**, which denotes excessively numerous and abnormally small gyri

- **Heterotopic nodules**, which are conglomerates of neurons of various cortical types that have differentiated without laminar organization

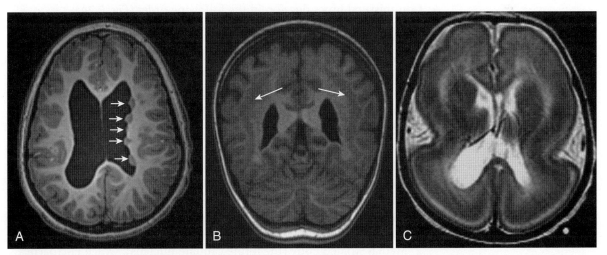

FIGURE 2.23   (A) Multiple nodular heterotopias protruding into a dilated ventricular system; (B) band heterotopia in both cerebral hemispheres; (C) lissencephaly characterized by a thickened agyric cortex.

Source: *(A) from Piña-Garza JE, MD. Disorders of cranial volume and shape. Fenichel's clinical pediatric neurology. p. 348–65, Chapter 18; (B) from Nalbantoglu M, MD. The diagnosis of band heterotopia. Pediatr Neurol 51(1):178–80; (C) from Kanekar S, MD. Malformations of cortical development. Semin Ultrasound, CT, MRI 32(3):211–27.*

As the cerebral cortex expands, the ventricular cavities progressively narrow due to parietal lobes' development.

- The lateral ventricles bend with the hemisphere.
- The original posterior aspect of the neural tube becomes the temporal horn rather than the occipital horn of the mature brain.
- Diverticula from the caudal end of the lateral ventricles develop into the occipital horns.

At **midgestation**, the brain is normally smooth, with only the interhemispheric, Sylvian and calcarine fissures formed (Fig. 2.20).

- **Gyri** and **sulci** develop between the **20th** and **36th weeks** of gestation.
- The **mature pattern** of gyration is evident **at term**.
- Gyri develop as a result of:
  - Continuous arrival of migrating neuroblasts and glial cells
  - Development of neurites (neuronal projections) and glial processes
- Progressive development of gyri helps accommodate the waves of migrating cells:
  - By increasing the surface of the cerebral cortex
  - Without a concomitant increase in cerebral volume

At **11 weeks** of gestation, fibres interconnecting the two cerebral hemispheres start to develop. These are collectively known as the **commissural fibres**.

- A **commissural plate** differentiates within the **lamina terminalis** at **day 39**.
- This plate serves as a **bridge** between the two hemispheres.
- Within the plate, preformed glial pathways provide a guide for decussating axons.
- Commissural fibres develop in the following order (Fig. 2.24):
  - **Anterior commissure**: connects the **olfactory bulbs** and **temporal lobes**
  - **Fornix**: connects the **hippocampi**
  - **Corpus callosum**: arches back over the roof of the third ventricle and connects the **frontal** and **parietal lobes**
  - The rest of the lamina terminalis between the corpus callosum and the fornix becomes stretched out to form a thin septum (**septum pellucidum**)

Active proliferation of the **matrix cells** lining the floor of the forebrain produces a large number of neuroblasts and gives rise to the primordia of the **striated nuclei**.

- The **striated nucleus** later differentiates into two parts (Fig. 2.25):
  1. **Lateral** striated body (the future **lentiform nucleus**)
  2. **Medial** striated body (the future **caudate nucleus**), which encroaches on the wall of the lateral ventricle

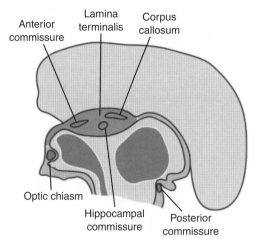

FIGURE 2.24   Midline section through the developing brain showing the cerebral commissures.

Source: *Fotos J, MD. Embryology of the brain and molecular genetics of central nervous system malformation. Semin Ultrasound, CT, MRI 32(3): 159–66.*

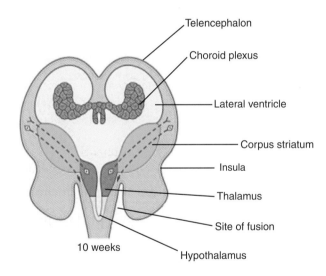

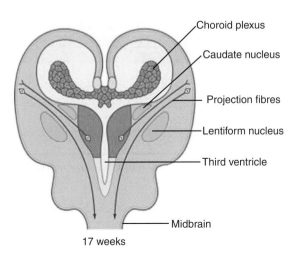

FIGURE 2.25   Coronal sections of the developing cerebrum. At 10 weeks, the corpus striatum is traversed by fibres projecting to and from the cerebral cortex. By the 17th week, the corpus striatum has already divided into the caudate nucleus medially and lentiform nucleus laterally.

Source: *Mtui E, MD. Embryology. Fitzgerald's clinical neuroanatomy and neuroscience. vol. 1, p. 1–5.*

- Nerve fibres to and from the developing cortex form a compact bundle of ascending and descending fibres known as the internal capsule. These fibres are forced to pass between the:
  - **Caudate** and **thalamus** medially
  - **Lentiform nucleus** laterally (Fig. 2.25)
- Rare cortical projections pass lateral to the lentiform nucleus and form the external capsule.

MYELINATION

Myelination is the process of acquiring a specialized insulating material around the axons, the **myelin sheath**.

- The main role of myelin is to **speed up nerve conduction**.
- Myelin is elaborated from the adjacent **oligodendrocytes** in the CNS and **Schwann cells** in the peripheral nervous system.
- The process of myelination is not a random process and follows a very precise order.

The overall period for myelination is **very long**. It stretches between **14 weeks** of gestation and continues to **past 30 years** of age in some areas.

- The **earliest tracts** to myelinate are as follows:
  - **Medial longitudinal fasciculus**
  - **Dorsal columns** of the spinal cord
- Myelination progresses to involve:
  - Brainstem structures
  - Basal ganglia
- However, the optic nerve and tract do not begin to acquire myelin until near term.
- Some structures do not acquire myelin until **after birth** (i.e. **corpus callosum**).
- Some association fibres connecting the frontal and parietotemporal lobe do not achieve full myelination until age 32.

CLINICAL INSIGHT

- **Myelination delay**
  - Many conditions can impede the myelination process. These include metabolic disorders such as hypothyroidism. Chronic hypoxia in premature infants is another cause of delayed myelination and contributes to delays in clinical neurological maturation. Delay of myelination can be reversible if the insult is removed as early as possible.

CASE STUDY DISCUSSION

PNH is the most common type of neuronal heterotopia, where neuroblasts fail to migrate during the expected developmental stages and eventually differentiate in the wrong place, forming **grey matter nodules** (clusters of **normal** neurons) that line and disrupt the normal outline of ventricular walls by protruding towards the lumen.

Clinical Presentation

The clinical presentation of PNH patients is highly variable; it depends on the number and location of heterotopic nodules, the presence of other brain malformations, and if it is in the context of a syndrome, i.e. diffuse PNH and Ehlers–Danlos syndrome due to mutations in the X-linked FLNA gene or diffuse PNH and congenital microcephaly, a rare autosomal recessive disease.

Isolated, single or multiple PNH are associated with:

- **Epilepsy:** most common presenting symptom (80–90%)
  - Age of onset is variable
  - Most of seizures are **focal**
  - Some seizures are easily controlled by anti-epileptic medications, while others are refractory

- **Cognitive impairment: increases greatly when other brain malformations are present**
  - Learning problems are common: difficulty in reading and spelling
  - Normal intelligence to borderline intellectual deficits

Diagnosis

- The diagnosis of PNH is established by detecting the lesions on brain MRI.
- In patients with intractable epilepsy, EEG is utilized to confirm that the nodules detected on MRI are causing the seizures.

Management and Prognosis

- Isolated PNH has a **stable course** where symptoms do not worsen if left untreated.
- Once a heterotopic nodule is confirmed to be epileptogenic in patients with **refractory epilepsy, surgical resection** is performed.
- Resection of epileptogenic nodules may partially or fully prevent the occurrence of seizures but does not improve the developmental disabilities if present.

CHAPTER 3

Meninges, Ventricles and Cerebrospinal Fluid Circulation

Mohammad Hassan A. Noureldine

CASE STUDY

Presentation and Physical Examination: A 72-year-old hypertensive man, otherwise not known to have any neurological disease, presented to the neurology unit complaining of balance and walking problems that started insidiously and progressively deteriorated over 14 months. Initially, the patient noticed difficulty in walking and turning on uneven surfaces, which evolved into difficulty in getting out of chair and need for the assistance of a cane. He also reported multiple falls over the last few months. Several physicians examined him and an extensive workup was done including blood tests, nerve conduction studies and electromyographic testing without reaching a diagnosis. His family reported that he started forgetting things more often during the last 2 months, and recently, he started having urinary urgency and incontinence. Parkinson medications were prescribed, but the symptoms persisted except for mild improvement in memory. On examination, the patient is wheelchair-bound and cannot stand and walk without the assistance of his son and daughter. His gait is profoundly abnormal and characterized by bradykinesia, broad-based and shuffling foot movements. His mini-mental state test points towards abnormal cognitive processing and cognitive slowing. Cognitive processing was tested by asking the patient to recite the months backwards, while slowing was documented by testing for verbal fluency where the patient was asked to name as many animals as possible in one minute.

Diagnosis, Management and Follow-Up: A brain magnetic resonance imaging (MRI) (Fig. 3.1) revealed enlarged ventricles out of proportion to sulci atrophy and transependymal flow of cerebrospinal fluid (CSF), but otherwise normal.

The preliminary diagnosis was **normal pressure hydrocephalus (NPH)**. Removal of a large quantity of CSF by lumbar puncture was performed.

After few days, the family reported improvement in memory and movement; he was able to stand by himself and walk with the help of a cane. Urinary incontinence resolved as early as day 2 post-lumbar puncture, but the patient was left with intermittent urinary urgency.

Try to guess what is the pathophysiology, clinical features, management and prognosis of NPH after studying this chapter!

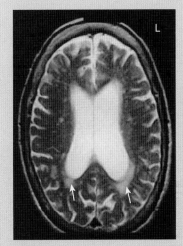

FIGURE 3.1 Brain magnetic resonance imaging (MRI) scan shows diffusely enlarged ventricles out of proportion to sulci atrophy and transependymal flow of cerebrospinal fluid (arrows).
Source: *Kelley RE, MD. Memory complaints and dementia. Med Clin North Am 93(2):389–406.*

BRIEF INTRODUCTION

The delicate structure and superior function of the CNS, the brain in particular, necessitate special protection measures and a highly regulated environment.

- The skull bones and vertebral column embrace the brain and spinal cord and provide a strong shield against traumatic injury.
- The meninges are three layers that isolate the CNS from the rest of the body tissues, thus preventing bodily processes from affecting the CNS function.
- The CSF provides the CNS with a distinct, highly regulated milieu.
- Any disruption of the CSF generation, circulation and absorption cycle is indicative of an ongoing pathological state and requires prompt investigation and a management plan.

The goal of this chapter is to introduce the neuroanatomy and the closely associated physiology of the meninges, ventricular system and CSF, and highlight important clinical correlations.

MENINGEAL STRUCTURE

The **meninges** strictly contain and separate the CSF from the extracellular spaces of body tissues other than that of the CNS (Figs. 3.2 and 3.3). The meninges comprise three coverings: **dura mater**, also called pachymeninx, **arachnoid mater** and **pia mater,** both of which are collectively known as leptomeninx.

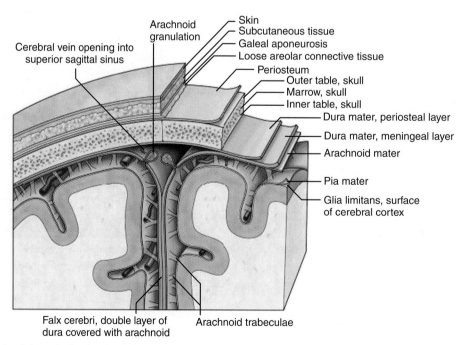

FIGURE 3.2 Schematic showing the skull and cranial meninges.

Source: *Bhattacharya JJ. Overview of anatomy, pathology and techniques; aspects related to trauma. Grainger & Allison's diagnostic radiology p. 1393–1427.e2, Chapter 60.*

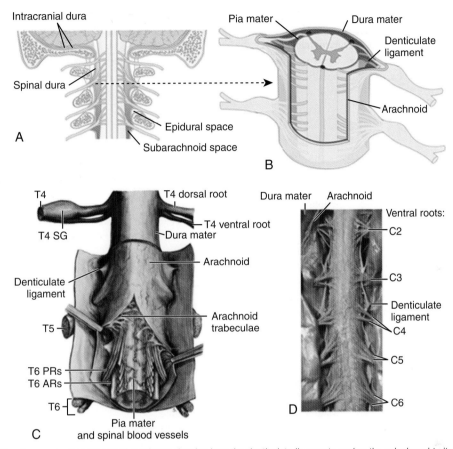

FIGURE 3.3 Arrangement of the spinal meninges showing how the denticulate ligaments anchor the spinal cord to its dural sheath through the arachnoid. (A and B) Show how the double-layered cranial dura mater is continuous with the single-layered dural sheath of the spinal cord. (A and C) Drawing of a posterior view. (D) Anterior view of a dissection in which the dural sheath was cut open longitudinally. ARs, anterior rootlets; PRs, posterior rootlets; SG, spinal ganglion.

Source: *A and B modified from Nolte J. Elsevier's integrated neuroscience. Philadelphia: Mosby/Elsevier; 2007. C from Mettler FA. Neuroanatomy, 2nd ed., St. Louis: Mosby, 1948. D courtesy Dr. Normal Koelling, University of Arizona College of Medicine.*

Dura Mater

- The outermost and strongest membrane consisting of dense connective tissue.
- It consists of two layers in the cranium, outer periosteal and inner meningeal, and one layer around the spinal cord.
- Cerebral venous blood flows through spaces or sinuses formed by separation of the periosteal and meningeal layers *(see chapter 4)*.

Epidural Space

The **epidural space** is located above the dura mater.

- A potential space in the cranium that is traversed by meningeal vessels.
- A true space around the spinal cord containing spinal nerve roots, loose connective and fatty tissue, lymphatic and small arterial vessels, and internal vertebral venous plexuses.

CLINICAL INSIGHT

- **Epidural injection**
  - A needle is inserted at a specific vertebral level, according to the type of procedure and the intended outcome, between the spinous processes of two vertebral bodies. The layers that it crosses are in the following order (Fig. 3.4):
    - Skin
    - Subcutaneous fat tissue
    - Supraspinous ligament
    - Interspinous ligament
    - Ligamentum flavum
  - It is important not to puncture the meninges, which is closely related to the ligamentum flavum, as this will result in intrathecal (inside spinal sheath) rather than epidural injection, a procedure with different indications and outcomes.
  - For anaesthetic purposes
    - An anaesthetic drug is injected into the epidural space of the spinal cord.
    - Applied before many surgical procedures and during childbirth, where it reliefs the associated pain but does not significantly affect muscle power necessary for uterine contractions.
  - For treatment purposes
    - Steroid injections may be utilized to manage radiculopathy associated with certain vertebral column related disorders such as disc herniation, spinal stenosis and degenerative disc disease.
- **Epidural haemorrhage**
  - Mostly encountered in young patients with a history of clearly identified head trauma and sometimes a skull fracture.
  - The clinical manifestations are often strongly suggestive of the diagnosis. If consciousness is disturbed by the trauma, patients usually regain normal level of consciousness, a period termed **'lucid interval'**, where they subsequently suffer from severe and persistent headaches and gradual decrease in the level of consciousness over the course of few hours.
  - The source of bleeding is a meningeal artery, the middle meningeal artery in the majority of cases (Fig. 3.5).
  - It appears as a characteristic hyperdense, **biconvex-shaped** and sharply demarcated lesion that is closely related to the skull bone on a computed tomography (CT) scan (Fig. 3.6).
  - Usually does not cross cranial sutures, but may cross venous sinuses (Fig. 3.7).
  - Can produce significant mass effect, midline shift and herniation of brain structures; cranial nerve (CN) III is often compressed by uncal herniation (Fig. 3.5), whereas if there is rise in intracranial pressure, CN VI is usually affected as it is the CN with the longest intracranial run.
  - A condition that must be managed promptly, otherwise patients are at risk of serious complications and death.

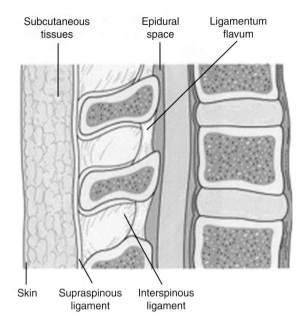

Subcutaneous tissues

Epidural space

Ligamentum flavum

Skin

Supraspinous ligament

Interspinous ligament

FIGURE 3.4   Layers crossed by the needle during an epidural injection.
Source: *O'Connor TC, MB FFARCSI. Atlas of pain injection techniques. vol. 3, p. 15–36.*

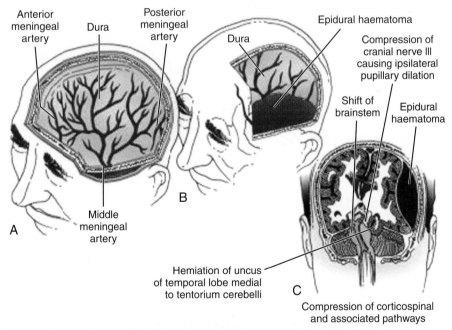

Anterior meningeal artery

Dura

Posterior meningeal artery

Dura

Epidural haematoma

Compression of cranial nerve III causing ipsilateral pupillary dilation

Shift of brainstem

Epidural haematoma

Middle meningeal artery

A

B

Hemiation of uncus of temporal lobe medial to tentorium cerebelli

C

Compression of corticospinal and associated pathways

FIGURE 3.5   Epidural haematoma. (A) The middle meningeal artery (MMA) extensively covers the lateral, external surface of the dura. (B) A tear in the MMA leads to rapid accumulation of high flow arterial blood in the epidural space. (C) A large epidural haematoma may cause a mass effect with midline shift, uncal herniation and compression of cranial nerve III and corticospinal pathways, among others.
Source: *Ferri FF, MD, FACP, Ferri's clinical advisor 2016, 475–6.e1.*

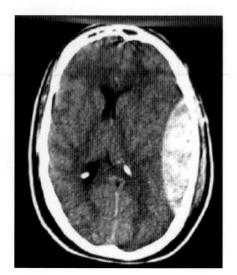

FIGURE 3.6 CT scan of a patient with a large left temporal epidural haematoma, with left to right midline shift.
Source: *Smith SW, MD. Emergency department skull trephination for epidural hematoma in patients who are awake but deteriorate rapidly. J Emergency Med 39(3):377–83.*

FIGURE 3.7 Coronal diagram of the epidural haema-toma (EDH) and subdural haematoma (SDH). The EDH is located above the outer dural layer (i.e. the periosteum), and the SDH is located beneath the inner (meningeal) dural layer. The EDH is located at the coup site, does not cross sutures, but can displace dural venous sinuses away from the inner table of the skull. The SDH is more often located at the contrecoup site, does not directly cross the falx or the tentorium, and cannot displace dural sinuses.
Source: *Reprinted with permission from Gean AD. Imaging of head trauma. Philadelphia: Williams & Wilkins-Lippincott; 1994. p. 76.*

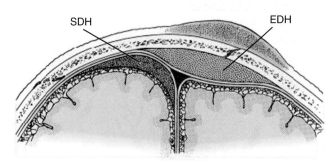

Subdural Space

The **subdural space** lies between the inner layer of the dura mater and arachnoid mater.

- A potential space
- Small **bridging veins** cross through the subdural space from arachnoid to dura mater in the cranium

---

CLINICAL INSIGHT

- **Subdural haemorrhage**
  - Occurs at any age, mostly after head trauma.
  - The source of bleeding is bridging veins, veins that cross the subdural space to drain cerebral blood into the venous sinuses; these veins are torn due to over-stretching forces following a trauma (Fig. 3.8).

- In elderly patients, head trauma is often mild or absent and usually occurs after falls. Minimal trauma to the head of an elderly patient may be sufficient to tear the already stretched bridging veins due to physiologic atrophic changes of the brain. Patients usually present with pseudodementia and gradual decrease in level of consciousness over several weeks. In this case, the subdural haemorrhage is referred to as subacute or chronic in nature.
- Can be classified as hyperacute, acute, subacute, chronic and acute on top of chronic.
- Has a characteristic **crescent-shape** on brain CT scan (Fig. 3.9). Density varies according to the chronicity of the bleed. It appears as hyperdense in hyperacute and acute, isodense in subacute, and hypodense in chronic lesions. The blood degradation process explains this change in density, where a fresh clot appears as hyperdense on CT scan.
- Is not limited by cranial sutures, but rather by dural reflections such as the falx cerebri, tentorium and falx cerebelli (Fig. 3.7).
- Subdural haematomas must be surgically evacuated once neurological symptoms appear.

Arachnoid Mater

- The middle, fine and nonvascular membrane.
- Projections of the arachnoid membrane into the dural sinuses are called **arachnoid or Pacchionian villi and granulations** (Fig. 3.2); they allow the CSF to escape from the subarachnoid space into the cerebral venous system *(see CSF Generation and Flow section)*.

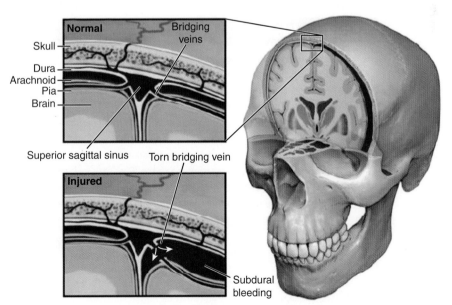

FIGURE 3.8   Acute subdural haemorrhage (SDH). Note the traumatic disruption of the bridging cortical vein traversing the subdural space. The SDH is located between the inner meningeal layer of dura and the arachnoid.
Source: *Gean AD. Head trauma. Neuroimag Clin North Am 20(4):527–56.*

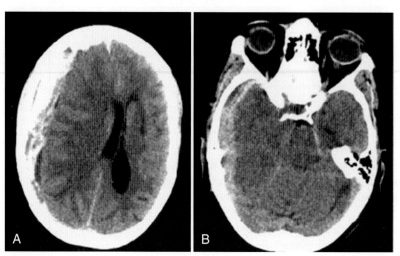

FIGURE 3.9   Axial brain CT scans showing (A) an extensive right hemispheric acute subdural haematoma, causing a 2 cm midline shift and (B) a right uncal herniation with deformation of both cerebral peduncles and obliteration of the perimesencephalic cisterns. Source: *Carrasco R. Kernohan-Woltman notch phenomenon caused by an acute subdural hematoma. J Clin Neurosci 16(12):1628–31.*

Subarachnoid Space

The **subarachnoid space** lies between the arachnoid and pia mater.

- CSF circulates around the CNS in this space.
- The intracranial subarachnoid space is continuous with the spinal subarachnoid space.
- The spinal subarachnoid space terminates at the level of the second sacral vertebra.

CLINICAL INSIGHT

- **Subarachnoid haemorrhage:**
    - Mostly occurs in older middle aged persons.
    - Patients present with sudden onset of **'the worst headache of their lives'**, photophobia and nuchal rigidity.
    - Almost 50% of patients lose consciousness, but the majority regain it soon after the event.
    - Can occur after brain trauma or spontaneously. In the latter case, a ruptured cerebral aneurysm is the most common cause (Fig. 3.10).
    - Risk factors include family history, hypertension and heavy alcohol consumption.
    - CT scan shows **hyperdense fluid in the subarachnoid space**, most commonly around the Circle of Willis where the majority of berry aneurysms occur (Figs. 3.10 and 3.11).
    - Complications such as acute elevation of intracranial pressure and delayed cerebral vasospasm may occur.
    - Early detection and treatment of a cerebral aneurysm are essential to prevent rebleed, which is associated with a high mortality rate.
    - Prognosis is variable and depends on the aetiology and severity of the haemorrhage.

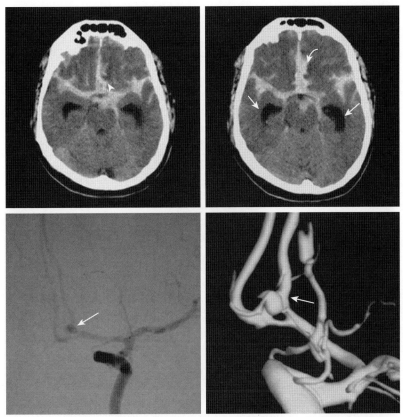

FIGURE 3.10   Upper row: brain CT scan showing subarachnoid haemorrhage with extensive and thick clot in the subarachnoid cisterns. Note focal clot in the interpeduncular cistern towards the left (arrowhead), early hydrocephalus signalled by dilatation of the temporal horns of the lateral ventricles (solid arrows) and left parasagittal intraparenchymal haemorrhage (curved arrow). Lower row: digital subtraction angiography (left panel) and three-dimensional (3D)-reconstructed images showing a saccular aneurysm arising from the left A1 segment of the anterior cerebral artery (open arrows).
Source: *Rabinstein AA. Subarachnoid hemorrhage. Practical neuroimaging in stroke. p. 293–319, Chapter 12.*

Pia Mater

- The innermost, thinnest, most delicate and highly vascularized membrane attaching directly to CNS tissue and following its outer terrain (gyri and sulci in the brain, and surface, grooves, and proximal part of nerve roots in the spinal cord).
- It is anchored to the brain by a sheet of star-shaped cells – astrocytes – and to the spinal cord through a series of small ligaments.
- **Dentate or denticulate ligaments** (21 pairs) extend from the pia mater of the spinal cord and attach it to the dura and arachnoid mater (Fig. 3.3).
- **Virchow–Robin (perivascular) spaces** are pia mater-lined interstitial fluid-filled structures that accompany penetrating vessels and project deeply into the brain cortex. They do not communicate with the subarachnoid space proximally; however, the pia mater progressively

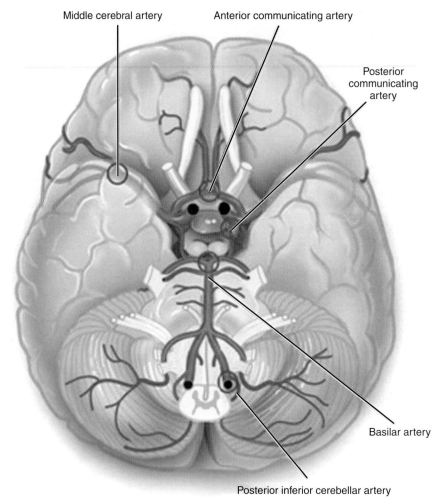

Middle cerebral artery

Anterior communicating artery

Posterior communicating artery

Basilar artery

Posterior inferior cerebellar artery

FIGURE 3.11   Base of brain, with most common sites of aneurysms (circles).
Source: *van Gijn J, Prof. Subarachnoid haemorrhage. The Lancet 369(9558):306–18.*

becomes perforated until it disappears at the capillary level distally. Veins are not usually lined by pia mater (Fig. 3.12).

Cisterns

Cisterns are CSF pools formed by the separation of pia from arachnoid membranes leading to enlarged subarachnoid spaces in certain areas around the brain.

CLINICAL INSIGHT

- **Decreased size** of one or more cisterns is a sign of increased intracranial pressure.
- **Loss of symmetry** of one or more cisterns is a sign of midline shift (Figs. 3.9 and 3.29).

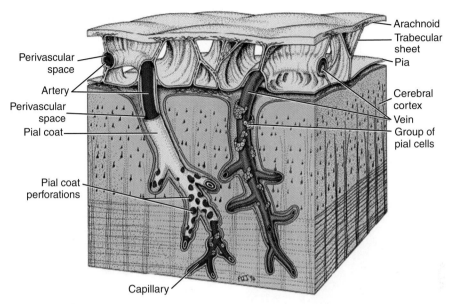

FIGURE 3.12   Virchow–Robin (perivascular) spaces.

Source: *Reproduced and modified from Zhang ET, Inman CBE, Weller RO. Interrelationships of the pia mater and the perivascular (Virchow–Robin) spaces in the human cerebrum. J Anat 1990;170:111–23, by permission from Blackwell Science.*

Cisterna Magna *(Fig. 3.13)*

- The largest cistern
- Between the dorsal surface of medulla oblongata and cerebellum

CLINICAL INSIGHT

- **Mega cisterna magna**
  - A normal anatomical variant; it refers to a focal enlargement of the subarachnoid space in the inferior and posterior portions of the posterior fossa.
  - Should be distinguished from pathological entities such as arachnoid, epidermoid and Blake's pouch cysts, cerebellar atrophy or hypoplasia and Dandy–Walker malformation *(see chapter 2)*.

Ambient Cistern *(Fig. 3.13)*

- Surrounds the midbrain laterally
- Acts as a connection between the quadrigeminal and interpeduncular cisterns
- Contains *(see chapters 4 & 8)*:
  - CN IV or trochlear nerve
  - Posterior cerebral arteries (PCAs)
  - Superior cerebellar arteries (SCAs)
  - Basal vein of Rosenthal

Interpeduncular (Basal) Cistern (Fig. 3.13)

- Between the anterior aspects of the temporal lobes and encloses structures within the interpeduncular fossa and the cerebral peduncles
- Closely related and opens to the pontine cistern inferiorly
- Contains:
  - CN III or oculomotor nerve
  - Distal basilar artery and its branches

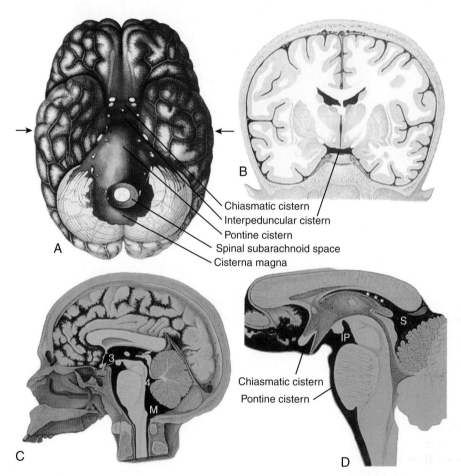

FIGURE 3.13 Subarachnoid cisterns. (A) Cisterns at the base of the brain, demonstrated by filling subarachnoid space with dyed gelatin. The dye fills prominent cisterns, as well as cerebral sulci, but is mostly excluded from the surface of gyri, where there is little subarachnoid space. (B) A coronal section of a similar specimen, in the plane indicated by the arrows in (A). Dye fills the ventricles and subarachnoid space, including the interpeduncular cistern. Low (C) and high (D) magnification views of the cisterns and ventricles near the midline, demonstrated by filling subarachnoid space (and in C, the ventricles as well) with dyed gelatin. As in (A) and (B), the dye fills prominent cisterns, as well as cerebral sulci, but is mostly excluded from the surface of gyri. *, transverse cerebral fissure; 3, third ventricle; 4, fourth ventricle; IP, interpeduncular cistern; M, cisterna magna (cerebellomedullary cistern); S, superior (quadrigeminal) cistern. Source: *From Key A, Retzius G. Studien in der anatomie des nervensystems und des bindegewebes. Stockholm: Norstad; 1875. vol. 1.*

Quadrigeminal (Superior) Cistern or Cistern of the Great Cerebral Vein (of Galen) (Fig. 3.13)

- Posterior to midbrain, at the angle between the colliculi, superior cerebellar surface and splenium (posterior segment) of the corpus callosum
- Contains:
  - CN IV
  - PCAs
  - SCAs
  - Posterior choroidal arteries
  - Venous confluence, i.e. the junction of the vein of Galen, inferior sagittal and straight sinuses

Pontine or Prepontine Cistern (Fig. 3.13)

- Large cavity in front of the pons
- Continuous with the cisterna magna, interpeduncular and quadrigeminal cisterns
- Contains:
  - CN V or trigeminal, CN VI or abducens, CN VII or facial, CN VIII or vestibulocochlear, CN IX or glossopharyngeal, CV X or vagal, CN XI or accessory and CN XII or hypoglossal nerves
  - Basilar artery

Other Cisterns (Fig. 3.13)

- **Suprasellar cistern:** Surrounding the infundibulum or stalk of the pituitary gland, between the uncus of the temporal lobes, under the hypothalamus, and above the sella turcica, which is a depression in the sphenoid bone containing the pituitary gland

---

CLINICAL INSIGHT

- **Obliterated suprasellar cistern**
  - Very high intracranial pressure and uncal herniation obliterates the suprasellar cistern on MRI scan

---

- **Cerebellopontine cistern:** Located at the angle between the pons and cerebellum
- **Premedullary cistern:** Located in front of the medulla oblongata

---

ADDITIONAL CLINICAL INSIGHTS

- **Meningiomas**
  - Most common tumours of the meninges.
  - Can grow anywhere the meninges are present.
  - Originate from meningocytes and arachnoid cap cells.

- Are typically benign, but some variants exhibit aggressive behaviour faster growth rate, and may recur.
- Risk factors include exposure to ionizing radiation and **neurofibromatosis type 2**.
- Symptoms are usually absent until the tumour becomes very large. The clinical manifestations also depend on the location of the meningioma. Signs and symptoms include, but are not limited to:
  - Headaches
  - Seizures
  - Changes in personality and behaviour
  - Progressive focal neurologic deficit
  - Muscle weakness
  - Visual disorders
  - Hearing loss
- Diagnosis is made by thorough neurological evaluation and brain imaging studies (CT scan or MRI) (Fig. 3.14).
- Optimal treatment is surgical resection of symptomatic tumours; otherwise, asymptomatic tumours are followed up until symptoms appear. Postoperative radiation therapy may be necessary in patients where complete resection is not possible.

■ **Herniation**
- Refers to shifting of brain tissue from one region to another as a result of mass effect exerted by a tumour, oedema, abscess or haemorrhage.
- Has several types depending on the shift pattern (Fig. 3.15).
  - **Transtentorial herniation** or bulging of brain tissue through the tentorial notch. Different patterns may occur:
    - **Descending or uncal herniation:** The uncus and adjacent temporal lobe tissue slide downwards through the tentorial notch and compress brainstem structures – may cause altered consciousness, haemiplegia, **oculomotor (CN III) weakness** and hemianopsia.
    - **Ascending herniation:** Superior cerebellar structures slide upwards through the tentorial notch due to a space occupying lesion in the posterior cranial fossa.
  - **Subfalcial herniation** or bulging of brain tissue, mostly the cingulate gyrus, below the free edge of the falx cerebri – may compress the anterior cerebral artery and cause contralateral leg paresis.
  - **Tonsillar herniation** or inferior bulging of cerebellar tonsils below the level of the foramen magnum – may be fatal by compression of brainstem and compromise of the functions of the respiratory and cardiac centres.

■ **Meningitis**
- Refers to **inflammation of meninges** of the brain and/or spinal cord, more frequently the pia and arachnoid mater – pachymeningitis refers to the condition where the dura mater is inflamed as well.
- Is a medical emergency and requires prompt management.
- Signs and symptoms include:
  - **Headache**
  - **Nuchal rigidity, i.e. neck stiffness**
  - **Fever**

- Altered level of consciousness and/or irritability
- Vomiting, mostly with projectile pattern
- Photophobia
- Phonophobia
- Rash, when caused by Neisseria meningitides bacteria
- **Kernig's sign:** Inability to completely extend the knee due to pain and resistance when the thigh is flexed at 90 degrees (Fig. 3.16)
- **Brudzinski's sign:** Involuntary flexion of the thighs and knees when the rigid neck is flexed (Fig. 3.16)

▪ Aetiologies include:
- Bacterial; most frequent organisms according to patients' age:
  - Newborns <1 month: Group B streptococcus, *Escherichia coli*, *Listeria monocytogenes*.
  - Infants between 1 and 23 months: *Streptococcus pneumoniae* and *Haemophilus influenzae* type B. However, *H. influenzae* meningitis is significantly reduced by early vaccination practices.
  - Children between 2 and 18 years: *Neisseria meningitides* and *Streptococcus pneumoniae*.
  - Adults >19 years: *Streptococcus pneumoniae*.
- Viral, including the following viruses:
  - **Herpes simplex type 2**
  - Mumps
  - Varicella zoster
  - Coxsackie
  - Echovirus
  - Epstein–Barr
  - HIV
  - Lymphocytic choriomeningitis virus (LCMV)
- Fungal, frequently associated with immunosuppression and advanced HIV infections. Some of the implicated fungi are as follows:
  - *Cryptococcus neoformans*, the most frequent cause of fungal meningitis
  - Candida species
  - *Coccidioides immitis*
  - *Blastomyces dermatitidis*
  - *Histoplasma capsulatum*
- Noninfectious aetiologies (aseptic meningitis):
  - Malignancy with meningeal metastasis
  - Drug-induced meningitis
  - Systemic diseases such as systemic lupus erythematosus, sarcoidosis and vasculitis
  - Cysts (epidermoid, dermoid) releasing contents that cause meningeal irritation

▪ Brain imaging and lumbar puncture are required to establish the diagnosis. CSF findings are summarized in Table 3.1.

▪ Prognosis depends on the cause and duration before starting treatment. Bacterial is more severe than viral meningitis and can be fatal if left untreated.

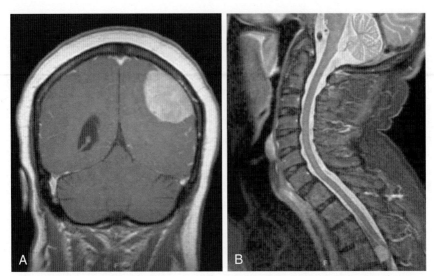

FIGURE 3.14 (A) Convexity meningioma on contrast T1-weighted MRI. Note the extraaxial location, uniform contrast enhancement and 'dural tail' sign, with mass effect causing compression of occipital horn of lateral ventricle. (B) Spinal cord meningioma on T2-weighted MRI. This thoracic cord meningioma (lower part of the image) pushes and compresses the spinal cord posteriorly. The normal rim of bright cerebrospinal fluid is displaced by the tumour and compressed cord.
Source: *Perry A. Meningiomas. Practical surgical neuropathology: a diagnostic approach. vol. 10, p. 185–217.*

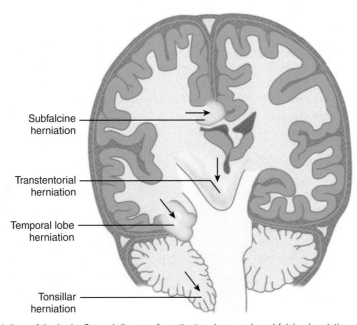

FIGURE 3.15 Herniations of the brain. Coronal diagram, from the top downwards, subfalcine herniation, central transtentorial herniation, downwards transtentorial temporal lobe (uncal) herniation and tonsillar herniation. Lines of force are demonstrated by the arrows. Note the pressure on the brainstem from these herniation patterns.
Source: *From Grossman RI, Yousem DM. Neuroradiology requisites. St. Louis: Mosby; 2004. p. 261.*

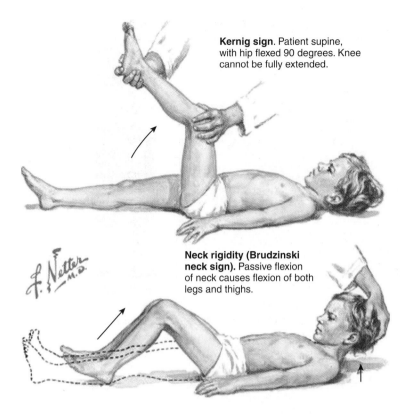

Kernig sign. Patient supine, with hip flexed 90 degrees. Knee cannot be fully extended.

Neck rigidity (Brudzinski neck sign). Passive flexion of neck causes flexion of both legs and thighs.

FIGURE 3.16   Kernig's and Brudzinski's signs.
Source: *Flynn SG. Neurologic emergencies. Netter's pediatrics. vol. 10, p. 62–66.*

Table 3.1 Composition of CSF in different meningeal infections in comparison to normal values

CSF	Appearance	Protein	Glucose	PMN Count	Lymphocyte Count
Normal	Clear	15–45 mg/dL	50–75 mg/dL	0	<5/mm³
Bacterial meningitis	Turbid and yellowish	↑↑↑	↓↓	↑↑↑	or ↑
Viral meningitis	Clear	↕ or ↑	↕	↕ or ↑	↑↑↑
Tuberculous meningitis	Viscous and yellowish	↑↑	↓↓	↕ or ↑	↑↑↑
Fungal meningitis	Viscous and yellowish	↕ or ↑	↕ or ↓↓	↕ or ↑	↑↑↑

Notes: PMN, polymorphonuclear cell; ↑↑↑, markedly increased; ↑↑, increased; ↑, slightly increased; ↕, normal; ↓↓, decreased.

VENTRICULAR SYSTEM

The cerebral **ventricles** are CSF-filled spaces located deep inside the brain core. Multiple openings or foramina connect these structures to each other and to the subarachnoid space. The brain ventricular system comprises the following spaces and foramina (Fig. 3.17):

Lateral Ventricles
- The largest of the ventricles.
- Two symmetrical C-shaped spaces; one in each cerebral hemisphere.

Ventricles of the brain

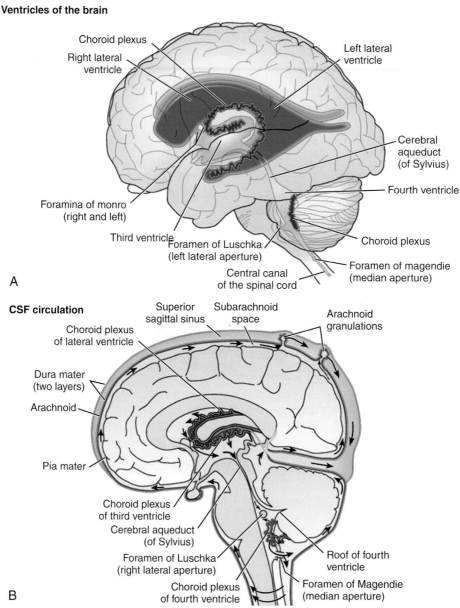

FIGURE 3.17 The brain ventricles and the cerebrospinal fluid. (A) This is a transparent view, looking from the left side of the brain. The two lateral ventricles communicate with the third ventricle, which in turn communicates with the fourth ventricle. (B) Each ventricle contains a choroid plexus, which secretes CSF. The CSF escapes from the fourth ventricle and into the subarachnoid space through the two lateral foramina of Luschka and the single foramen of Magendie.

Source: *Ransom BR. The neuronal microenvironment. Medical physiology. p. 289–309, Chapter 11.*

- Has a body and atrium in the frontal and parietal lobes respectively, from which anterior, inferior and posterior horns extend into the frontal, temporal and occipital lobes respectively (Fig. 3.18).
- Surfaces:
  - Dorsal: Corpus callosum
  - Ventral: Basal ganglia
  - Medial: Septum pellucidum
- **Foramina of Monro:**
  - Two interventricular foramina each connecting one lateral ventricle to the third ventricle medially.

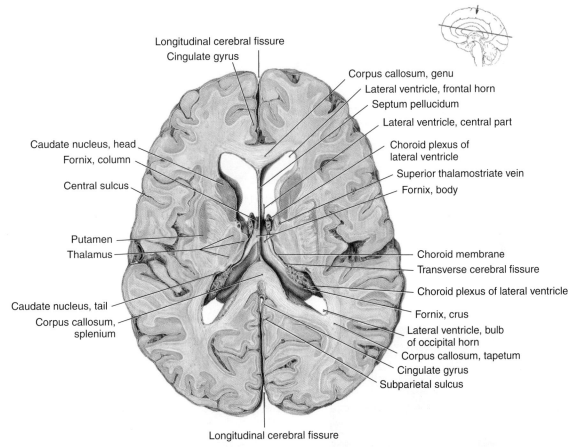

Longitudinal cerebral fissure
Cingulate gyrus

Corpus callosum, genu
Lateral ventricle, frontal horn
Septum pellucidum
Lateral ventricle, central part

Caudate nucleus, head
Fornix, column

Choroid plexus of lateral ventricle
Superior thalamostriate vein
Fornix, body

Central sulcus

Putamen
Thalamus

Choroid membrane
Transverse cerebral fissure
Choroid plexus of lateral ventricle

Caudate nucleus, tail
Corpus callosum, splenium

Fornix, crus
Lateral ventricle, bulb of occipital horn
Corpus callosum, tapetum
Cingulate gyrus
Subparietal sulcus

Longitudinal cerebral fissure

FIGURE 3.18 Brain; horizontal section at the level of the floor of the central part of the lateral ventricles; superior view. This central section shows parts of the thalamus lateral to the lateral ventricles. Anterior and posterior to the thalamus, the head and tail of the caudate nucleus are visible respectively. The genu of the corpus callosum locates to the anterior midline and its splenium is visible in the posterior midline.

Source: *Paulsen F. Brain and spinal cord. Sobotta atlas of human anatomy. vol. 3, p. 211–342, Chapter 12.*

■ Bounded by the fornix anteriorly and the thalamus posteriorly
(Fig. 3.19).
■ Structures passing through it (Fig. 3.20):
- Choroid plexus
- Branches of the medial posterior choroidal artery
- Thalamostriate, superior choroidal, septal and caudate veins

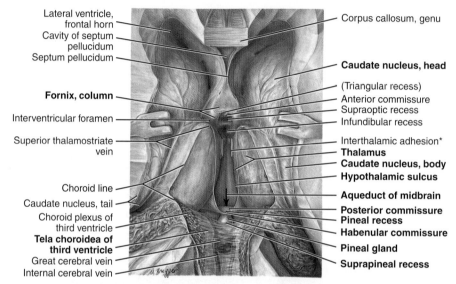

FIGURE 3.19   Lateral ventricles and third ventricle; superior view; parts of the cerebral hemispheres, the central part of the corpus callosum as well as the fornix and the choroid plexus have been removed; the choroid membrane of the third ventricle has been reflected. The margins of the third ventricle: roof – choroid membrane and choroid plexus; anterior wall – columna of fornix, anterior commissure, lamina terminalis, triangular recess and supraoptic recess; lateral wall – thalamus, stria medullaris of thalamus, hypothalamic sulcus and hypothalamus (wall); posterior wall – habenular commissure, posterior commissure, suprapineal recess and pineal recess; floor – infundibular recess. *Interthalamic adhesion (massa intermedia) cut in the median plane.

Source: *Paulsen F. Brain and spinal cord. Sobotta atlas of human anatomy. vol. 3, p. 211–342, Chapter 12.*

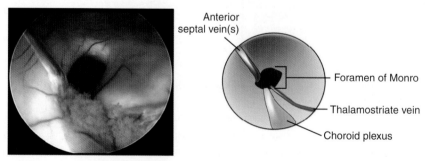

FIGURE 3.20   Endoscopic third ventriculostomy. Intraoperative view and corresponding schematic representation. View of foramen of Monro from right lateral ventricle. The choroid plexus (centre), anterior septal vein (medial) and thalamostriate vein (lateral) are seen. Care must be taken not to damage these structures when entering the foramen of Monro in order to prevent haemorrhage or venous infarcts. *Source: Recinos PF. Endoscopic third ventriculostomy. Schmidek and Sweet's operative neurosurgical techniques. p. 1143–50, Chapter 96.*

CLINICAL INSIGHT

- **Increase in size and volume of ventricles**
  - The size and volume of lateral ventricles physiologically increase with age due to brain tissue atrophy. However, several pathological states may be associated with enlarged ventricles such as Alzheimer disease, bipolar disorder, schizophrenia, major depressive disorder (also associated with enlarged third ventricle) and hydrocephalus *(see the Additional Clinical Insights subsection)*.

Third Ventricle (Figs. 3.19 and 3.20)

- Located at the core of the diencephalon, midline below the lateral ventricles and between the two thalami.
- **Massa intermedia** or interthalamic adhesion is a neuronal connection between both thalami crossing through the third ventricle – absent in 20–30% of humans and more likely to be found in females compared to males.
- Surfaces:
  - Lateral: Thalami and hypothalami
  - Roof: Ependymal layer of tela choroidea and choroid plexus *(see Choroid Plexus subsection)*
  - Floor: Hypothalamic structures (optic chiasm, tuber cinereum, infundibulum, mammillary bodies and posterior perforated substance) and subthalami
  - Anterior: Anterior commissure, column of fornix and lamina terminalis
  - Posterior: Stalk of pineal gland, posterior commissure and habenular commissures
- **Recesses** extending from the third ventricle (Figs. 3.19 and 3.21):
  - Anterior: Triangular recess between the anterior commissure and columns of the fornix, and supraoptic and infundibular recesses above the optic chiasm and pituitary stalk respectively
  - Posterior: Suprapineal and pineal recesses above and into the pineal gland respectively
- **Aqueduct of Sylvius (or cerebral aqueduct)**
  - Situated at the centre of the midbrain separating the posterior tectal from the anterior tegmental midbrain segments *(see chapter 7)*
  - Connects the third and fourth ventricles and drains CSF generated in the lateral and third ventricles (Fig. 3.21)

CLINICAL INSIGHT

- **Aqueductal stenosis**
  - Stenosis of the cerebral aqueduct due to congenital or acquired causes (midbrain tumours, gliosis) leads to obstructive hydrocephalus. Third ventriculostomy is the treatment of choice in many cases *(see Additional Clinical Insights subsection)*.

Fourth Ventricle (Figs. 3.21–3.23)

Anatomical Structure and Components

The fourth ventricle is a laterally rotated, **tent-shaped** space.

- Dorsally, the roof is formed by an upper and lower part; their point of convergence at the midline is called the **Fastigium**
  - The upper part of the roof consists of
    - Superior cerebellar peduncles
    - Superior medullary velum
    - *Lingula*, a tongue-shaped superior extension of the cerebellar vermis *(see chapter 9)*
  - The lower part of the roof consists of
    - Inferior medullary velum
    - Choroid plexus and tela choroidea
  - Ventrally, the floor has a **rhomboid or diamond shape** and is divided into two triangles by a horizontal strip called the **junctional part**
    - The larger, superior triangle extends over the pons with its apex directed towards the aqueduct of Sylvius
    - The smaller, inferior triangle extends over the medulla with its apex directed towards the **obex**, the caudal tip of the fourth ventricle

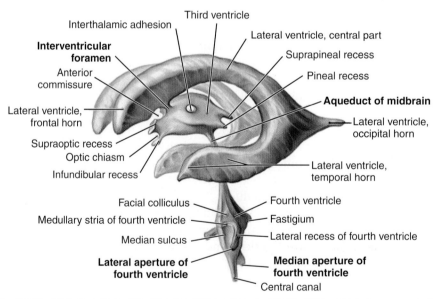

FIGURE 3.21 Ventricular system. Each of the lateral ventricles connects with the third ventricle by a separate interventricular foramen (foramen of Monro). The third ventricle communicates with the fourth ventricle through the aqueduct of midbrain. The fourth ventricle contains three openings to the outer subarachnoid space: the median aperture (foramen of Magendie) and the paired lateral apertures (foramina of Luschka). Important recesses extending from the third ventricle include supraoptic and infundibular anteriorly, suprapineal and pineal posteriorly.

Source: *Paulsen F. Brain and spinal cord. Sobotta atlas of human anatomy. vol. 3, p. 211–342, Chapter 12.*

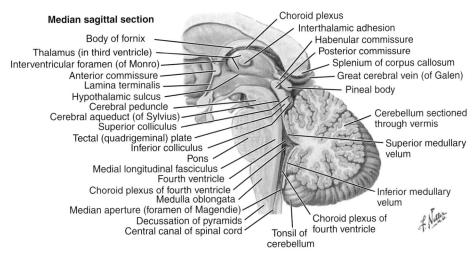

FIGURE 3.22 Sagittal section of the brainstem showing the fourth ventricle.

Source: *Netter illustration from www.netterimages.com.*

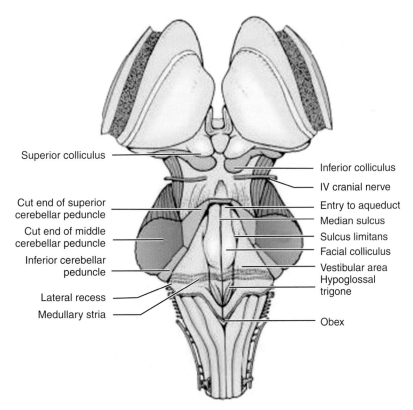

FIGURE 3.23 Fourth ventricle after removal of the cerebellum.

Source: *Modified from Cohen AR. Surgical disorders of the fourth ventricle. Cambridge, MA: Blackwell Science; 1996.*

- Other important structures appearing on the floor surface include:
  - Median sulcus: Runs vertically from the superior apex to the obex and divides the surface into two symmetrical halves
  - Sulcus limitans: Divides each half into two raised longitudinal strips, the **median eminence** and the lateral **'area vestibularis'**, under which the vestibular (part of CN VIII) nucleus lies
  - **Facial colliculi:** Located in the superior triangle along the median eminence – consists of facial nerve (CN VII) fibres looping around the abducens (CN VI) nucleus
  - Superior fovea: A triangular indentation located at the lateral limit of the facial colliculus along the sulcus limitans
  - **Hypoglossal trigone:** Overlies the hypoglossal (CN XII) nucleus in the inferior triangle
  - **Inferior fovea:** An indentation located at the lateral limit of the hypoglossal trigone along the sulcus limitans
  - **Vagal trigone:** Overlies the vagus (CN X) nucleus in the inferior triangle
  - **Area postrema:** Located in the midline at the inferior limit, slightly above the obex

CLINICAL INSIGHT

- **Area postrema:** The area postrema belongs to the group of circumventricular organs – a set of highly vascularized structures situated at strategic locations in the brain and lacking the blood–brain barrier. The specialized ependymal cells of the **chemoreceptor trigger zone** located within the area postrema detect blood-circulating toxins, drugs and hormones, and induce vomiting after relaying the information to the **vomiting centres**, such as the dorsal motor nucleus of the vagus nerve and nucleus of the solitary tract.

Foramina of Luschka (Figs. 3.17 and 3.21)
- Two apertures situated at the lateral walls of the fourth ventricle
- Form a link between the ventricle and the quadrigeminal cistern
- Allow CSF flow from the ventricular system to the subarachnoid space

Foramen of Magendie (Figs. 3.17 and 3.21)
- A median aperture situated at the dorsal wall of the fourth ventricle
- Forms a link between the ventricle and the cisterna magna
- Allows CSF flow from the ventricular system to the subarachnoid space

CLINICAL INSIGHT

- **Foraminal atresia**
  - Atresia of the foramina of Luschka and Magendie as part of the Dandy–Walker malformation, a congenital posterior fossa syndrome, causes noncommunicating hydrocephalus (see Additional Clinical Insights subsection).

ADDITIONAL CLINICAL INSIGHTS

- **Hydrocephalus**
  - Is the abnormal increase in CSF volume and subsequent enlargement of the brain ventricles (Fig. 3.24).
  - Can be classified into two categories: communicating, which is further subclassified into obstructive or nonobstructive, and noncommunicating hydrocephalus.
    - **Communicating,** which refers to the ability of CSF to freely move out from the brain ventricles to the subarachnoid space.
      - **Obstructive,** which refers to the inability of CSF from being absorbed into the venous sinuses due to any of the following conditions:
        - Scarring of the arachnoid granulations and/or subarachnoid space
        - Meningitis, mostly bacterial or tuberculous
        - Malignancy with meningeal metastases
      - **Nonobstructive,** where CSF absorption is not disturbed; however, there is abnormal CSF dynamics or apparent ventriculomegaly that is related to conditions other than increased CSF volume.
        - Choroid plexus papillomas, which are thought to increase CSF production out of proportion to the absorption rate.
        - **Hydrocephalus ex-vacuo,** where the apparent ventriculomegaly on imaging is due to adjacent brain tissue loss rather than increased CSF volume.
        - NPH; although it can sometimes be classified as obstructive when the aetiology is scarring of arachnoid granulations (see Case Study Discussion).
    - **Noncommunicating**, which refers to the inability of CSF to freely move out from the brain ventricles to the subarachnoid space, is by definition due to an obstructive aetiology.
      - Ventricles proximal to the obstruction are enlarged and exert mass effect on adjacent brain tissue.
      - Obstruction due to various aetiologies (tumours, congenital anomalies, infarcts or interventricular haemorrhage) can occur at any level of the ventricular system.
        - At the foramen of Monro, which leads to enlargement of the ipsilateral ventricle if unilateral or both ventricles if bilateral obstruction. Sizes of the third and fourth ventricles appear normal.
        - At the aqueduct of Sylvius, which leads to enlargement of both lateral ventricles and the third ventricle.
- **Ventriculoperitoneal (VP) Shunting (Fig. 3.25)**
  - A surgical procedure for the treatment of hydrocephalus, whereby a shunt is introduced into an enlarged lateral ventricle, passed under the skin from the skull to the abdomen and then introduced through a small opening into the peritoneal cavity.
  - High intracranial pressure drains accumulating CSF through the shunt.
  - After the procedure, intracranial pressure can be regulated noninvasively by controlling CSF flow through a preinstalled valve.

- **Endoscopic third ventriculostomy (Figs. 3.20 and 3.26)**
  - A surgical procedure whereby an endoscope is inserted through a burr hole into a lateral ventricle and then advanced into the third ventricle through one of the foramina of Monro.
  - The goal of the procedure is to treat hydrocephalus, mainly noncommunicating type, by creating an opening in the floor of the third ventricle, which is made of a thin membrane separating the ventricular space from the basal cistern.
- **Ependymomas (Fig. 3.27)**
  - Account for one third of all brain tumours in patients < 3 years.
  - Originate from the ependymal cells lining the brain ventricles and central canal of the spinal cord.
  - In paediatric patients, the commonest location is the posterior fossa in contrast to adult patients where it grows supratentorially.
  - The most common presentation includes signs of elevated intracranial pressure, although other symptoms such as ataxia, seizures and focal neurological deficits may be present.
    - Associated with **neurofibromatosis type 2**, 50% are **glial fibrillary acidic protein (GFAP) positive**, and form **ependymal rosettes** and **perivascular pseudorosettes** on histology (Fig. 3.28).
    - Can be benign or malignant, and can be complicated by haemorrhage.
    - Diagnosis is suspected on imaging studies and confirmed on pathologic studies.
    - Prognosis is not favourable in many cases due to the challenge of completely resecting the tumour.

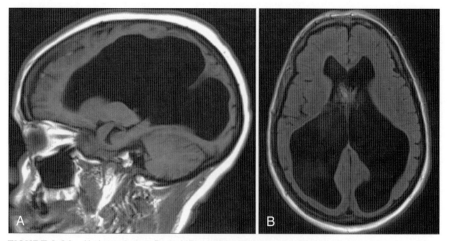

FIGURE 3.24   Hydrocephalus. Brain MRI, sagittal (A) and axial (B), showing prominent ventriculomegaly.
Source: *Alvin DM, Dr. Compensated hydrocephalus. The Lancet 387(10036):2422.*

Ventriculoperitoneal (VP) Shunt

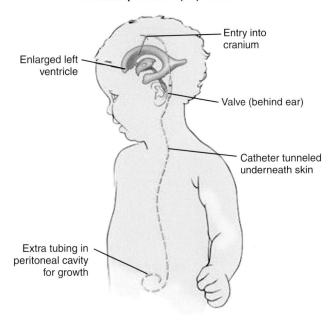

FIGURE 3.25   VP shunt anatomy.
Source: *Horton C, MD. Emergency care of children with high-technology neurologic disorders. Clin Pediatr Emergency Med 13(2):114–24.*

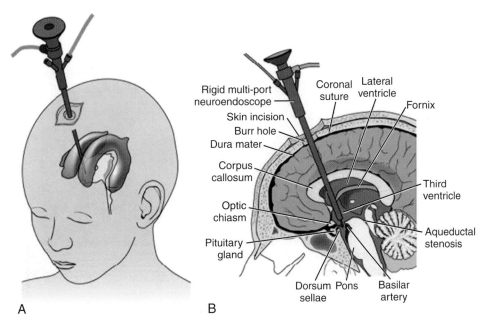

A   B

FIGURE 3.26   Schematic demonstrating the surgical trajectory for endoscopic third ventriculostomy (ETV) using a rigid endoscope. (A) Oblique view showing the endoscope passing through the lateral ventricle and foramen of Monro and into the third ventricle. (B) Sagittal view depicting the perforation of the floor of the third ventricle. It is important to understand the close relationship of the floor of the third ventricle to the anterior structures (optic chiasm and infundibulum) and posterior structures (basilar artery and brainstem) to avoid undesired complications. Source: *Recinos PF. Endoscopic third ventriculostomy. Schmidek and Sweet's operative neurosurgical techniques. vol. 1143–50, Chapter 96.*

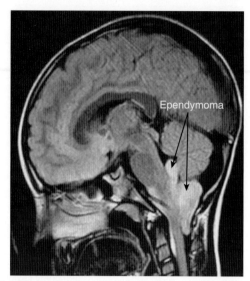

FIGURE 3.27   Brain MRI of a child presenting with headache, vomiting and gait ataxia. The image is typical of posterior fossa ependymomas, which have a propensity to grow through the foramen of Magendie and into the cervical canal. These tumours are also likely to progress through the lateral foramina and grow out the skull base foramina.
Source: *Duntsch CD. Ependymoma. Youmans neurological surgery. p. 2086–94, Chapter 200.*

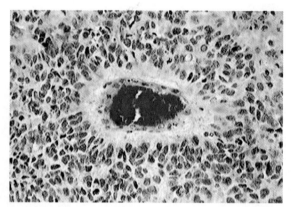

FIGURE 3.28   Perivascular rosette in an ependymoma.
Source: *Smith AB. Cerebellopontine angle and internal auditory canal neoplasms. Imaging of the brain. p. 802–25, Chapter 36.*

CSF GENERATION AND FLOW

CSF is the interstitial environment bathing the CNS and its delicate structures. Its main functions are as follows:

- Provides an optimal milieu for the CNS by buffering the pH and circulating the nutrients, electrolytes, hormones and hormone-releasing factors.

- Acts as a shock absorber and cushions the brain and spinal cord.
  - Interestingly, the floating effect of the brain in the CSF bath produces a 50 g net effective weight instead of the real weight, which is approximated at 1400 g.
- Removes waste products from cerebral metabolism.

CLINICAL INSIGHT

- **Types of traumatic brain injury**
  - **Concussion**
    - Most common type, also known as mild traumatic brain injury
    - Usually follows direct head trauma and does not cause damage to brain structures
    - Signs and symptoms are due to transient disturbance of neuronal function; they include:
      - Confusion
      - Loss of consciousness, followed by rapid return to normal function
      - **Amnesia**, a hallmark of concussion injury
    - CT scan is normal
  - **Contusion**
    - Differs from concussion by the presence of structural abnormalities that are detected on brain imaging, i.e. oedema and haemorrhages in brain areas impacted by nearby bony prominences such as temporal, frontal and occipital poles (Fig. 3.29)
    - Surgical intervention, decompressive craniectomy (Fig. 3.29B), may be required to relieve the augmented intracranial pressure (due to oedema or haemorrhage) and prevent herniation
  - **Coup-Contrecoup (Fig. 3.30)**
    - Occurs when the brain receives a force strong enough to cause two contusions: one at the site of the impact and another on the opposite side where the brain moves rapidly and hits the skull bones
  - **Diffuse Axonal (Fig. 3.31)**
    - Occurs after **shaking** or **rotational acceleration/deceleration injury** to the brain, leading to extensive tearing of neural axons in the white matter
    - Can cause temporary or permanent widespread brain damage, coma or even death

---

Choroid Plexus

CSF is synthesized and secreted by a network of fenestrated capillaries contained within granular meningeal protrusions that are covered with columnar and cuboidal epithelial layers. They are strategically located at specific areas within the ventricular system and organized into structures collectively known as the **choroid plexuses**.

Each ventricle contains a choroid plexus that buds from the **tela choroidea** layer, which is a highly vascularized, loose connective tissue arising from the thin pia mater (Fig. 3.17).

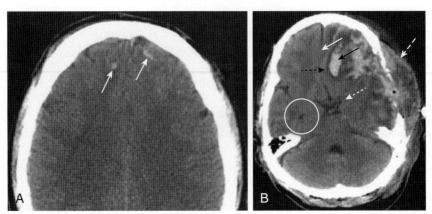

FIGURE 3.29 Cerebral contusions. (A) Cerebral contusions are usually the result of trauma and can manifest by multiple areas of high-attenuation haemorrhage (white arrows) within the brain parenchyma on CT scan. (B) Contusions (solid black arrow) are frequently surrounded by a rim of hypoattenuation from oedema (dotted black arrow), and mass effect is common, as it is demonstrated here by amputation of the ipsilateral basal cisterns (dotted white arrow), midline displacement (solid white arrow) representing subfalcine herniation and dilatation of the contralateral temporal horn (circle). A portion of the left side of the skull has been surgically removed, and there is a large scalp haematoma present (dashed white arrow).
Source: *Herring W, MD, FACR, Recognizing some common causes of intracranial pathology. Learning radiology. vol. 279–302, Chapter 27.*

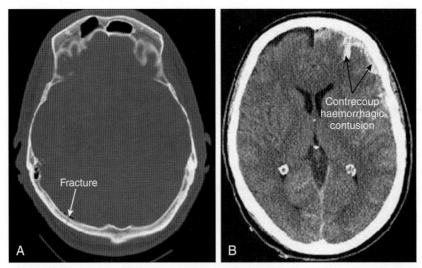

FIGURE 3.30 (A) Axial CT image in bone window and level settings showing a fracture in the right side of the occipital bone indicating the location of direct impact. (B) Axial CT image in brain window and level settings showing a contrecoup haemorrhagic contusion in the left frontal lobe with associated extra-axial haemorrhage.
Source: *Hijaz TA, MD. Imaging of head trauma. Radiol Clin North Am 49(1):81–103.*

- In the lateral ventricles, the plexus originates from the superior part of the temporal horn and climbs upwards to eventually cross the foramina of Monro.
  - Frontal and occipital horns are relatively far and thus not covered by the plexus.

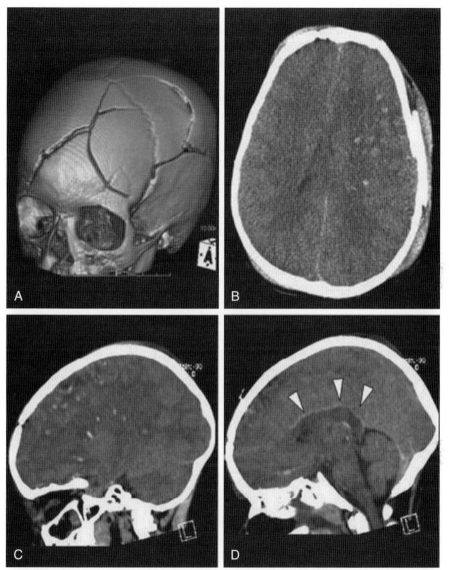

FIGURE 3.31   Different images from a severe craniocerebral trauma showing multiple complex skull fractures, multiple punctuate haemorrhagic diffuse axonal injury in the deep and subcortical white matter, predominantly of the left hemisphere, and extensive, but more subtle, nonhaemorrhagic shearing injuries of the corpus callosum (arrowheads in D). The corpus callosum appears irregularly swollen and hypodense, with bumpy contours, on the midline sagittal reformatted image (D).
Source: *Cianfoni A. Brain trauma. Problem solving in neuroradiology. p. 427–72, Chapter 12.*

- The tela choroidea settles on the choroidal fissure, a C-shaped cleft running between the fornix and thalamus along the medial wall, and is supplied by the:
  - **Anterior choroidal artery**
  - Medial and lateral posterior choroidal arteries, which are branches of the PCA

- In the third ventricle, the plexus is continuous with that of the lateral ventricles and *is located at the roof.*
  - The floor of the third ventricle and the aqueduct of Sylvius have no choroid plexus extensions.
  - The tela choroidea is supplied by the
    - **Medial posterior choroidal arteries**
    - Superior posterior choroidal artery, if present
- In the fourth ventricle, the tela choroidea and choroid plexus stand on their own and *are located at the lower segment of the roof.*
  - The choroid plexus has a T shape with two vertical bars: the horizontal bar extends towards the cerebellopontine angles bilaterally.
  - The tela choroidea is supplied by:
    - **Posterior inferior cerebellar artery**
    - **Anterior inferior cerebellar artery**

Cerebrospinal Fluid (Fig. 3.32)
Production

The total volume of CSF markedly varies between normal adults, is approximated at 125–150 mL and is distributed as the following:

- Lateral, third and fourth ventricles: 25 mL
- Spinal subarachnoid space: 30 mL
- Cranial subarachnoid space and major cisterns: 70–95 mL

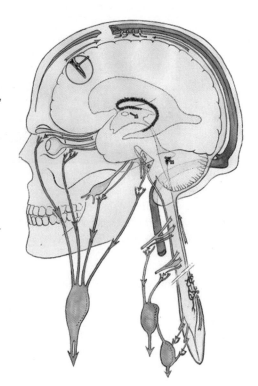

FIGURE 3.32   Cerebrospinal fluid (CSF) 'secretion-circulation-absorption' process. CSF is mainly secreted by the choroid plexus and, to a lesser extent, by the interstitial compartment. It circulates rostrocaudally inside the ventricles and drains into the cerebellomedullary cistern (cisterna magna) through the median aperture (foramen of Magendie) of the fourth ventricle. CSF circulates in cranial and spinal subarachnoid spaces. In the cranial subarachnoid space, CSF flows towards arachnoid villi in the wall of venous sinuses from which it is absorbed. Part of the CSF is absorbed by the olfactory mucosa and cranial nerve (optic, trigeminal, facial and vestibulocochlear nerves) sheaths and is drained by the lymphatic system. In the spinal subarachnoid space, the part of the CSF absorbed by the epidural venous plexus and spinal nerve sheaths enters the lymphatic system, while the remaining CSF circulates rostrally towards the cranial subarachnoid space. CSF communicates with interstitial fluid via Virchow–Robin perivascular spaces.
Source: *Sakka L. Anatomy and physiology of cerebrospinal fluid. Eur Ann Otorhinolaryngol, Head Neck Dis 128(6):309–16.*

In the lateral recumbent position, the physiological values of CSF pressure are estimated at **10–15 mm Hg** (approx. 135–200 mm H_2O) in adults and 3–4 mm Hg (approx. 40–55 mm H_2O) in infants.

The rate of production is **0.3–0.4 mL per minute** or **400–600 mL per day**, accounting for a turnover rate of four to five times per day.

The choroid plexuses produce 60–75% of the CSF. Less significantly, extrachoroidal secretion contributes to the final CSF volume as well.

- Choroidal secretion: The microstructure of the choroid plexus allows effective two-step secretion of CSF.
  - Passive transport of plasma filtrate across the fenestrated capillaries due to pressure gradient.
  - Active transport from the choroidal interstitial compartment to the ventricular lumen.
- Extrachoroidal secretion: Plays a minimal role under physiologic states.
  - Derived from extracellular fluid, ependymal epithelium and cerebral capillaries across the blood–brain barrier.
  - Facilitated by Virchow–Robins spaces that extend deeply inside the brain cortex, which allow small solutes to diffuse between the interstitial fluid and CSF.

Circulation and Absorption

In a very similar, yet slower and less complicated manner than the systemic blood circulation, CSF circulation is dynamic and ensures proper cerebral homeostasis under physiologic conditions.

The CSF flow pattern is a simple consequence of ventricular anatomy and the strategic location of the choroid plexuses.

- CSF produced in the lateral ventricles flows to the third ventricle through the foramina of Monro, then to the fourth ventricle through the aqueduct of Sylvius and finally to the subarachnoid space through the foramina of Luschka and Magendie.
- Outside the ventricular system, CSF flows rostrally to the cranial and caudally to the spinal subarachnoid space.
- Several factors contribute to the continuous flow of CSF.
  - **Cardiovascular waves,** which are associated with rhythmical rises and falls in cerebral arterial blood volume and pressure.
  - **Respiratory waves,** which increase and decrease cerebral arterial pressure during exhalation and inhalation respectively.
  - **Upright posture,** which facilitates passive production of CSF inside the ventricles and decreases cerebral venous pressure by the effect of gravity.

The relatively high CSF production rate is compensated by an almost identical absorption rate to ensure an intracranial pressure that is well tolerated by the CNS. Similar in structure to the granulations of the production site, i.e. choroid plexuses, the CSF absorption site is composed of **arachnoid granulations**, also called Pacchioni's (Pacchionian) granulations.

- Macroscopically, arachnoid granulations protrude through the dura mater as finger-like structures or villi to reach the lumen of large venous sinuses, mostly the superior sagittal sinus (Figs. 3.2, 3.17 and 3.32).
- Microscopically, villi are lined by an endothelial layer on top of the primary epithelioid layer of the arachnoid and dura mater (Fig. 3.33).
- Pressure gradient between CSF and venous blood is the driving force of CSF flow through the granulations and is estimated to be 3–5 mm Hg under normal conditions.
- Arachnoid granulations act as **one-way valves**, thus preventing backflow of CSF/plasma to the subarachnoid space (Fig. 3.34).
- Fluid is transported through the granulation layer in large vacuoles that may contain all CSF constituents, including red blood cells.

Accessory pathways of CSF absorption have been suggested to account for normal absorption rates in certain conditions such as neonatal underdeveloped and elderly dysfunctional arachnoid granulations, where the capacity of circulation–absorption pathways has been exceeded.

- Cranial and spinal nerve meningeal sheaths absorb CSF, which is subsequently drained by the lymphatic system and/or nearby venous plexuses (Fig. 3.33).

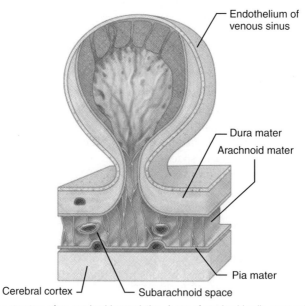

Endothelium of venous sinus

Dura mater
Arachnoid mater

Pia mater

Cerebral cortex

Subarachnoid space

FIGURE 3.33   Diagram of the structure of an arachnoid granulation. A cap of arachnoid cells surrounds the core. The arachnoid cap is thin laterally and thickest at the apex of the granulation.

Source: *From Standring S, et al. editors. Gray's anatomy: the anatomical basis of clinical practice, 40th ed. Philadelphia: Elsevier; 2009.*

Mechanism of CSF absorption

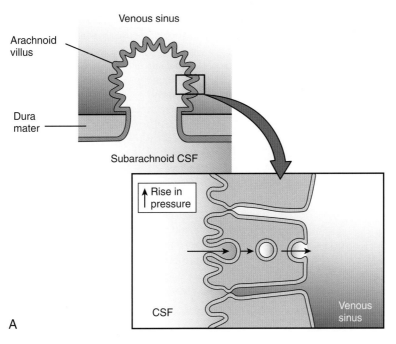

A

Rate of CSF absorption

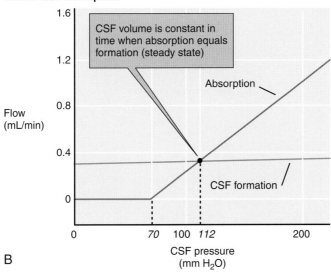

B

FIGURE 3.34 Absorption of CSF. (A) Arachnoid villi. The absorption of CSF may involve transcytosis. Note that arachnoid villi and granulations serve as one-way valves; fluid cannot move from the vein to the subarachnoid space. (B) The rate of CSF formation is virtually insensitive to changes in the pressure of the CSF. However, the absorption of CSF increases steeply at CSF pressures above ~70 mm H₂0.

Source: *Ransom BR. The neuronal microenvironment. Medical physiology. p. 289–309, Chapter 11.*

CASE STUDY DISCUSSION

NPH is an idiopathic, complex and progressive CSF circulation disorder affecting **elderly patients** in the majority of cases.

Clinical Features (the Three Ws: Wet, Wacky and Wobbly)

- **Abnormal gait:** Broad-based, shuffling/magnetic with difficulty initiating movement
- **Dementia:**
  - Early: Cognitive impairment, spatial memory and perception deficits
  - Late: Abulia, disorientation and emotional lability
- **Incontinence:**
  - Early: Urinary urgency and frequency, then urinary incontinence
  - Late: Faecal incontinence

Pathophysiology: Two Theories

- Reduced CSF absorption due to obstructive communicating hydrocephalus
  - Mainly due to scarring of the arachnoid granulations and subarachnoid space
- Ventricular wall weakening due to periventricular white matter ischaemic changes
  - Slowing of CSF flow through extracellular spaces leading to back pressure effect and subsequent ventricular enlargement

Management

VP shunting is the treatment of choice. Short duration symptom relief after CSF drainage with lumbar puncture usually predicts a positive effect of CSF shunting and is frequently performed before surgery.

Prognosis

The following factors point towards a favourable prognosis:

- Short-term improvement in symptoms post-lumbar puncture
- Short duration of symptoms before performing the VP shunting
- Appearance of gait disturbances before cognitive symptoms (dementia)
- Absence of significant cerebral vascular disease

CHAPTER 4

Blood Circulation

Abeer J. Hani

CASE STUDY

Presentation and Physical Examination: A 60-year-old right-handed man was brought to the emergency room due to sudden onset of inability to speak and right face, arm and leg paralysis. He was having his lunch with his wife when he suddenly started looking only to the left and was unable to speak and follow commands or move his right arm and leg. Past medical history was significant for hypertension and hyperlipidaemia, for which he was taking medications. On examination, the patient was alert and would occasionally utter unintelligible sounds; he would not repeat or follow commands. He had left gaze preference and did not cross the midline to the right. He had markedly decreased movement of the right face with sparing of the forehead. He had no movement of his right arm and leg, with hyperreflexia noted on the right side. He had markedly decreased sensation in the right arm and leg.

Diagnosis, Management and Follow-Up: Initial head computed tomography (CT) done within 1 h of symptom onset was negative, except for a hyperdensity in the proximal left middle cerebral artery (MCA), consistent with a blood clot. This was further documented via CT angiography (Fig. 4.1).

The preliminary diagnosis was left MCA embolic stroke. Further workup showed evidence of atrial fibrillation. Thrombolysis was performed.

After few days, the patient continued to have marked right-sided weakness with minimal improvement in his speech. He required extensive rehabilitation services afterwards.

After studying this chapter, try to guess how the clinical findings on examination fit the vascular territory involved in the stroke!

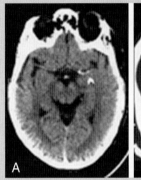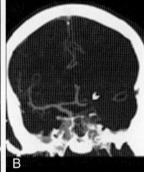

FIGURE 4.1 Acute ischaemic stroke. A 60-year-old male presented with right hemiparesis and aphasia. (A) Noncontrast CT at the level of the temporal lobes reveals a hyperdense clot is present within the left MCA stem (arrowhead). (B) Coronal CTA image depicts absent enhancement of the left MCA stem due to embolic occlusion (arrowhead) and absent enhancement within the collateral arteries supplying the cortex in the left MCA territory.
Source: *Boulter DJ, MD. Stroke and stroke mimics: a pattern-based approach. Semin Roentgenol 2014;49(1):22–38.*

BRIEF INTRODUCTION

The brain and the spinal cord are supplied by an intricate array of blood vessels that ensure their proper functioning. The goal of this chapter is to introduce the blood supply of the brain and spinal cord as well as provide a brief review of the regional brain anatomy that would help us make the clinical–anatomical correlations that can be made when the blood supply is transiently or permanently disrupted.

REVIEW OF THE MAIN FUNCTIONAL AREAS IN THE CENTRAL NERVOUS SYSTEM (CNS)

The **functional areas** of the CNS involve those areas present in the cerebral cortices, brainstem, cerebellum and spinal cord.

Cerebral Cortex (Fig. 4.2)
- The **face** and **hand** areas of the sensorimotor homunculi are on the **lateral convexities** of the hemisphere.
- The **leg** areas are present in the **interhemispheric fissure**.
- **Broca's** area is present in the **dominant** hemisphere (**usually left**) in the **inferior frontal gyrus**. This area constitutes the **motor speech** area.
- **Wernicke's** area lies in the **superior temporal gyrus**. This area is important for **speech articulation**.
- The **association cortex** lies in the **nondominant (usually right)** hemisphere, especially **parietal lobe**, and is important for **attention to the contralateral body** and **space**.
- The **primary visual cortex** for the **contralateral visual hemifields** lies along the **calcarine fissure** of the **occipital lobe**.
- **Optic radiations** and white matter trajectories that carry **visual information** from the thalamus to the visual cortex pass under the **parietal** and **temporal cortices**.

Brainstem (Fig. 4.3)
- Cranial nerve nuclei and related structures, lesions of which cause cranial nerve abnormalities.
- Long tracts, lesions of which cause long tract findings.
- **Cerebellar** circuitry, lesions of which cause **ataxia**.
- **Reticular formation** and related structures, lesions of which cause **impaired consciousness** and **autonomic dysregulation**.

Cerebellum (Fig. 4.4)
- **Lateral hemispheres** are responsible for **motor planning for extremities**.
- **Intermediate hemispheres** control **distal limb coordination**.
- **Vermis** and **flocculonodular lobe** control **proximal limb** and **trunk coordination** and **balance**, as well as **vestibuloocular reflexes**.

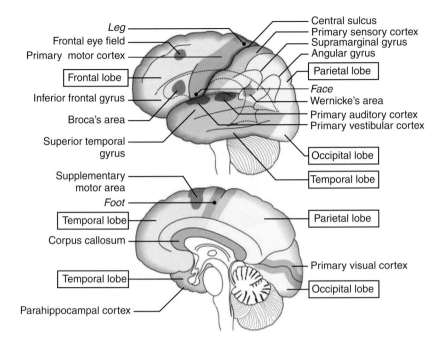

FIGURE 4.2 Anatomy of the cerebral cortex.
Source: *Leach JP. Neurological disease. Davidson's principles and practice of medicine. vol. 26, p. 1137–230.*

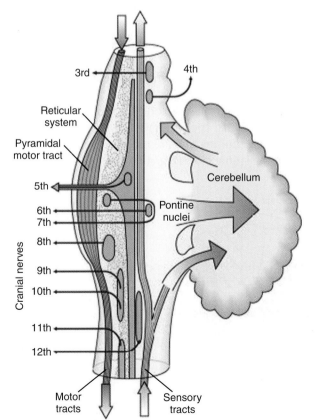

FIGURE 4.3 Anatomy of the brainstem.
Source: *Leach JP. Neurological disease. Davidson's principles and practice of medicine. vol. 26, p. 1137–230.*

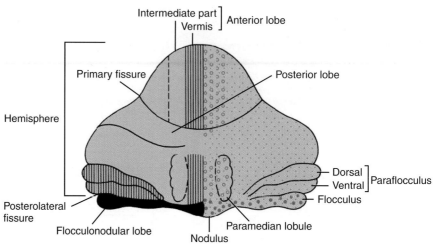

FIGURE 4.4 Anatomy of the cerebellum. Vermis and flocculonodular lobe (hatched and black areas), intermediate part (lateral to vermis; lateral open circles) and lateral hemispheres (lateral to intermediate part; small dots) are responsible for proximal limb/trunk coordination and balance, distal limb coordination and motor planning for extremities respectively.
Source: *Redrawn from Brodal A. Neurological anatomy, 3rd ed. New York: Oxford University Press; 1981.*

Spinal Cord (Fig. 4.5)

The spinal cord consists of a butterfly-shaped central grey matter surrounded by ascending and descending white matter tracts.

- **Dorsal (posterior) horn** of the grey matter is mainly involved in **sensory processing**.
- **Intermediate zone** of the grey matter contains **interneurons** and **specialized nuclei**.
- **Ventral (anterior) horn** of the grey matter contains **motor neurons**.
- The white matter consists of dorsal (posterior) columns, lateral columns and ventral (anterior) columns that are made of the ascending and descending tracts of the spinal cord (Fig. 4.6).

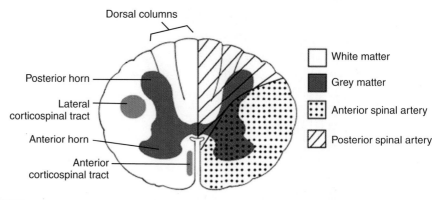

FIGURE 4.5 Spinal cord anatomy.
Source: *Jenkins TJ, MD. Neuromonitoring for cervical disc surgery: concepts and controversies. Semin Spine Surg 28(2):90–6.*

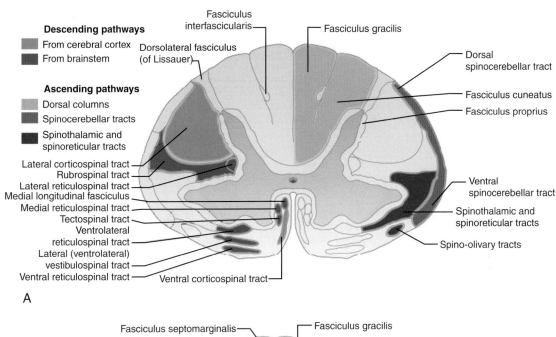

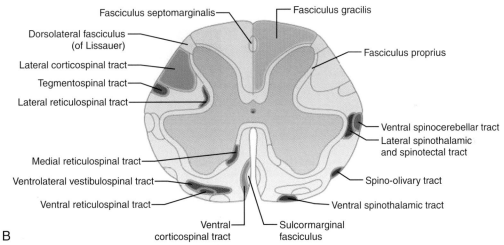

FIGURE 4.6   White matter pathways in the spinal cord. The approximate positions of nerve fibre tracts in the spinal cord at midcervical (A) and lumbar (B) levels.

Source: *Figure 18.9 from Gray's anatomy 2014. Cohen-Adad J. Annex: anatomy of the spinal cord, Quantitative MRI of the spinal cord, 291–305.*

ARTERIAL SUPPLY OF THE BRAIN

Arterial Supply of the Cerebral Hemispheres

The **anterior** circulation, which constitutes the **bilaterally paired internal carotid arteries (ICAs)**, as well as the **posterior** circulation, which constitutes the **bilateral vertebral arteries**, provide the arterial supply of the **cerebral cortex** (Figs. 4.7 and 4.8).

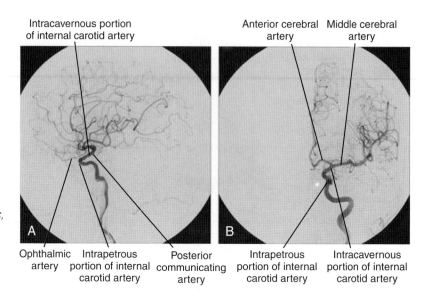

Intracavernous portion
of internal carotid artery

Anterior cerebral   Middle cerebral
artery   artery

A

B

Ophthalmic   Intrapetrous   Posterior   Intrapetrous   Intracavernous
artery   portion of internal communicating portion of internal portion of internal
             carotid artery   artery   carotid artery   carotid artery

FIGURE 4.7   Internal carotid arteriograms. (A) Lateral projection; (B) Towne's (angled anteroposterior) projection.
Source: *Standring S, MBE, PhD, DSc, FKC, Hon FAS, Hon FRCS. Vascular supply and drainage of the brain. Gray's anatomy. p. 280–90.e1, Chapter 19.*

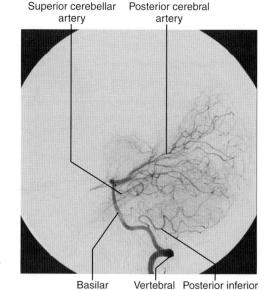

Superior cerebellar   Posterior cerebral
artery   artery

Basilar   Vertebral   Posterior inferior
artery   artery   cerebellar artery

FIGURE 4.8   Vertebral arteriogram, lateral projection.
Source: *Standring S, MBE, PhD, DSc, FKC, Hon FAS, Hon FRCS. Vascular supply and drainage of the brain. Gray's anatomy. p. 280–90.e1, Chapter 19.*

- The main arteries supplying the cerebral hemispheres are the **anterior cerebral** arteries (ACAs), MCAs and **posterior cerebral** arteries (PCAs).
- The ACAs and MCAs are the terminal branches of the ICAs. The **anterior communicating** artery (AComm) joins the ACAs anteriorly.
- The PCAs arise from the top of the **basilar** artery, which is formed by the **convergence of the two vertebral** arteries.

Anterior Circulation

- It arises from the common carotid arteries that originate at the aorta or at the brachiocephalic arteries (Fig. 4.9A).
- The **common carotid** artery splits at the carotid bifurcation into the **internal** carotid and **external** carotid arteries. Each of these vessels has its own branches (Fig. 4.9B and C).
- The ICA has several segments along its course: the **vertical cervical** segment in the neck, the **petrous** segment as the ICA enters the temporal

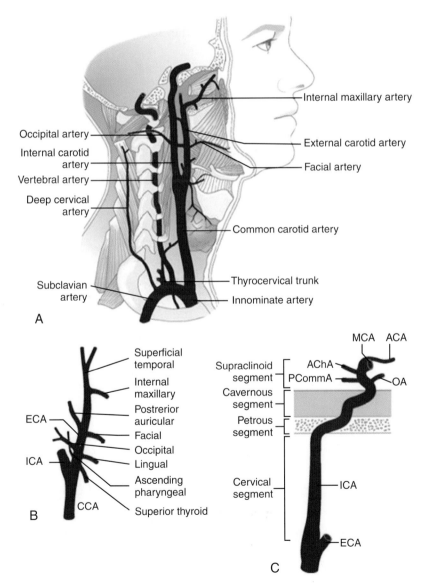

FIGURE 4.9 Drawings of the major right-sided neck arteries. (A) The innominate artery gives rise to subclavian and common carotid artery branches. The right vertebral artery is shown originating from the right subclavian artery. The common carotid artery bifurcation into internal and external carotid arteries is also shown. The external carotid artery and its branches (B) and (C) the segments of the internal carotid artery are shown in relation to their relationships with the adjacent skull structures. ACA, anterior cerebral aretry; AChA, anterior choroidal artery; CCA, common carotid artery; ECA, external carotid artery; ICA, internal carotid artery; MCA, middle cerebral artery; OA, ophthalmic artery; PCommA, posterior communicating artery.
Source: *Caplan LR, MD. Basic pathology, anatomy, and pathophysiology of stroke. Caplan's stroke p. 22–63, Chapter 2.*

bone, the **cavernous** segment and then the **supraclinoid** or **intracranial** segment as the ICA pierces the dura and enters the subarachnoid space (Fig. 4.9C).

- The main branches of the **intracranial ICA** are the **ophthalmic, posterior communicating, anterior choroidal, anterior cerebral** and MCAs (Fig. 4.9C).

Posterior Circulation

- The **vertebral** arteries arise from the **subclavian** arteries, ascend through **foramina** in the **transverse processes** of the **cervical vertebrae** before entering the **foramen magnum** and then ascend rostrally to join at the junction of the medulla and pons where they form the **basilar** artery (Fig. 4.10).

Circle of Willis

- The anterior and posterior circulations meet in a ring-like vascular structure referred to as **circle of Willis**.

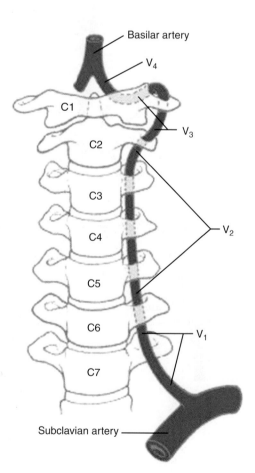

FIGURE 4.10   The origin and course of the vertebral artery and the landmarks that are used to divide it into segments V1 to V4.
Source: *Haines DE. A survey of the cerebrovascular system. Fundamental neuroscience for basic and clinical applications. p. 109–23.e1, Chapter 8.*

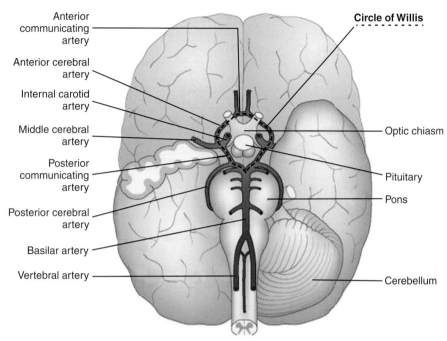

FIGURE 4.11   Anatomy of the circle of Willis (dotted black line).
Source: *Talke P. Central nervous system disease. Basics of anesthesia; 2011. p. 476–85, Chapter 30.*

- The **posterior communicating** arteries (PComms) join the anterior and posterior circulation together (Fig. 4.11).
- The PComm connects the ICA to the PCA.
- This circle is **complete in only 25%** of individuals.
- The circle allows for **collateral flow**.

Vascular Supply of the Superficial Cerebral Hemispheres
(Figs. 4.12 and 4.13)

- The **ACA** travels in the interhemispheric fissure and supplies most of the cortex on the **anterior medial surface** of the brain from the frontal to the anterior parietal lobes.
- The **MCA** enters the depths of the Sylvian fissure and bifurcates into a superior and inferior division. Branches of the MCA pass around the insula, then over and around the operculum and finally exit onto the lateral convexity.
    - The **superior** division supplies the **cortex above the Sylvian fissure**, including the **lateral frontal lobe**.
    - The **inferior** division supplies the **cortex below the Sylvian fissure**, including the **lateral temporal lobe** and a **portion of the parietal lobe**.
- The **PCA**, after arising from the top of the basilar artery, supplies the **inferior** and **medial temporal lobe** and the **medial occipital cortex**.

A-P view

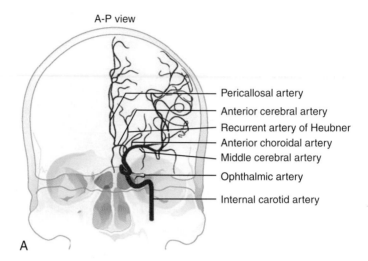

Pericallosal artery
Anterior cerebral artery
Recurrent artery of Heubner
Anterior choroidal artery
Middle cerebral artery
Ophthalmic artery
Internal carotid artery

A

Lateral view

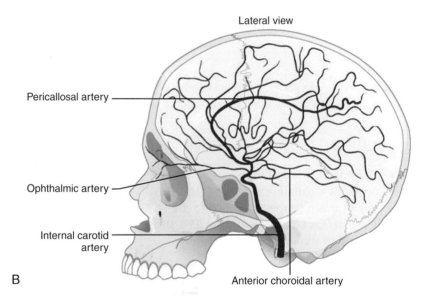

Pericallosal artery

Ophthalmic artery

Internal carotid artery

Anterior choroidal artery

B

FIGURE 4.12   The intracranial branches of the internal carotid artery. (A) Anteroposterior (A-P) and (B) lateral view.
Source: *Caplan LR, MD. Basic pathology, anatomy, and pathophysiology of stroke. Caplan's stroke; 2009. p. 22–63, Chapter 2.*

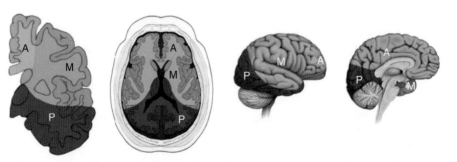

FIGURE 4.13   Arterial territories of the cerebral hemispheres. Coronal image is shown on the left, axial in the middle and sagittal on the right. A, anterior cerebral artery territory; M, middle cerebral artery territory; P, posterior cerebral artery territory.
Source: *Rabinstein AA. Clinical-anatomical syndromes of ischemic infarction. Practical neuroimaging in stroke; 2009. p. 19–69, Chapter 2.*

Vascular Supply of the Deep Cerebral Structures

- The penetrating **lenticulostriate** arteries, which branch off the MCA, supply large regions of the **basal ganglia** and **internal capsule** (Fig. 4.14).
- The **anterior** choroidal artery arises from the ICA and supplies portions of the **globus pallidus, putamen, thalamus** and the **posterior limb of the internal capsule** (Fig. 4.15).
- The recurrent artery of Heubner comes off the initial portion of the ACA to supply portions of the **head of the caudate, anterior putamen, globus pallidus** and **internal capsule.**
- Small penetrating arteries, which arise from the proximal PCA, include the thalamoperforator arteries (as well as the **thalamogeniculate** and **posterior choroidal** arteries); these supply the **thalamus** and sometimes a **portion of the posterior limb of the internal capsule**, as well as the **midbrain** (Fig. 4.16).

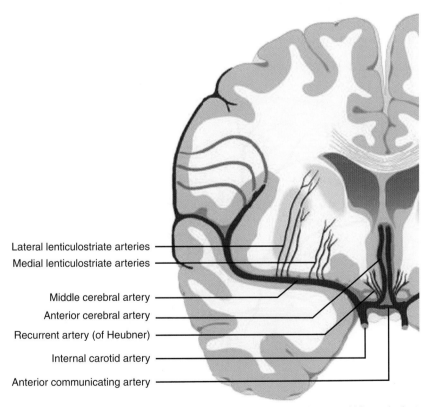

Lateral lenticulostriate arteries
Medial lenticulostriate arteries

Middle cerebral artery
Anterior cerebral artery
Recurrent artery (of Heubner)
Internal carotid artery
Anterior communicating artery

FIGURE 4.14   Drawing of a coronal section of the cerebral hemispheres showing one main stem middle cerebral artery and its lenticulostriate artery branches.

Source: *Caplan LR, MD. Basic pathology, anatomy, and pathophysiology of stroke. Caplan's stroke; 2009. p. 22–63, Chapter 2.*

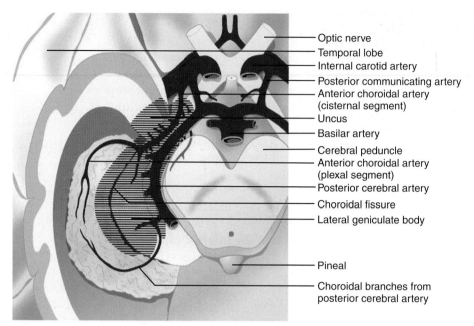

Optic nerve
Temporal lobe
Internal carotid artery
Posterior communicating artery
Anterior choroidal artery
(cisternal segment)
Uncus
Basilar artery
Cerebral peduncle
Anterior choroidal artery
(plexal segment)
Posterior cerebral artery
Choroidal fissure
Lateral geniculate body

Pineal

Choroidal branches from
posterior cerebral artery

FIGURE 4.15 Drawing of vascular supply of the anterior choroidal artery.
Source: *Caplan LR, MD. Basic pathology, anatomy, and pathophysiology of stroke. Caplan's stroke; 2009. p. 22–63, Chapter 2.*

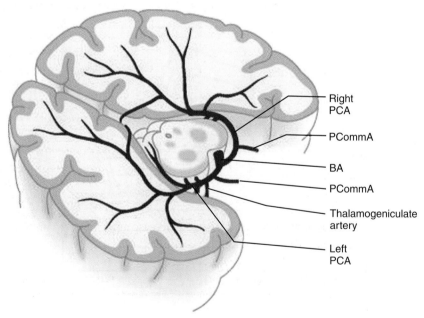

Right
PCA
PCommA
BA
PCommA
Thalamogeniculate
artery
Left
PCA

FIGURE 4.16 Drawing shows the course and branching of the PCAs as they course around the midbrain, and branches to the temporal and parietooccipital lobes. BA, basilar artery; PCA, posterior cerebral artery; PCommA, posterior communicating artery.
Source: *Caplan LR, MD. Basic pathology, anatomy, and pathophysiology of stroke. Caplan's stroke; 2009. p. 22–63, Chapter 2.*

CLINICAL INSIGHTS

- **Clinical syndromes produced by infarcts of the MCA, ACA and PCA (Table 4.1)**
  - MCA infarcts are more common than ACA or PCA infarcts.
  - Proximal MCA occlusions, also called MCA stem infarcts, cause large infarcts.
  - MCA infarcts occur in the regions of the superior division, inferior division and deep territory (Table 4.1).
  - Infarcts of the **superior** division of the **MCA** cause **contralateral face** and **arm weakness**, whereas infarcts of the **ACA** cause **contralateral leg more than face** or **arm weakness**.
  - Infarcts of the **PCA** typically cause a **contralateral homonymous haemianopia**.
- **Watershed infarcts (Fig. 4.17)**
  - **Watershed** infarcts occur when blood supply to the **region supplied by two adjacent cerebral arteries** is compromised.
  - **ACA–MCA watershed infarcts** may occur due to **sudden occlusion of the ICA or a drop in blood pressure of a patient** with carotid stenosis.
  - ACA–MCA watershed infarcts can produce proximal arm and leg weakness (**'man in the barrel' syndrome**).
- **Transient ischaemic attacks and strokes**
  - A **transient ischaemic attack (TIA)** is defined as a **transient episode of neurologic dysfunction** caused by focal brain, spinal cord or retinal ischaemia without acute infarction.
  - A **stroke** is defined as an **infarction (tissue injury)** of the CNS tissue.
  - Stroke could be **ischaemic** or **haemorrhagic**. Watershed infarcts are often due to systemic hypoperfusion (Fig. 4.18).
  - **Ischaemic** stroke is due to **inadequate blood supply** to an area of the brain that lasts enough to cause tissue infarcts. There are two mechanisms for ischaemic strokes.
    - An **embolic** infarct is caused by a blood clot that **forms in one place** and then **travels through the bloodstream** to **occlude a blood vessel in the brain**. Usually these infarcts involve the cerebral cortex and have **sudden onset of maximal deficits**.
    - A **thrombotic** infarct is caused by blood clot that **forms locally** in a blood vessel wall **inside the brain** at the site of an underlying atherosclerotic plaque, causing the vessel to occlude. There infarcts have a **slower course** than embolic infarcts.
  - Ischaemic infarcts could be large vessel or small vessel.
    - **Large-vessel** infarcts involve **major** blood vessels on the surface of the brain.
    - **Small-vessel** infarcts, also known as **lacunar** infarcts, involve **small penetrating** vessels that supply **deep structures** such as the basal ganglia, thalamus and medial brainstem structures.
    - **Lacunar** infarcts are often caused by **chronic hypertension** and lead to lacunar syndromes, some of which are summarized in Table 4.2.
  - TIAs need to be addressed emergently to identify causes and risk factors and to prevent stroke.
  - Common stroke risk factors include hypertension, diabetes, hypercholesterolaemia, tobacco smoking, cardiac disease, prior history of stroke or other vascular diseases and conditions leading to hypercoagulability in some cases.
  - Diagnosis of stroke is done using brain imaging, with CT scan showing hypodensity in the infarcted region few hours after the stroke, while magnetic resonance imaging (MRI) shows acute infarcts using specific diffusion sequences.

- In the absence of brain haemorrhage, patients with ischaemic strokes may be eligible for treatment with **thrombolytic agents** such as tissue plasminogen activator if they present within **4.5 hours** of onset of stroke symptoms.
- **Carotid stenosis**
    - ICA stenosis is often seen beyond the aortic bifurcation in the setting of atherosclerotic disease. Thrombi may form at the site of stenosis and embolize to the brain (Fig. 4.19).
    - **Carotid stenosis** is often associated with **MCA territory** infarcts and may also cause ophthalmic artery symptoms such as **monocular ipsilateral visual loss**, also known as **amaurosis fugax**.
    - Carotid stenosis is often clinically silent and may be suspected on examination if a **carotid bruit** is heard.
    - Treatment of symptomatic carotid stenosis is **carotid endarterectomy**, where the vessel is cut and the atheroma is removed, or **carotid stenting**.
- **Dissection of the carotid or vertebral arteries**
    - **Dissection** of these vessels may occur in the setting of **head** or **neck trauma** (Fig. 4.20).
    - It involves a **small tear on the intimal surface** of the artery, allowing blood to flow into the vessel wall and produce a dissection.
    - An **ipsilateral Horner syndrome** is often seen with a **carotid** dissection.
    - In a vertebral **dissection**, there is often **posterior neck** and **occipital pain**.
    - **Anterior circulation** infarcts may occur following a **carotid** dissection, whereas **posterior circulation** infarcts may occur following a **vertebral** dissection.
    - Diagnosis is via vessel imaging using **MR angiography** or **CT angiography** of neck vessels or **digital subtraction angiography** (Fig. 4.21).
    - Treatment often involves the use of **antiplatelets** and **anticoagulants**.
- **Brain haemorrhages**
    - Bleeds in the brain could be **intracerebral, subarachnoid, subdural** or **epidural** (Fig. 4.22).
    - **Subarachnoid** bleeds are often due to **aneurysmal ruptures**. An aneurysm is an abnormal balloon-like swelling of an artery. They often present with **sudden severe headache** and **neck stiffness** and may be followed by neurological deficits and coma.
    - An **angioma** or **arteriovenous malformation** is a **congenital** collection of blood vessels that **can rupture** and cause cerebral haemorrhage.

Table 4.1 Major clinical syndromes of MCA, ACA and PCA

Location of Infarct	Affected Territory	Deficits
Left MCA superior division		Right face and arm weakness of the upper motor neuron type and a nonfluent, or Broca's, aphasia. In some cases there may also be some right face and arm cortical-type sensory loss.
Left MCA inferior division		Fluent, or Wernicke's, aphasia and a right visual field deficit. There may also be some right face and arm cortical-type sensory loss. Motor findings are usually absent, and patients may initially seem confused or crazy but otherwise intact, unless carefully examined. Some mild right-sided weakness may be present, especially at the onset of symptoms.
Left MCA deep territory		Right pure motor hemiparesis of the upper motor neuron type. Larger infarcts may produce 'cortical' deficits, such as aphasia as well.

Table 4.1 Major clinical syndromes of MCA, ACA and PCA—cont'd

Location of Infarct	Affected Territory	Deficits
Left MCA stem		Combination of the above, with right hemiplegia, right hemianaesthesia, right homonymous hemianopia, and global aphasia. There is often a left gaze preference, especially at the onset, caused by damage to left hemisphere cortical areas important for driving the eyes to the right.
Right MCA superior division		Left face and arm weakness of the upper motor neuron type. Left hemineglect is present to a variable extent. In some cases, there may also be some left face and arm cortical-type sensory loss.
Right MCA inferior division		Profound left hemineglect. Left visual field and somatosensory deficits are often present; however, these may be difficult to test convincingly because of the neglect. Motor neglect with decreased voluntary or spontaneous initiation of movements on live left side can also occur. However, even patients with left motor neglect usually have normal strength on the left side, as evidenced by occasional spontaneous movements or purposeful withdrawal from pain. Some mild, left-sided weakness may be present. There is often a right gaze preference, especially at onset.
Right MCA deep territory		Left pure motor hemiparesis of the upper motor neuron type. Larger infarcts may produce 'cortical' deficits, such as left hemineglect as well.
Right MCA stem		Combination of the above, with left hemiplegia, left hemianaesthesia, left homonymous hemianopia and profound left hemineglect. There is usually a right gaze preference, especially at the onset, caused by damage to right hemisphere cortical areas important for driving the eyes to the left.
Left ACA		Right leg weakness of the upper motor neuron type and right leg cortical-type sensory loss. Grasp reflex, frontal lobe behavioural abnormalities and transcortical aphasia can also be seen. Larger infarcts may cause right hemiplegia.
Right ACA		Left leg weakness of the upper motor neuron type and left leg cortical-type sensory loss. Grasp reflex, frontal lobe behavioural abnormalities, and left hemineglect can also be seen. Larger infarcts may cause left hemiplegia.
Left PCA		Right homonymous hemianopia. Extension to the splenium of the corpus callosum can cause alexia without agraphia. Larger infarcts, including the thalamus and internal capsule, may cause aphasia, right hemisensory loss and right hemiparesis.
Right PCA		Left homonymous hemianopia. Larger infarcts including the thalamus and internal capsule may cause left hemisensory loss and left hemiparesis.

Source: *Adapted from Blumenfeld, Neuroanatomy through clinical cases, 2nd ed. 2010. Sinauer Associates Inc.: Sunderland, MA.*

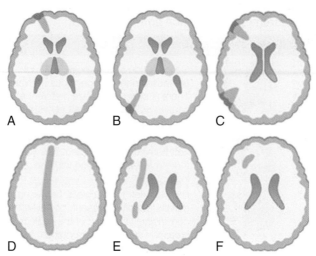

FIGURE 4.17 Most common CT locations of infarcts in the watershed areas (infarcts are shown by hatched grey): (A) wedge-shaped anterior watershed infarct; (B) wedge-shaped posterior watershed infarct; (C) anterior and posterior watershed infarcts; (D) linear watershed infarct; (E) ovular deep watershed infarct and (F) small white-matter watershed infarct.

Source: *Caplan LR, MD. Large artery occlusive disease of the anterior circulation, Caplan's stroke; 2009. p. 221–57, Chapter 6.*

Table 4.2 Common lacunar syndromes

Syndrome	Clinical Features	Possible Locations for Infarct	Possible Vessels Involved
Pure motor hemiparesis or dysarthria hemiparesis	Unilateral face, arm and leg upper motor neuron-type weakness, with dysarthria	Posterior limb of internal capsule (common)	Lenticulostriate arteries (common), anterior choroidal artery or perforating branches of posterior cerebral artery
		Ventral pons (common)	Ventral penetrating branches of basilar artery
		Corona radiata	Small middle cerebral artery branches
		Cerebral peduncle	Small proximal posterior cerebral artery branches
Ataxic hemiparesis	Same as pure motor hemiparesis, but with ataxia on same side as weakness	Same as pure motor hemiparesis	Same as pure motor hemiparesis
Pure sensory stroke (thalamic lacune)	Sensory loss to all primary modalities in the contralateral face and body	Ventral posterior lateral nucleus of the thalamus (VPL)	Thalamoperforator branches of the posterior cerebral artery
Sensorimotor stroke (thalamocapsular lacune)	Combination of thalamic lacune and pure motor hemiparesis	Posterior limb of the internal capsule, and either thalamic VPL or thalamic somatosensory radiation	Thalamoperforator branches of the posterior cerebral artery, or lenticulostriate arteries
Basal ganglia lacune	Usually asymptomatic, but may cause hemiballismus	Caudate, putamen, globus pallidus or subthalamic nucleus	Lenticulostriate, anterior choroidal or Heubner's arteries

Source: *Adapted from Blumenfeld, Neuroanatomy through clinical cases, 2nd ed. 2010. Sinauer Associates Inc.: Sunderland, MA.*

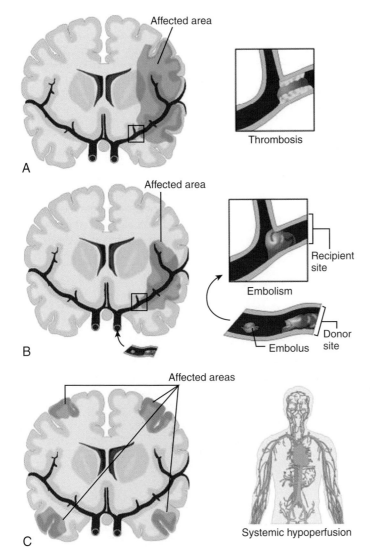

A

Affected area

Thrombosis

B

Affected area

Embolism

Recipient site

Embolus

Donor site

C

Affected areas

Systemic hypoperfusion

FIGURE 4.18 Illustrations of the three major causes of brain ischaemia. (A) Thrombosis: The inset shows a thrombus in an atherosclerotic artery leading to a brain infarct. (B) Embolism: A thrombus that originated in a donor source embolized to the recipient site (shown in the inset) causing an embolic brain infarct. (C) Systemic hypoperfusion: Infarcts are in border-zone regions.
Source: *Caplan LR, MD. Basic pathology, anatomy, and pathophysiology of stroke, Caplan's stroke; 2009. p. 22–63, Chapter 2.*

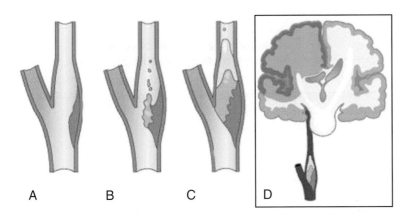

A   B   C   D

FIGURE 4.19 Internal carotid artery atherosclerotic lesions: (A) plaque; (B) plaque with platelet-fibrin emboli; (C) plaque with occlusive thrombus; (D) recent ischaemic cerebral infarct due to embolization of the internal carotid artery thrombus.
Source: *Caplan LR, MD. Basic pathology, anatomy, and pathophysiology of stroke. Caplan's stroke; 2009. p. 22–63, Chapter 2.*

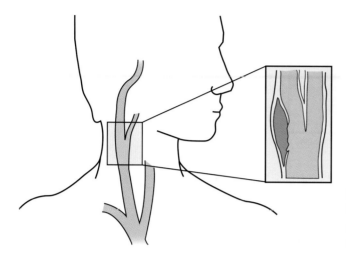

FIGURE 4.20 Schematic of a carotid artery dissection. Source: *Vilke GM, MD. Evaluation and management for carotid dissection in patients presenting after choking or strangulation, J Emerg Med 2011;40(3):355–8.*

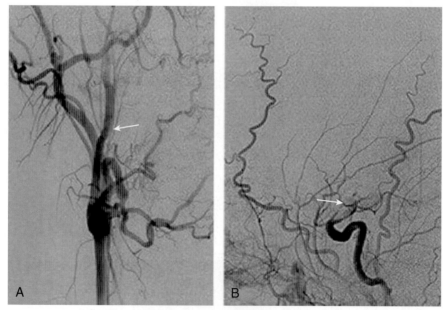

FIGURE 4.21 Selective right common carotid arteriogram showing: (A) irregularity (arrow) of the right internal carotid artery (ICA) distal to the common carotid bifurcation without significant focal stenosis, typical of a carotid dissection and (B) a large filling defect completely occluding the M1 segment of the right middle cerebral artery and the supraclinoid segment of the right ICA (arrow). Source: *Fridley J. Internal carotid artery dissection and stroke associated with wakeboarding. J Clin Neurosci 2011;18(9):1258–60.*

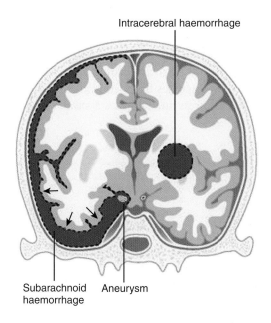

Intracerebral haemorrhage

Subarachnoid haemorrhage   Aneurysm

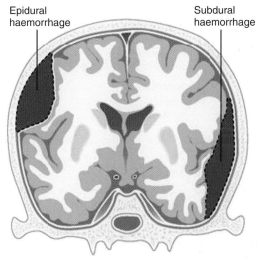

Epidural haemorrhage

Subdural haemorrhage

FIGURE 4.22 Illustrations of the main types of brain haemorrhages: intracerebral, subarachnoid, subdural and epidural.
Source: *Caplan LR, MD. Basic pathology, anatomy, and pathophysiology of stroke. Caplan's stroke; 2009. p. 22–63, Chapter 2.*

Arterial Supply of the Brainstem and Cerebellum

- The **vertebrobasilar** system consists of the vertebral arteries that arise from the subclavian arteries and join at the pontomedullary junction to form a single basilar artery. The **basilar** artery splits at the ponto-mesencephalic junction into the **two** PCAs, which connect via the PComms to the ICAs of the anterior circulation (Figs. 4.23 and 4.24).
- The following branches of the vertebrobasilar system supply the brainstem and cerebellum:
  - The **posterior–inferior cerebellar artery (PICA)** arises from the vertebral artery at the level of the medulla and supplies the **lateral medulla, inferior cerebellum** and **inferior vermis**.

▦ The **anterior–inferior cerebellar artery (AICA)** arises from the proximal basilar artery at the level of the caudal pons and supplies the **lateral caudal pons, middle cerebellar peduncle** and a strip of the **ventral (anterior) cerebellum**, including the **flocculus**.

▦ The **superior cerebellar artery (SCA)** arises from the top of the basilar artery at the level of the rostral pons and supplies a **small region**

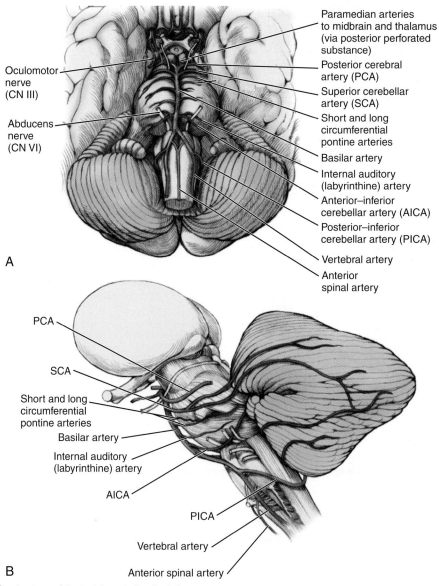

FIGURE 4.23 Anatomy of the brain's posterior circulation.

Source: *Reprinted with permission Reddy CC, MD. Stroke and neurodegenerative disorders: 1. Stroke management in the acute care setting. PM&R 2009;1(3 Suppl):S4–12.*

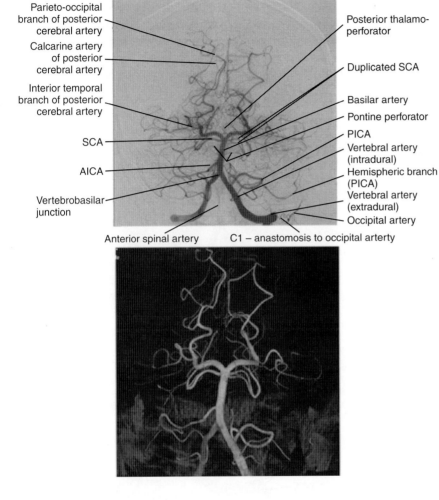

Parieto-occipital branch of posterior cerebral artery

Calcarine artery of posterior cerebral artery

Interior temporal branch of posterior cerebral artery

SCA

AICA

Vertebrobasilar junction

Anterior spinal artery

Posterior thalamo-perforator

Duplicated SCA

Basilar artery

Pontine perforator

PICA

Vertebral artery (intradural)

Hemispheric branch (PICA)

Vertebral artery (extradural)

Occipital artery

C1 – anastomosis to occipital artery

FIGURE 4.24 Posterior circulation, frontal view on conventional angiogram (top) and three-dimensional angiogram (bottom). PICA, posterior–inferior cerebellar artery; AICA, anterior–inferior cerebellar artery; SCA, superior cerebellar artery.
Source: *Rabinstein AA. Clinical-anatomical syndromes of ischemic infarction. Practical neuroimaging in stroke; 2009. p. 19–69, Chapter 2.*

of the rostral laterodorsal pons, superior cerebellar peduncle and most of the superior half of the cerebellar hemisphere, including the deep cerebellar nuclei and the superior vermis.

- The PCA arises from the top of the basilar artery as well, just beyond the SCA. The oculomotor nerves (CN III) usually pass between the SCA and the PCA. The PCA wraps around the midbrain, supplying it, as well as most of the thalamus, medial occipital lobes and inferomedial temporal lobes.
- Paramedian branches arising from these main vessels supply the paramedian regions.
- Short circumferential arteries and long circumferential arteries (including PICA, AICA, as well as smaller branches) give rise to penetrating branches that supply the more lateral portions of the brainstem.

Vascular Territories of the Brainstem and the Cerebellum (Fig. 4.25)

- The **medial medulla** is supplied by **paramedian** branches of the **anterior spinal** artery in more **caudal** regions and by **paramedian** branches of the **vertebral** arteries in more **rostral** regions.
- The **lateral medulla** is supplied by **penetrating** branches from the **vertebral** artery and the **PICA**.

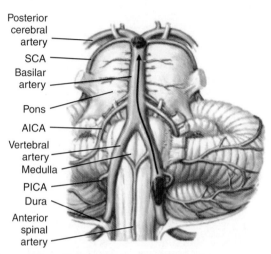

Intracranial obstruction of vertebral artery proximal to origin of posterior–inferior cerebellar artery (PICA) may be compensated by preserved flow from contralateral vertebral artery. If PICA origin is blocked, lateral medullary syndrome (shown above) may result. Clot also may extend to block anterior spinal artery branch, causing hemiplegia, or embolization to basilar bifurcation may cause 'top of basilar' syndrome.

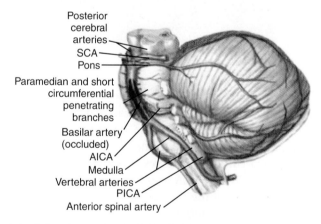

FIGURE 4.25   Vascular supply of the brainstem and cerebellum. Source: *Felten DL, MD, PhD. Netter's atlas of neuroscience 2016;7:93–124.*

Collateral circulation via superior cerebellar (SCA), anterior–inferior cerebellar (AICA) and posterior–inferior cerebellar (PICA) arteries may partially compensate for basilar occlusion. Basilar artery has paramedian, short circumferential and long circumferential (AICA) and (SCA) penetrating branches. Occlusion of any or several of these branches may cause pontine infarction. Occlusion of AICA or PICA may also cause cerebellar infarction.

- The medial pons is supplied by **paramedian** branches from the **basilar** artery.
- The lateral pons is supplied by **circumferential** branches of the **basilar** artery. In the more **caudal** regions, the lateral pons is supplied by the **AICA**.
- The **inner ear** is supplied by the internal auditory (labyrinthine) artery, which usually arises as a branch of the **AICA**, but occasionally comes directly off the **basilar** artery.
- The midbrain is supplied by **penetrating** branches arising from the **top of the basilar** artery and from the **proximal PCAs**.
- The **inferior half** of the **cerebellum** is supplied by the **PICA**.
- The **superior half** of the **cerebellum** is supplied by the **SCA**.

CLINICAL INSIGHT

- **Vertebrobasilar vascular disease**
  - **Vertebrobasilar ischaemia** may present with vertigo, dizziness, nausea, diplopia, ataxia, dysarthria, dysphagia, somnolence, occipital headaches and bilateral or perioral numbness.
  - There may be symptoms of brainstem involvement such as **crossed signs** (e.g. decreased sensation or weakness on one side of the face and contralateral body) and cranial nerve involvement causing **eye movement abnormalities**.
  - Table 4.3 shows signs of dysfunction in case of infarcts involving the midbrain, pons, medulla and cerebellum.
  - The vertebrobasilar system is also susceptible to strokes, infarcts and dissection similar to the anterior circulation system detailed above. Tables 4.4–4.6 detail focal vascular syndromes of the midbrain, pons and medulla (Fig. 4.26).
  - **Cerebellar ischaemia** causing **ipsilateral ataxia with no brainstem signs** are more common with **SCA** infarcts.
- **Cerebellar haemorrhage (Fig. 4.27)**
  - Cerebellar haemorrhage, **similar to spontaneous intraparenchymal haemorrhage (Fig. 4.28) in other brain regions,** is seen in the setting of chronic hypertension, arteriovenous malformation, haemorrhagic conversion of an ischaemic infarct and metastases, among other causes.
  - A large haemorrhage may cause obstruction of the fourth ventricle resulting in **hydrocephalus**, accompanied by **sixth-nerve (abducens nerve) palsies** and **impaired consciousness** and may eventually cause brainstem compression and **death**.
  - Proper identification and treatment (via **decompression**) are often needed.

Table 4.3 Signs of dysfunction of the various brainstem regions

Brainstem Region	Signs of Dysfunction
Midbrain	Third nerve palsy
	Unilateral or bilateral pupil dilation
	Ataxia
	Flexor (decorticate) posturing
	Impaired consciousness

Continued

Table 4.3 Signs of dysfunction of the various brainstem regions—cont'd

Brainstem Region	Signs of Dysfunction
Pons	Bilateral Babinski signs
	Perioral numbness or facial tingling
	Bilateral upper or lower visual loss or blurring; ocular bobbing (quick downwards dip of the eyes)
	Irregular respirations
	Abducens palsy or horizontal gaze palsy
	Bilateral small but reactive pupils
	Extensor (decerebrate) posturing
	Impaired consciousness
Medulla	Vertigo
	Ataxia
	Nystagmus
	Nausea and vomiting
	Hiccups
	Autonomic instability
	Respiratory arrest
Cerebellum	Vertigo
	Nausea and vomiting
	Horizontal nystagmus
	Limb ataxia
	Unsteady gait
	Headache (occipital, frontal or cervical)

Table 4.4 Focal vascular syndromes of the midbrain

Region	Syndrome Name(s)	Vascular Supply	Structure(s)	Anatomical Clinical Feature(s)
Midbrain basis	Weber syndrome	Branches of PCA and top of basilar artery	Oculomotor nerve fascicles Cerebral peduncle	Ipsilateral third nerve palsy Contralateral hemiparesis
Midbrain tegmentum	Claude syndrome	Branches of PCA and top of basilar artery	Oculomotor nerve fascicles	Ipsilateral third nerve palsy
			Red nucleus, superior cerebellar peduncle fibres	Contralateral ataxia
Midbrain basis and tegmentum	Benedikt syndrome	Branches of PCA and top of basilar artery	Oculomotor nerve fascicles	Ipsilateral third nerve palsy
			Cerebral peduncle Red nucleus, substantia nigra, superior cerebellar peduncle fibres	Contralateral hemiparesis Contralateral ataxia, tremor and involuntary movements

Source: Adapted from Blumenfeld, *Neuroanatomy through clinical cases,* 2nd ed. 2010. Sinauer Associates Inc.: Sunderland, MA.

Table 4.5 Focal Vascular syndromes of the pons

Region	Syndrome Name	Vascular Supply	Structure(s)	Anatomical Clinical Feature(s)
Medial pontine basis	Dysarthria hemiparesis (pure motor hemiparesis)	Paramedian branches of basilar artery, ventral territory	Corticospinal and corticobulbar tracts	Contralateral face, arm and leg weakness; dysarthria
	Ataxic hemiparesis	Same as above	Corticospinal and corticobulbar tracts	Contralateral face, arm and leg weakness; dysarthria
			Pontine nuclei and pontocerebellar fibers	Contralateral ataxia (occasionally, ipsilateral ataxia)
Medial pontine basis and tegmentum	Foville syndrome	Paramedian branches of basilar artery, ventral and dorsal territories	Corticospinal and corticobulbar tracts	Contralateral face, arm and leg weakness; dysarthria
			Facial colliculus	Ipsilateral face weakness; ipsilateral horizontal gaze palsy
	Pontine wrong-way eyes	Same as above	Corticospinal and corticobulbar tracts	Contralateral face, arm and leg weakness; dysarthria
			Abducens nucleus or paramedian pontine reticular formation	Ipsilateral horizontal gaze palsy
	Millard–Gubler syndrome	Same as above	Corticospinal and corticobulbar tracts	Contralateral face, arm and leg weakness; dysarthria
	Other regions variably involved	Same as above	Medial lemniscus	Contralateral decreased position and vibration sense
			Medial longitudinal fasciculus	Internuclear ophthalmoplegia (INO)
Lateral caudal pons	AICA syndrome	AICA	Middle cerebellar peduncle	Ipsilateral ataxia
			Vestibular nuclei	Vertigo, nystagmus
			Trigeminal nucleus and tract	Ipsilateral facial decreased pain and temperature sense
			Spinothalamic tract	Contralateral body decreased pain and temperature sense
			Descending sympathetic fibres	Ipsilateral Horner syndrome
	Other regions variably involved	Labyrinthine artery	Inner ear	Ipsilateral hearing loss
Dorsolateral rostral pons	SCA syndrome	SCA	Superior cerebellar peduncle and cerebellum	Ipsilateral ataxia
			Other lateral tegmental structures (variable)	Variable features of lateral tegmental involvement (see AICA syndrome)

Source: Adapted from Blumenfeld, Neuroanatomy through clinical cases, 2nd ed. 2010. Sinauer Associates Inc.: Sunderland, MA.

Table 4.6 Focal vascular syndromes of the medulla

Region	Syndrome Name	Vascular Supply	Structure(s)	Anatomical Clinical Feature(s)
Medial medulla	Medial medullary syndrome	Paramedian branches of vertebral and anterior spinal arteries	Pyramidal tract Medial lemniscus	Contralateral arm or leg weakness Contralateral decreased position and vibration sense
			Hypoglossal nucleus and exiting CN XII fascicles	Ipsilateral tongue weakness
Lateral medulla	Wallenberg syndrome (lateral medullary syndrome)	Vertebral artery (more commonly than PICA)	Inferior cerebellar peduncle, vestibular nuclei	Ipsilateral ataxia, vertigo, nystagmus, nauseaw
			Trigeminal nucleus and tract	Ipsilateral facial decreased pain and temperature sense
			Spinothalamic tract	Contralateral body decreased pain and temperature sense
			Descending sympathetic fibres Nucleus ambiguus Nucleus solitarius	Ipsilateral Horner syndrome Hoarseness, dysphagia Ipsilateral decreased taste

Source: Adapted from Blumenfeld, Neuroanatomy through clinical cases, 2nd ed. 2010. Sinauer Associates Inc.: Sunderland, MA.

MIDBRAIN

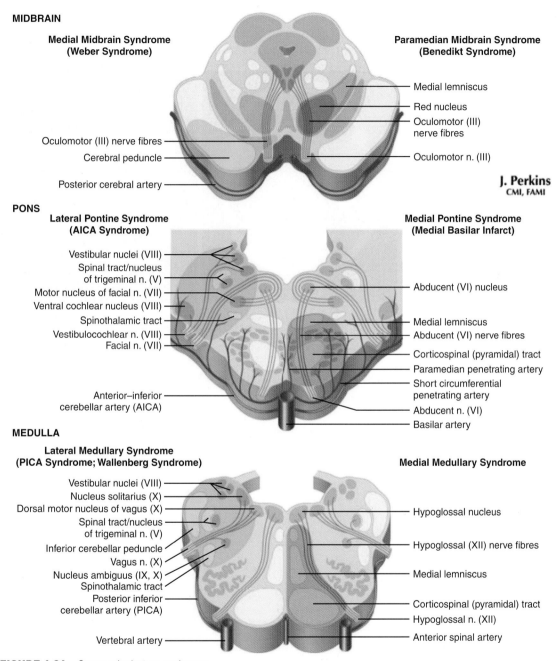

Medial Midbrain Syndrome
(Weber Syndrome)

Paramedian Midbrain Syndrome
(Benedikt Syndrome)

Medial lemniscus

Red nucleus

Oculomotor (III)
nerve fibres

Oculomotor n. (III)

Oculomotor (III) nerve fibres

Cerebral peduncle

Posterior cerebral artery

J. Perkins
CMI, FAMI

PONS

Lateral Pontine Syndrome
(AICA Syndrome)

Medial Pontine Syndrome
(Medial Basilar Infarct)

Vestibular nuclei (VIII)
Spinal tract/nucleus
of trigeminal n. (V)
Motor nucleus of facial n. (VII)
Ventral cochlear nucleus (VIII)
Spinothalamic tract
Vestibulocochlear n. (VIII)
Facial n. (VII)

Abducent (VI) nucleus

Medial lemniscus
Abducent (VI) nerve fibres

Corticospinal (pyramidal) tract
Paramedian penetrating artery
Short circumferential
penetrating artery

Anterior–inferior
cerebellar artery (AICA)

Abducent n. (VI)

Basilar artery

MEDULLA

Lateral Medullary Syndrome
(PICA Syndrome; Wallenberg Syndrome)

Medial Medullary Syndrome

Vestibular nuclei (VIII)
Nucleus solitarius (X)
Dorsal motor nucleus of vagus (X)
Spinal tract/nucleus
of trigeminal n. (V)
Inferior cerebellar peduncle
Vagus n. (X)
Nucleus ambiguus (IX, X)
Spinothalamic tract
Posterior inferior
cerebellar artery (PICA)

Hypoglossal nucleus

Hypoglossal (XII) nerve fibres

Medial lemniscus

Corticospinal (pyramidal) tract
Hypoglossal n. (XII)
Anterior spinal artery

Vertebral artery

FIGURE 4.26 Common brainstem syndromes.
Source: *Felten DL, MD, PhD. Netter's atlas of neuroscience; 2016. vol. 11, p. 247–87.*

FIGURE 4.27   Cerebellar haemorrhage. Left: CT scan of a right hemispheric cerebellar haematoma in a 51-year-old woman with a history of headache and dysarthria 30 min before admission. Right: CT scan of a 78-year-old patient who was last seen healthy 2 h before admission. Twenty minutes before admission he was found comatose (GCS 3), brainstem reflexes were absent and Babinski signs were positive on both sides. CT scan shows a massive cerebellar haematoma involving both hemispheres.

Source: *Witsch J. Primary cerebellar haemorrhage: complications, treatment and outcome. Clin Neurol Neurosurg 2013;115(7):863–9.*

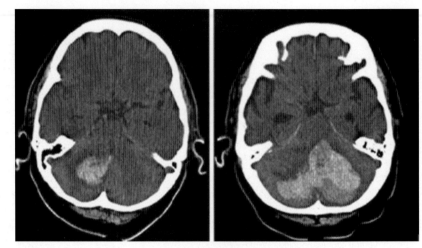

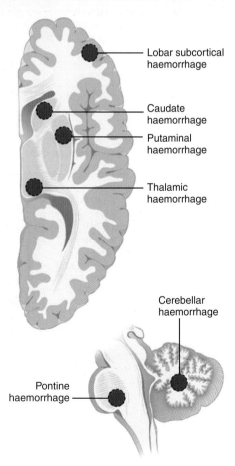

Lobar subcortical
haemorrhage

Caudate
haemorrhage

Putaminal
haemorrhage

Thalamic
haemorrhage

Cerebellar
haemorrhage

Pontine
haemorrhage

FIGURE 4.28   The most common sites of intracerebral haemorrhage.
Source: *Caplan LR, MD. Basic pathology, anatomy, and pathophysiology of stroke. Caplan's stroke; 2009. p. 22–63, Chapter 2.*

ARTERIAL SUPPLY OF THE SPINAL CORD (Fig. 4.29)

- The blood supply to the spinal cord arises from branches of the vertebral arteries and spinal radicular arteries and is provided by the **anterior spinal** artery and the **two posterior spinal** arteries.
- The anterior spinal artery arises from both vertebral arteries and runs along the ventral surface of the spinal cord. It supplies approximately the **anterior two-thirds** of the cord, including the **anterior horns** and **anterior** and **lateral white matter columns**.
- The two posterior spinal arteries arise from the vertebral or PICAs and supply the **dorsal surface** of the cord. They supply the **posterior columns** and **part of the posterior horns**.
- The anterior and posterior spinal arteries form a spinal arterial plexus that surrounds the spinal cord.
- Thirty-one segmental arterial branches enter the spinal canal along its length; most of the branches arise from the aorta and supply the meninges. Only six to ten of these reach the spinal cord as radicular arteries, which arise at variable levels.
- The great radicular artery of Adamkiewicz (artery of the lumbar enlargement) is a prominent radicular artery most frequently arising from the

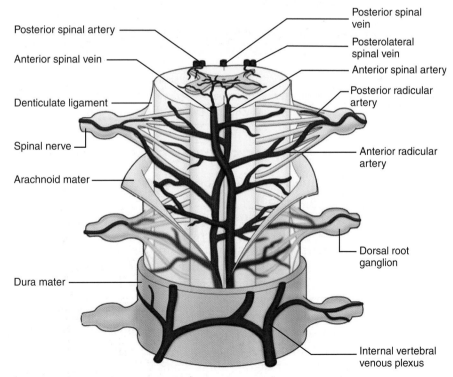

FIGURE 4.29   The arterial supply and venous drainage of the spinal cord.

Source: *Crossman AR, PhD, DSc. Vasculature of the central nervous system. Neuroanatomy: an illustrated colour text; 2015. p. 61–8, Chapter 7.*

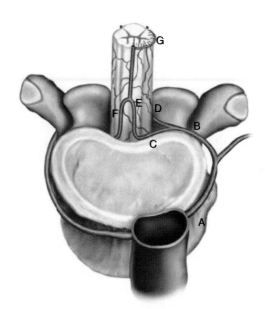

FIGURE 4.30   An illustration shows the normal anatomy of the arterial supply of the spinal cord: (A) intercostal artery; (B) radiculomedullary artery; (C) anterior radicular artery, the great anterior radicular artery called the Adamkiewicz artery (AKA); (D) posterior radicular artery; (E) hairpin-curve connection to the anterior spinal artery (F) anterior spinal artery and (G) pial network.
Source: *Domoto S, MD. Intraspinal collateral circulation to the artery of Adamkiewicz detected with intra-arterial injected computed tomographic angiography. J Vasc Surg 63(6):1631–34.*

left side between **T9** and **T12**. It provides the major blood supply to the **lumbar** and **sacral cord** (Fig. 4.30).

CLINICAL INSIGHT

■ The midthoracic area lying between T4 and T8 levels, i.e. midway between vertebral and lumbar arterial supplies, has a relatively decreased perfusion and is referred to as the **vulnerable zone**. This area is susceptible to ischaemia during major thoracic surgeries and other conditions associated with decreased aortic pressure.

VENOUS DRAINAGE OF THE BRAIN

- The venous drainage of the brain has superficial and deep territories (Figs. 4.31–4.33).
- The superficial **veins** drain mainly into the superior sagittal sinus and the cavernous sinus (Fig. 4.34).
- The deep **structures** drain into the internal cerebral **veins**, the basal veins of Rosenthal and other veins to reach the great cerebral vein of Galen. The great vein of Galen joins the inferior sagittal sinus to form the straight sinus.
- All venous drainage for the brain reaches the internal jugular **veins**.
- The major cerebral venous sinuses lie enclosed within folds of the two layers of dura.
- The **superior sagittal sinus** drains into the **two** transverse sinuses.
- The **transverse sinus** turns downwards to become a sigmoid sinus that exits the skull through the jugular foramen, forming the **internal jugular vein**.

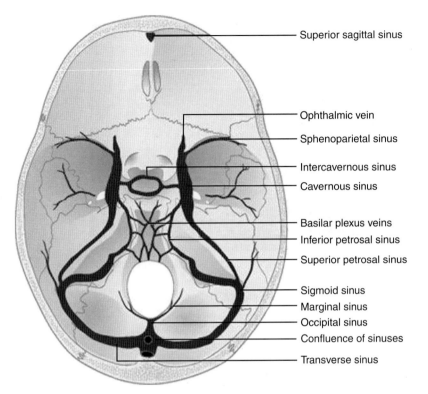

Superior sagittal sinus

Ophthalmic vein

Sphenoparietal sinus

Intercavernous sinus

Cavernous sinus

Basilar plexus veins

Inferior petrosal sinus

Superior petrosal sinus

Sigmoid sinus

Marginal sinus

Occipital sinus

Confluence of sinuses

Transverse sinus

FIGURE 4.31 Drawing of the base of the skull with the brain removed showing the various dural sinuses.
Source: *Caplan LR, MD. Basic pathology, anatomy, and pathophysiology of stroke. Caplan's stroke; 2009. p. 22–63, Chapter 2.*

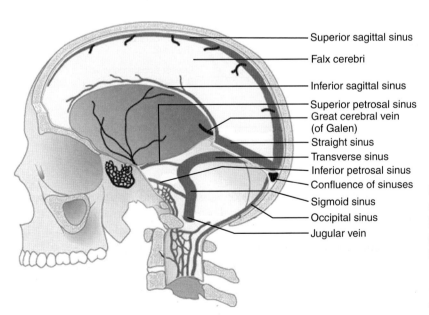

Superior sagittal sinus

Falx cerebri

Inferior sagittal sinus

Superior petrosal sinus

Great cerebral vein (of Galen)

Straight sinus

Transverse sinus

Inferior petrosal sinus

Confluence of sinuses

Sigmoid sinus

Occipital sinus

Jugular vein

FIGURE 4.32 Drawing of a midsagittal view of the skull showing the major large veins and dural sinuses.
Source: *Caplan LR, MD. Basic pathology, anatomy, and pathophysiology of stroke. Caplan's stroke; 2009. p. 22–63, Chapter 2.*

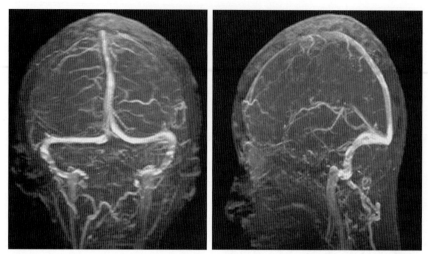

FIGURE 4.33   Magnetic resonance (MR) venogram showing the superior and inferior sagittal sinuses, the lateral and sigmoid sinuses and the jugular veins.

Source: *Caplan LR, MD. Basic pathology, anatomy, and pathophysiology of stroke. Caplan's stroke; 2009. p. 22–63, Chapter 2.*

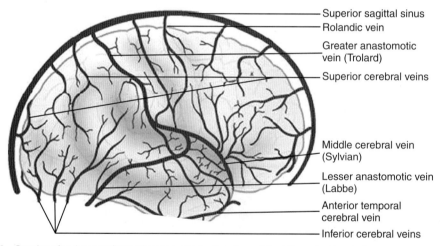

FIGURE 4.34   Drawing of major superficial veins seen on lateral surface of the left cerebral hemisphere.

Source: *Caplan LR, MD. Basic pathology, anatomy, and pathophysiology of stroke. Caplan's stroke; 2009. p. 22–63, Chapter 2.*

- The cavernous sinus is a plexus of veins located on either side of the sella turcica. The cavernous sinus drains via the superior petrosal sinus into the **transverse sinus** and via the inferior petrosal sinus into the **internal jugular vein**.

- The ICAs and cranial nerves III, IV (trochlear), V_1 (first branch of trigeminal), V_2 (second branch of trigeminal) and VI all pass through the cavernous sinus.

- The confluence of the sinuses, torcular herophili (or more simply, the torcular), occurs where the superior sagittal, straight and occipital sinuses join together and are drained by the transverse sinuses.

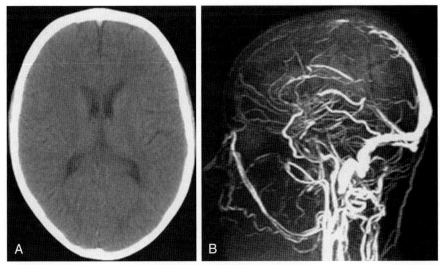

FIGURE 4.35   Superior sagittal sinus thrombosis. Thrombosis of the superior sagittal sinus is easily appreciated on CT (A) due to the marked difference in the density of the thrombosed anterior part of the sinus compared with the patent posterior part. Thrombus of different ages may also explain this differential density, but magnetic resonance venography (B) confirmed the CT findings in this case. Source: *Downer JJ. Symmetry in computed tomography of the brain: the pitfalls. Clin Radiol 2008;64(3):298–306.*

- The inferior anastomotic vein of Labbe drains into the **transverse sinus**.
- The superior anastomotic vein of Trolard drains into the **superior sagittal sinus**.
- The superficial middle cerebral vein drains into the **cavernous sinus**.
- The anterior cerebral veins and deep middle cerebral **veins** drain into the basal veins of Rosenthal, which then join the **internal cerebral** veins to form the **great vein of Galen**.

CLINICAL INSIGHT

- **Sagittal sinus thrombosis (Fig. 4.35)**
    - It is often due to **hypercoagulable states**.
    - It occurs more in **pregnant women** and within the **first few weeks postpartum**.
    - Obstruction of venous drainage usually leads to **elevated intracranial pressure** causing headaches, papilloedema, seizures and sometimes alteration of consciousness.
    - The increased venous pressure may limit cerebral perfusion, leading to **infarcts**.
    - The more definitive diagnostic imaging modality is a **magnetic resonance venography (MRV)**.
    - Treatment usually involves **anticoagulation** therapy.

VENOUS DRAINAGE OF THE SPINAL CORD

- Venous return from the spinal cord occurs via a plexus of veins located in the epidural space before reaching systemic circulation (Fig. 4.29).
- These epidural veins are called Batson plexus and do not contain valves (Fig. 4.36).

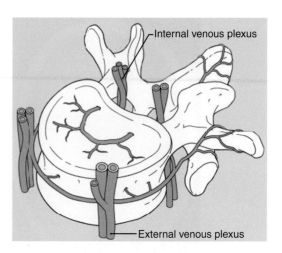

Internal venous plexus

External venous plexus

FIGURE 4.36   Venous plexuses in the spinal cord. The veins of the vertebral column form intricate plexuses around the column, along the spinal canal, and through the bone substance. These venous plexuses, also known as Batson plexus, communicate freely with the segmental systemic veins and portal system. Because of these anastomoses and the lack of valves in these veins, retrograde flow frequently occurs and may result in metastatic infection, as well as metastatic tumours, affecting the vertebral bodies, spinal cord, brain and skull.
Source: *Bullough PG, MB, ChB. Bone and joint infection. Orthopaedic Pathology; 2010. p. 109–39, Chapter 5.*

CLINICAL INSIGHT

■ **Batson venous plexus**

   ■ In the absence of valves in the spinal venous plexus, elevated intra-abdominal pressure can cause reflux of blood carrying metastatic cells or pelvic infections into the epidural space. The Batson plexus is continuous with the cerebral venous system and can be a root of **infection** and **metastasis** to the **cranium**.

CASE STUDY DISCUSSION

Left **MCA stem infarcts** tend to produce **large territory infarcts** with extensive symptoms. The sudden onset of maximal deficits suggests a possible **embolic stroke**.

Clinical Features

- **Right hemiplegia** with upper motor neuron signs (right hyperreflexia) are caused by a large lesion affecting the **entire left motor cortex** or by a lesion to the **corticobulbar** or **corticospinal tracts**.
- Loss of response to pain on the right side could be due to a **right hemisensory loss** as a result of a large lesion in the **left somatosensory cortex**, lesion of the **left thalamus** or **thalamosensory radiations**.
- **Global aphasia** may be caused by **large dominant hemisphere** infarcts.
- **Ipsilateral gaze preference** may be seen in **large cortical** lesions where eyes are unable to move to the side **opposite** to the lesion.

The aggregation of these four clinical signs suggests that the most likely localization is a large lesion affecting the **entire left cerebral cortex**. A left MCA stem infarct could produce these deficits as well as a **massive left hemisphere haemorrhage** if there is an acute onset of the symptoms. To help identify the cause, **neuroimaging** is often warranted.

Management

Initial head CT brain done within few hours was negative except for a **hyperdensity** in the **proximal left MCA**, consistent with a **blood clot**. This suggested an **embolic stroke**. Workup for embolic stroke showed evidence of atrial fibrillation, suggesting that an embolus had formed in the left atrium and travelled to the left MCA stem.

Thrombolysis via tissue plasminogen activator was given with minimal improvement in the patient's symptoms.

A repeat **head CT** 1 day after admission again showed a hyperdensity in the left MCA stem, but also showed a **massive area of hypodensity** consistent with infarction of the **entire left MCA territory**, involving both the superficial and deep MCA territories (Fig. 4.37), while sparing the thalamus, inferior temporal lobe and medial occipitoparietal cortex (PCA territory), in addition to sparing the medial frontoparietal cortex (ACA territory).

The patient showed minimal improvement in his deficits and required extensive rehabilitation after being discharged home few weeks later.

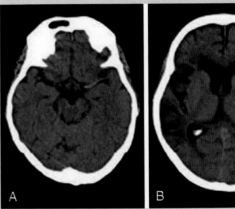

FIGURE 4.37   Progression of features of left MCA stem infarct on head CT. (A) A simple transverse CT scan performed when the patient arrived at the emergency department displays spontaneous hyperdense left MCA. (B) Simple transverse CT scan performed 24 h after stroke demonstrating an extensive hypodense area in the cortical–subcortical region affecting most of the territory of the left MCA, compatible with extensive subacute infarction in that area with a discrete mass effect on the left lateral ventricle.

Source: *Iglesias-Mohedano AM. Is the fogging effect related to futile recanalisation? Neurology (Neurología, English ed.) 2013;30(7): 447–9.*

CHAPTER 5

Peripheral Nerves

Mohammad Hassan A. Noureldine

CASE STUDY

Presentation and Physical Examination: A 32-year-old woman presented to the outpatient clinic complaining of numbness, tingling and weakness in her legs. She was initially seen for diarrhoea 2 weeks prior to presentation and was managed with a course of antibiotics. Her diarrhoea improved, but a week later, she started having tingling and numbness in her feet that progressively ascended to her legs and thighs. She was referred to the emergency room (ER); her workup included blood cultures and a lumbar puncture (LP). A neurologist was consulted, but the patient left the ER against medical advice. Her sensory symptoms continued to worsen, and she started having leg weakness and gait disturbances. Her past medical history was negative except for diarrhoea 2 weeks earlier. She denied fever, chills, upper and lower respiratory and gastrointestinal symptoms, and swallowing difficulties. Neurologic examination was positive for motor deficits in bilateral wrist extensors and flexors (4/5), deltoids (4/5), hip flexors, quadriceps and hamstrings (4/5) and plantar flexors and dorsiflexors (3/5). Her deep tendon reflexes were 1+ in triceps, brachioradialis and biceps, and absent in knees and ankles. Decreased sensation to light touch and pinprick was noted in the lower extremities bilaterally and the abdomen. She had bilateral dysmetria on finger-to-nose and rapid alternating movements, and her gait was ataxic.

Diagnosis, Management and Follow-Up: Previous LP results showed increased cerebrospinal fluid (CSF) proteins (220 mg/dL) and normal cell count. Electromyography (EMG) studies revealed slow nerve conduction velocities and delayed distal latencies in the legs more than the arms.

The patient was diagnosed with **Guillain–Barre syndrome (GBS)** and admitted to the intensive care unit (ICU) for close monitoring. She was managed with a 5-day course of intravenous immunoglobulins (IVIG). Symptoms progressively improved over 10 days and the patient was discharged home.

BRIEF INTRODUCTION

The **peripheral nervous system (PNS)** includes all the nervous system components that reside outside the boundaries of the central nervous system (CNS).

- In general, the PNS is classified as the following:
  - **Somatic** nervous system, which consists of spinal sensory nerves and ganglia, spinal motor nerves and cranial nerves (CNs) except for CNs I and II. It is concerned with the **conscious** control of **voluntary** movements and the facilitation of the involuntary **somatic reflexes**.
  - **Autonomic** nervous system, which consists of sympathetic and parasympathetic pre- and postganglionic nerves and ganglia. It is the regulatory centre of **unconscious**, **involuntary** bodily functions.

- Peripheral nerves contain sensory (afferent), motor (efferent) or mixed (sensory and motor) fibres.
- Spinal nerve roots provide **sensation** and **muscular innervation** at specific sites; these are known as **dermatomes** and **myotomes**, respectively.
- **Ventral rami** from different spinal nerve roots join with each other to form **nerve plexuses**.
- Somatic reflexes play an integral role in protecting the body against damage from external factors, in addition to other essential functions such as maintaining posture and equilibrium.

This chapter focuses on the spinal sensory and motor nerves, whereas cranial and autonomic nerves will be discussed in separate chapters that will follow.

GENERAL ORGANIZATION AND ANATOMY

The anatomy of a single **spinal nerve** is best described as the following (Fig. 5.1):

- A layer of connective tissue, called the **endoneurium**, surrounds **nerve fibres**, which consist of axons of motor neurons and dendrites of sensory neurons.
- Nerve fibres are organized into bundles called **fasciculi**. Another layer of connective tissue known as the **perineurium** surrounds every fasciculus.
- Multiple fasciculi are stacked inside a layer called the **epineurium** to form a **nerve** or a **nerve root**.
- Fat, small arteries and veins may be dispersed inside the connective tissue layers and between the fasciculi.
- In close proximity to the spinal cord, a **posterior (dorsal; sensory)** root meets an **anterior (ventral; motor)** root to form a spinal nerve (Fig. 5.2).

Spinal nerves emerge as pairs from the **lateral aspects** of the spinal cord. The union of a ventral root and a dorsal root forms a single spinal nerve that leaves the vertebral column through the **intervertebral foramen**. In total, there are **31 pairs** of spinal nerves; these are divided into five **groups** according to the spinal cord and vertebral levels they arise from (Fig. 5.3).

- **Cervical: Eight pairs** emerging **above** the corresponding cervical vertebrae, i.e. C1 nerve above C1 vertebra (atlas), C2 nerve above C2 vertebra (axis). Since the human body contains **seven cervical vertebrae** only, C8 nerve emerges below C7 and above T1 vertebra.
- **Thoracic: Twelve pairs** emerging **below** the corresponding thoracic vertebrae.
- **Lumbar: Five pairs** emerging **below** the corresponding lumbar vertebrae.
- **Sacral: Five pairs**, four of which emerge from the anterior sacral foramina formed by the fusion of the sacral vertebrae and one emerging below the fifth sacral vertebra.
- **Coccygeal: One pair** emerging **below** the first piece of the coccyx.

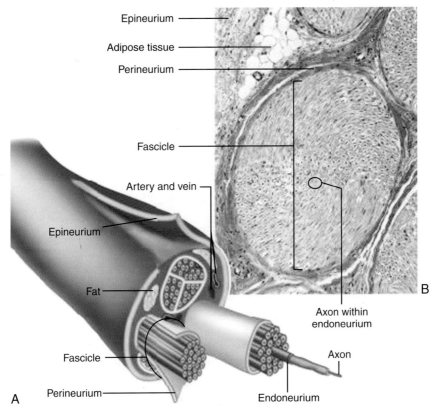

Epineurium
Adipose tissue
Perineurium
Fascicle
Artery and vein
Epineurium
Fat
Fascicle
Perineurium
Axon within endoneurium
Axon
Endoneurium
A
B

FIGURE 5.1 (A) Schematic representation of nerve organization. (B) Low-power cross section of polyfascicular nerve showing the organization of the nerve, with individual nerve fibres surrounded by endoneurium, fascicles surrounded by perineurium and the investing epineurium. The mesoneurium is visible surrounding the entire nerve sheath at the periphery, with adipose tissue (upper left).
Source: *(A from Patton K, Thibodeau G. Anatomy and physiology, 7th ed., St. Louis: Mosby; 2010) Miloro M. Traumatic injuries of the trigeminal nerve. Oral and maxillofacial trauma. p. 650–82, Chapter 25.*

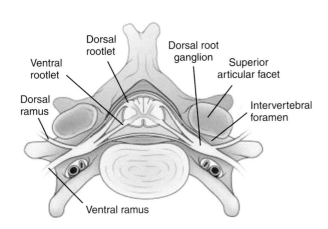

Dorsal rootlet
Ventral rootlet
Dorsal ramus
Dorsal root ganglion
Superior articular facet
Intervertebral foramen
Ventral ramus

FIGURE 5.2 Anatomy of a spinal nerve. Dorsal and ventral rootlets combine within the intervertebral foramen to form mixed spinal nerves, which further divide on exiting the foramen into the dorsal and ventral rami.
Source: *(Image courtesy Cleveland Clinic, 2006. Illustrator, David Schumick, BS, CMI.) Tsao B. Trauma of the nervous system: peripheral nerve trauma. Bradley's neurology in clinical practice. p. 903–19.e2, Chapter 64.*

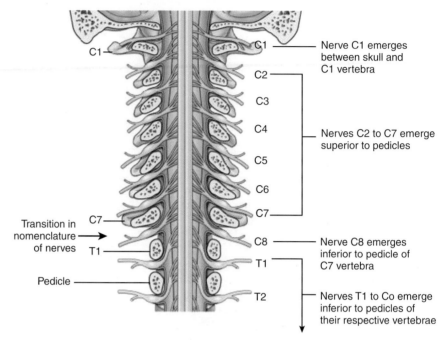

FIGURE 5.3   Nomenclature of the spinal nerves.
Source: *From Drake RL, Vogl W, Mitchell AWM. Gray's anatomy for students, 2nd ed., Philadelphia: Elsevier; 2010.*

CLINICAL INSIGHT

- **Nerve Root Damage in Lumbar Disc Disease**
  - A nerve root assumes an **anterolateral path** before exiting through its corresponding intervertebral foramen. To note, intervertebral foramina are located **immediately above** the horizontal level of intervertebral discs found between the same two vertebrae.
  - In **lumbar disc disease**, a nerve root is vulnerable to compression by a bulging disc that protrudes laterally from vertebral levels above the vertebral level of the exit foramina of nerve roots; this occurs because a laterally protruding disc will not reach the nerve root that have exited through the same-level intervertebral foramen located above the disc. The nerve root, however, may be compressed by same level vertebral disc that is protruding in an upward direction.
    - For example, an L4/L5 laterally protruding disc would compress the L5 root before it reaches its exit point: the L5/S1 intervertebral foramen.
    - Large discs, however, may compress not only the nerve root crossing it but also the nerve root emerging through the same level intervertebral foramen (Fig. 5.4).
    - On the other hand, **stenosis** of an intervertebral foramen would damage the root exiting through it. Thus, a L4/L5 stenotic foramen would damage the L4 nerve root.

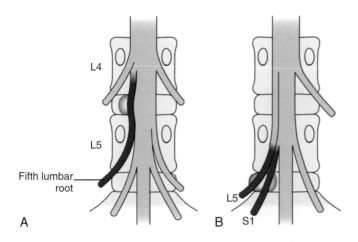

L4

L5

Fifth lumbar
root

A

L5

B   S1

FIGURE 5.4   Possible effects of disc herniation. (A) Herniation of the disc between L4 and L5 compresses the fifth lumbar root. (B) Large herniation of the L5–S1 disc compromises not only the nerve root crossing it (first sacral nerve root) but also the nerve root emerging through the same foramen (fifth lumbar nerve root).

Source: *Redrawn from MacNab I. Backache. Baltimore: Williams & Wilkins; 1977. p. 96–7.*

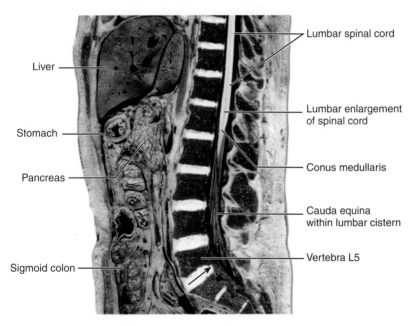

Liver

Stomach

Pancreas

Sigmoid colon

Lumbar spinal cord

Lumbar enlargement of spinal cord

Conus medullaris

Cauda equina within lumbar cistern

Vertebra L5

FIGURE 5.5   Midline sagittal section of embalmed cadaver displaying thoracic, lumbar and sacral spinal cord and cauda equina. Arrow indicates most frequent intervertebral disc to prolapse.

Source: *Reproduced, with permission, from the Liu S, et al. editors. Atlas of human sectional anatomy. Jinan: Shantung Press of Science and Technology; 2003.*

Spinal nerve roots arising from **L2 spinal segment level to the caudal end of the spinal cord**, also known as the **conus medullaris**, are arranged next to each other and form the **cauda equina** (Fig. 5.5).

After exiting from the intervertebral foramina, a spinal nerve divides into the following branches (Fig. 5.6):

- **Posterior (dorsal)** ramus: conveys somatic sensory, somatic motor and visceral motor information to and from the **posterior trunk**.

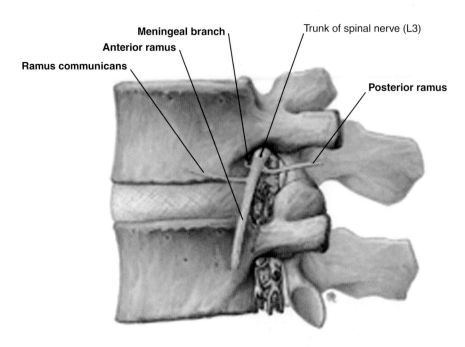

FIGURE 5.6   Spinal nerve in the lumbar region of the vertebral column; view from the left side. Upon its passage through the intervertebral foramen, the spinal nerve divides into the anterior ramus, posterior ramus, meningeal branch and ramus communicans *(See chapter 16).*
Source: *Paulsen F. Trunk. Sobotta atlas of human anatomy. vol. 1, p. 39–126, Chapter 2.*

- **Anterior (ventral)** ramus: conveys somatic sensory, somatic motor and visceral motor information to and from the **anterior** and **lateral trunk** and the **upper** and **lower limbs**.
- **Meningeal** branch: re-enters the foramen immediately after branching off the spinal nerve and conveys information to and from structures inside the vertebral column (periosteum, facet joints, ligaments, intervertebral discs, dura mater, etc.).

A **spinal (dorsal root) ganglion**, which is located outside the CNS, houses cell bodies of **afferent sensory** nerve fibres. These are situated on the **posterior root** of the spinal nerves in close proximity to the spinal cord (Fig. 5.2).

DERMATOMAL AND MYOTOMAL INNERVATION OF SPINAL NERVE ROOTS

A 'dermatome' is the **skin area** supplied by the **sensory** component of a **single spinal nerve root**, whereas a 'myotome' is the **group of muscles** innervated by the **motor** component of a **single spinal nerve root**.

- Most dermatomes and myotomes overlap.
- 'Autonomous zones' refers to distinct skin areas that are **solely innervated** by a **single** nerve root. These zones do not exist in myotomes as no muscle is supplied by only one nerve root. Thus,

complete paralysis of a single muscle from a single nerve root injury is extremely rare.

■ Table 5.1 summarizes the dermatomal autonomous zones and myotomal innervation of every spinal nerve root, whereas Fig. 5.7 demonstrates the full dermatomal map of the human body.

Table 5.1 Dermatomal autonomous zones and myotomal innervation of spinal nerves

Spinal Nerve Root	Approximated Dermatomal Autonomous Zones	Myotome Function
Cervical		
C1	No dermatome	Neck flexion and extension
C2	Occipital protuberance	Neck flexion and extension
C3	Supraclavicular fossa	Diaphragm contraction; neck lateral flexion
C4	Acromioclavicular joint	Diaphragm contraction; shoulder elevation
C5	Lateral (radial) antecubital fossa	Diaphragm contraction; shoulder abduction and flexion; elbow flexion
C6	Thumb	*Mainly:* wrist extension; *Also:* elbow flexion
C7	Middle finger	*Mainly:* elbow extension; *Also:* wrist flexion
C8	Little finger	Finger flexion
Thoracic		
T1	Medial (ulnar) antecubital fossa	Finger abduction
T2	Inner arm, apex of axilla	Contraction of chest wall and/or abdominal muscles
T3	Intersection between midclavicular line and 3rd intercostal space	Contraction of chest wall and/or abdominal muscles
T4	Nipple; Intersection between midclavicular line and 4th intercostal space	Contraction of chest wall and/or abdominal muscles
T5	Intersection between midclavicular line and 5th intercostal space	Contraction of chest wall and/or abdominal muscles
T6	Intersection between midclavicular line and level of xiphoid process	Contraction of chest wall and/or abdominal muscles
T7	Intersection between midclavicular line and area at one quarter the distance between T6 and T10 landmarks	Contraction of chest wall and/or abdominal muscles
T8	Intersection between midclavicular line and area at midway between T6 and T10 landmarks	Contraction of chest wall and/or abdominal muscles
T9	Intersection between midclavicular line and area at three quarters the distance between T6 and T10 landmarks	Contraction of chest wall and/or abdominal muscles
T10	Umbilicus; Intersection between midclavicular line and horizontal level of umbilicus	Contraction of chest wall and/or abdominal muscles
T11	Intersection between midclavicular line and area at midway between T10 and T12 landmarks	Contraction of chest wall and/or abdominal muscles
T12	Intersection between midclavicular line and midpoint of inguinal ligament	Contraction of chest wall and/or abdominal muscles

Continued

Table 5.1 Dermatomal autonomous zones and myotomal innervation of spinal nerves—cont'd

Spinal Nerve Root	Approximated Dermatomal Autonomous Zones	Myotome Function
Lumbar		
L1	Upper anterior thigh	Hip flexion
L2	Mid anterior thigh	Hip flexion and adduction
L3	Knee, medial femoral condyle	Knee extension
L4	Medial malleolus	*Mainly:* Ankle dorsiflexion and inversion; *Also:* hip extension/abduction and knee extension
L5	Dorsum of foot, over 3rd metatarsophalangeal joint	*Mainly:* Great toe extension; *Also:* hip extension/abduction, knee flexion, and ankle dorsiflexion
Sacral		
S1	Lateral malleolus	*Mainly:* Ankle plantar flexion; *Also:* hip extension, ankle eversion, and knee flexion
S2	Popliteal fossa	*Mainly:* Knee flexion; *Also:* toe flexion and ankle plantar flexion
S3	Ischial tuberosity, infragluteal fold	*Mainly:* Toe abduction/adduction; *Also:* anal wink and contraction of bladder, bowel, genital, among other pelvic muscles
S4	Perianal area (within a 2 cm radius)	*Mainly:* Anal wink; *Also:* contraction of bladder, bowel, genital, among other pelvic muscles
S5	Perianal area (within a 1 cm radius)	*Mainly:* Anal wink; *Also:* contraction of bladder, bowel, genital, among other pelvic muscles
Coccygeal		
Co	Anal triangle, overlapping with S4 and S5 dermatomes (no autonomous zone)	No significant myotome

Note: *See Fig. 5.7 for the full dermatomal map*

NERVE PLEXUSES

A **nerve plexus** is formed by intercommunication between **ventral rami** of spinal nerves.

- **Afferent (sensory)** and **efferent (motor)** fibres travel along the plexuses. Nerve fibres may join and separate on multiple tracks but are eventually allocated to specific peripheral nerves.
- **Four major** nerve plexuses (**cervical**, **brachial**, **lumbar** and **sacral**) and **one minor** plexus (**coccygeal**) exist in the human body.
- Interestingly, a **thoracic plexus does not exist**; intercostal nerves and the subcostal nerve arise independently from the ventral rami of thoracic spinal roots (T1–T12) and innervate the thoracic and abdominal wall muscles, parietal pleura of the thorax, abdominal peritoneum and skin over the chest, abdomen and part of the pelvis and groin.
- Table 5.2 lists the nerve plexuses, somatic peripheral nerves and their sensory/motor innervation pattern.

Table 5.2 Nerve plexuses, somatic peripheral nerves and their motor/sensory innervations

Nerve Plexus	Plexus Location	Peripheral Nerves	Nerve Root Supply	Innervation
Cervical (C1–C5) (Fig. 5.8)	Neck, deep to sternocleidomastoid	Ansa cervicalis	C1–C3	■ **Motor:** Geniohyoid; sternohyoid; omohyoid; sternothyroid; thyrohyoid
		Lesser (small) occipital	C2	■ **Sensory:** Skin of neck and scalp superior and posterior to the auricle
		Greater auricular	C2, C3	■ **Sensory:** Skin over parotid gland and mastoid process; deep layer of parotid fascia
		Superficial (transverse) cervical	C2, C3	■ **Sensory:** Skin over anterior cervical region
		Supraclavicular	C3, C4	■ **Sensory:** Skin over upper chest and shoulders
		Phrenic	C3–C5	■ **Motor:** Diaphragm ■ **Sensory:** Mediastinal and central diaphragmatic pleura; pericardium; peritoneum; diaphragm
Brachial (C5–T1) (Figs. 5.9–5.12)	Neck, extending into axilla	Axillary	C5, C6	■ **Motor:** Deltoid; teres minor ■ **Sensory:** Skin over deltoid by superior lateral cutaneous nerve of the arm
		Musculocutaneous	C5-C7	■ **Motor:** Muscles of anterior compartment of arm (coracobrachialis, biceps brachii, part of brachialis) ■ **Sensory:** Lateral aspect of forearm by lateral cutaneous branch
		Radial	C5–T1	■ **Motor:** Muscles of posterior compartment of arm (triceps brachii, anconeus); part of brachialis; brachioradialis and extensor muscles of the forearm by posterior interosseous nerve, a continuation of the deep branch ■ **Sensory:** Skin over dorsal hand, dorsal 1st to 3rd fingers, and dorsolateral 4th finger
		Median	C5–T1	■ **Motor:** Pronator teres; pronator quadratus; flexor muscles of forearm except for flexor carpi ulnaris and ulnar half of flexor digitorum profundus; abductor pollicis brevis; thenar muscles; 1st and 2nd (radial) lumbricals ■ **Sensory:** Palmar skin over 1st to 3rd and medial aspect of 4th fingers
		Ulnar	C8, T1	■ **Motor:** Flexor carpi ulnaris; medial half of flexor digitorum profundus; hypothenar muscles; 3rd and 4th (ulnar) lumbricals; adductor pollicis flexor; other intrinsic hand muscles ■ **Sensory:** Skin over palmar and dorsal aspects of hand on ulnar side, 5th and medial 4th fingers
Lumbar (T12–L5) (Figs. 5.13 and 5.14)	Lumbar region, within psoas major muscle	Iliohypogastric	L1	■ **Sensory:** Skin over the upper part of buttocks by the lateral cutaneous branch, and lower part of the rectus abdominis and mons pubis by the anterior cutaneous branch

Continued

Table 5.2 Nerve plexuses, somatic peripheral nerves and their motor/sensory innervations—cont'd

Nerve Plexus	Plexus Location	Peripheral Nerves	Nerve Root Supply	Innervation
		Ilioinguinal	L1	■ **Motor:** Internal oblique; transversus abdominis ■ **Sensory:** Skin over superior medial thigh, anterior one-third of scrotum and root of penis in men, and anterior one-third of labium majus and root of clitoris in women
		Genitofemoral	L1, L2	■ **Motor:** Cremaster and dartos muscles in men by the genital branch ■ **Sensory:** Spermatic fasciae, tunica vaginalis of the testis, skin over upper anterior scrotum in men, and skin over mons pubis and labium majus in women, by the genital branch; skin over femoral triangle at the groin by the femoral branch
		Lateral femoral cutaneous	L2, L3	■ **Sensory:** Skin over anterolateral and posterolateral surfaces of thigh by anterior and posterior branches, respectively
		Femoral	L2–L4	■ **Motor:** Pectineus; sartorius; iliacus; muscles of anterior compartment of thigh (rectus femoris; vastus lateralis; vastus medialis; vastus intermedius) ■ **Sensory:** Skin over anterior and medial surface of thigh by intermediate and medial femoral cutaneous nerves, branches of the superficial division, and medial leg by saphenous nerve, a continuation of the deep division
		Obturator	L2–L4	■ **Motor:** Muscles of medial compartment of thigh (gracilis, adductors longus and brevis by anterior division; adductor magnus [pubic segment] by posterior division); obturator externus by posterior branch ■ **Sensory:** Skin over medial aspect of thigh by cutaneous branch, part of the anterior division
Sacral (L4–S4) (Fig. 5.15)	Lumbar and sacral region, on anterior belly of the piriformis muscle	Quadratus femoris	L4–S1	■ **Motor:** Quadratus femoris; inferior gemellus
		Superior gluteal	L4–S1	■ **Motor:** Gluteus medius and minimus; tensor fasciae latae
		Common peroneal (fibular)	L4–S2	■ **Motor:** Short head of biceps femoris; peroneus longus and brevis by superficial peroneal branch; muscles of anterior compartment of leg (tibialis anterior; extensor hallucis longus; extensor digitorum longus; peroneus tertius) by deep peroneal branch ■ **Sensory:** Skin over posterolateral leg and lateral foot by lateral sural cutaneous branch, distal anterior leg and dorsal foot by superficial peroneal branch, and 1st and 2nd toes by deep peroneal branch

Table 5.2 Nerve plexuses, somatic peripheral nerves and their motor/sensory innervations—cont'd

Nerve Plexus	Plexus Location	Peripheral Nerves	Nerve Root Supply	Innervation
		Tibial	L4–S3	■ **Motor:** Muscles of posterior compartment of thigh (biceps femoris; semitendinosus; semimembranosus), superficial posterior (gastrocnemius; soleus; plantaris) and deep posterior (popliteus; tibialis posterior; flexor digitorum longus; flexor hallucis longus) compartments of leg, and sole of foot by medial plantar, lateral plantar and medial calcaneal nerves ■ **Sensory:** Skin over posterolateral leg and lateral foot by medial sural cutaneous branch, heel by medial calcaneal branch, and sole of foot by medial and lateral branches
		Internal obturator	L5–S2	■ **Motor:** Obturator internus; superior gemellus
		Inferior gluteal	L5–S2	■ **Motor:** Gluteus maximus
		Piriformis	S1, S2	■ **Motor:** Piriformis
		Posterior femoral cutaneous	S1–S3	■ **Sensory:** Skin over posterior thigh by cutaneous branch, inferior half of buttocks by gluteal branch (inferior cluneal nerve) and posterior part of scrotum or labium majus by perineal branch
		Pudendal	S2–S4	■ **Motor:** External anal sphincter by inferior rectal branch and perineal muscles (bulbospongiosus; ischiocavernosus; superficial transverse perinei; deep transverse perinei; sphincter urethra; levator ani) by deep branch of perineal nerve, a large branch of the pudendal ■ **Sensory:** Mucosa of anal canal below the pectinate line by inferior rectal branch, clitoris and skin over penis by dorsal nerve of clitoris or penis, skin over scrotum or labium majus by superficial branch of the perineal nerve and urethral mucosa by bulbospongiosus branch of perineal nerve
Coccygeal (S4, S5, Co) (Fig. 5.15)	Sacral region, within ischiococcygeal muscle	Anococcygeal	S4, S5, Co (?)	■ **Sensory:** Skin over anal triangle
		Ischiococcygeus branch	(S3), S4, S5	■ **Motor:** Ischiococcygeus
		Levator ani branch	(S3), S4, S5	■ **Motor:** Levator ani (also receives innervation from pudendal)

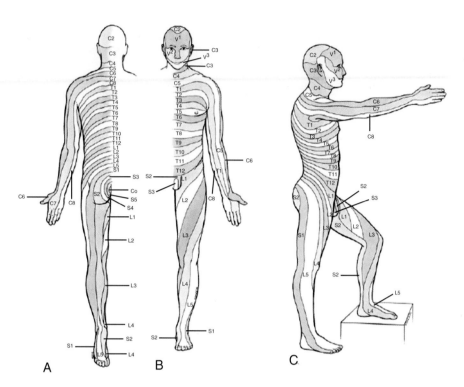

FIGURE 5.7   Dermatome map. A, posterior view; B, anterior view; C, lateral view.
Source: *From Agur AMR, Lee MJ, Anderson JE. Dermatomes. In: Grant's atlas of anatomy. 9th ed. Philadelphia: Lippincott Williams & Wilkins; 1991. p. 252.*

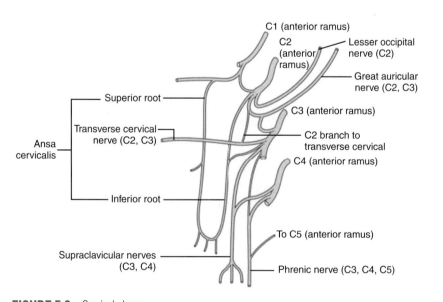

FIGURE 5.8   Cervical plexus.
Source: *Drake RL, PhD, FAAA. Head and neck. Gray's atlas of anatomy. p. 475–608, Chapter 8.*

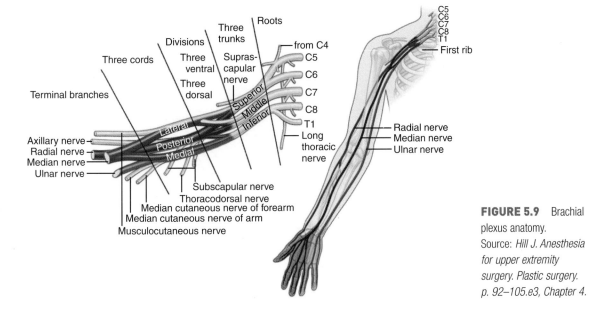

FIGURE 5.9 Brachial plexus anatomy.
Source: *Hill J. Anesthesia for upper extremity surgery. Plastic surgery. p. 92–105.e3, Chapter 4.*

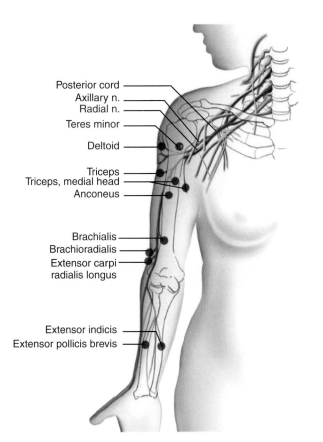

FIGURE 5.10 Muscles innervated by the nerves from the posterior cord of the brachial plexus.
Source: *Boezaart AP, MBChB, MPraxMed, DA (SA), FFA(CMSA), MMed (Anaesth), PhD. Distal brachial plexus: applied anatomy. Atlas of peripheral nerve blocks and anatomy for orthopaedic anesthesia. p. 72, Chapter 5.*

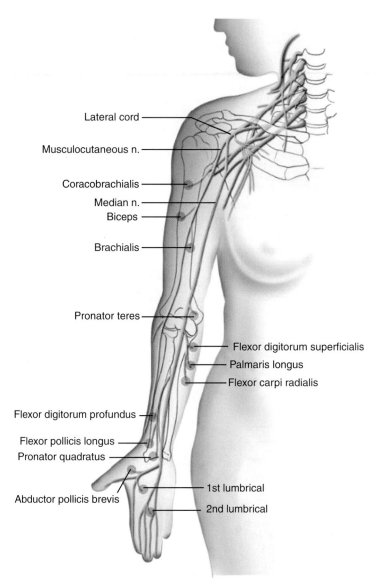

FIGURE 5.11   Muscles innervated by the nerves from the lateral cord of the brachial plexus.
Source: *Boezaart AP, MBChB, MPraxMed, DA (SA), FFA(CMSA), MMed (Anaesth), PhD. Distal brachial plexus: applied anatomy. Atlas of peripheral nerve blocks and anatomy for orthopaedic anesthesia. p. 67, Chapter 5.*

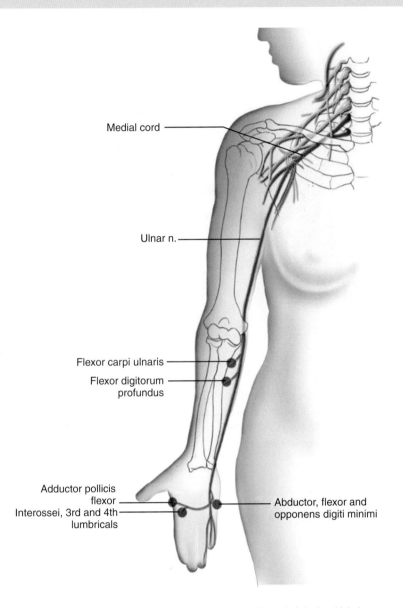

Medial cord

Ulnar n.

Flexor carpi ulnaris

Flexor digitorum
profundus

Adductor pollicis
flexor

Interossei, 3rd and 4th
lumbricals

Abductor, flexor and
opponens digiti minimi

FIGURE 5.12   Muscles innervated by the nerve from medial cord of the brachial plexus.
Source: *Boezaart AP, MBChB, MPraxMed, DA (SA), FFA(CMSA), MMed (Anaesth), PhD. Distal brachial
plexus: applied anatomy. Atlas of peripheral nerve blocks and anatomy for orthopaedic anesthesia.
p. 70, Chapter 5.*

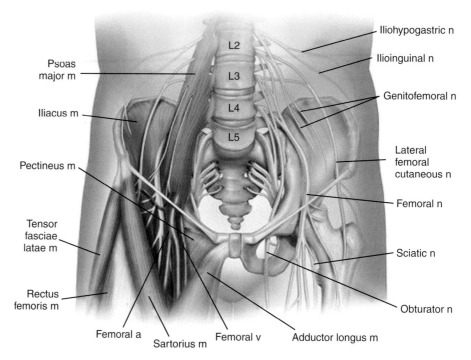

FIGURE 5.13 Anatomy of the lumbar plexus.

Source: *From Hebl JR, Lennon RL, editors. Mayo Clinic atlas of regional anesthesia and ultrasound-guided nerve blockade. Rochester, MN: Mayo Clinic Scientific Press; 2009. Used with permission of Mayo Foundation for Medical Education and Research.*

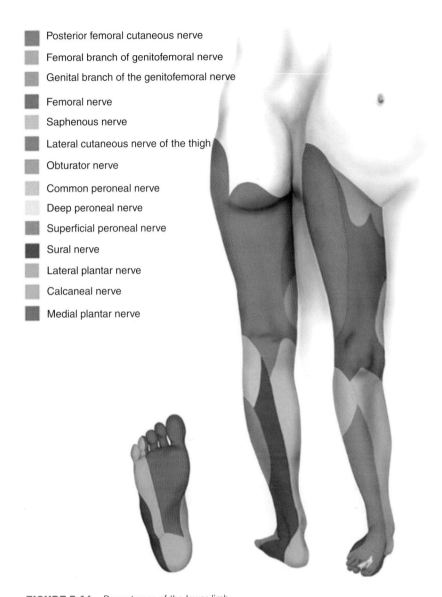

Posterior femoral cutaneous nerve

Femoral branch of genitofemoral nerve

Genital branch of the genitofemoral nerve

Femoral nerve

Saphenous nerve

Lateral cutaneous nerve of the thigh

Obturator nerve

Common peroneal nerve

Deep peroneal nerve

Superficial peroneal nerve

Sural nerve

Lateral plantar nerve

Calcaneal nerve

Medial plantar nerve

FIGURE 5.14   Dermatomes of the lower limb.
Source: *Boezaart AP, MBChB, MPraxMed, DA (SA), FFA(CMSA), MMed (Anaesth), PhD, Lumbar plexus: applied anatomy. Atlas of peripheral nerve blocks and anatomy for orthopaedic anesthesia. p. 136, Chapter 11.*

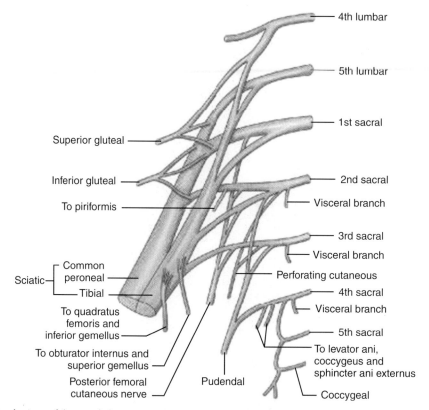

FIGURE 5.15 Anatomy of the sacral plexus.
Source: *Pruthi S. Imaging of the sacral plexus. Imaging of the spine. p. 567–88, Chapter 27.*

CLINICAL INSIGHTS

- **Lesser occipital nerve**
  - **Occipital neuralgia**: Chronic burning, aching and throbbing **pain** that is often associated with shooting episodes, starting at the **base of the skull** and spreading inferiorly to the back and anteriorly to the lateral and frontal head.
- **Supraclavicular nerve**
  - May be injured during surgical approach to clavicular shaft fractures; nerve injury leads to incisional and chest wall **numbness**.
- **Phrenic nerve**
  - **Phrenic nerve palsy**: Although idiopathic in the majority of cases, it can result from any lesion along the nerve course (from the neck to the diaphragm). Unilateral palsy is usually asymptomatic. **Bilateral** palsy causes **dyspnoea/orthopnoea**.
- **Radial nerve**
  - **Radial tunnel syndrome**: **Pain** and **tenderness** over the dorsal upper forearm due to compression of the **posterior interosseous nerve**, a continuation of the deep branch of the radial nerve, as it passes through the lateral intermuscular septum of the arm.

- **Median nerve**
  - **Carpal tunnel syndrome (CTS)** (Fig. 5.16): **Pain** and **paraesthesia** over the palmar surface of the **radial three and a half fingers** (fingers located on the radial side of the hand) due to compression of the median nerve at the carpal tunnel, the fibro-osseous canal at the anterior wrist. Positive **Tinel's** and **Phalen's tests** are highly suggestive of CTS (Fig. 5.17), i.e. tingling sensation or pain elicited by **tapping** the median nerve at the wrist (for the former test) and by **wrist flexion** for 1 min or less (for the latter test).
  - **Pronator teres syndrome**: Pain, **tenderness** and/or **paraesthesia** over the ventral surface of the forearm and the **radial three and a half digits** due to compression of the median nerve near the elbow. Symptoms are augmented by resisted pronation.
- **Ulnar nerve**
  - **Cubital tunnel syndrome** (Fig. 5.18): **Tingling** and **sensory loss** over the **4th and 5th fingers** due to compression of ulnar nerve in the cubital tunnel, a channel situated along the dorsomedial elbow, in which the nerve passes to the forearm. **Hand clumsiness** and **wasting of ulnar muscles** are noted in advanced cases.
  - **Ulnar nerve dislocation** (Fig. 5.18): **Pain** and **paraesthesia** along the ulnar nerve territory due to anterior dislocation of the nerve along the anterior medial epicondyle during elbow flexion and extension.
- **Lateral cutaneous nerve of thigh**
  - **Meralgia paraesthetica**: **Tingling, pain** and **paraesthesia** over the lateral aspect of the thigh due to compression of the lateral cutaneous nerve of the thigh under the inguinal ligament (Fig. 5.19) or when it penetrates the fascia lata.
- **Femoral nerve**
  - **Femoral nerve neuropathy**: The femoral nerve is susceptible to compression under the inguinal ligament due to iatrogenic causes such as femoral artery catheterization, arterial bypass and improper positioning in long surgeries. In addition, hematomas, pseudoaneurysms and muscle tears impinge on the femoral nerve and could lead to its dysfunction.
- **Superior gluteal nerve**
  - **Trendelenburg** or **gluteal gait** (Fig. 5.20): Injury to the superior gluteus nerve leads to weakness in the **gluteus medius** and **minimus** muscles, which are leg abductors. The patient's **pelvis tilts down** on the side **contralateral** to the lesion due to inability of the weak abductors to stabilize it. The **trunk**, however, attempts to compensate for the contralateral droop by **tilting to the side ipsilateral** to the lesion. **Bilateral** lesions lead to **waddling gait**.
- **Peroneal nerve**
  - **Peroneal nerve injury**: Tingling, **paraesthesia, pain** and/or **foot drop** due to injury of the peroneal nerve at the knee where it is exposed the most (Fig. 5.21). The majority of aetiologies are due to direct trauma or prolonged pressure such as knee trauma/dislocations, fibular fractures and lower extremity casts.
- **Posterior tibial nerve**
  - **Tarsal tunnel syndrome**: **Pain** and **paraesthesia** over the heel, sole and plantar aspect of the toes due to compression of the posterior tibial nerve at the tarsal tunnel, the fibro-osseous canal at the medial side of the ankle. Tapping over the damaged nerve elicits distal paraesthesia, also known as positive Tinel's sign.

- **Inferior gluteal nerve**
  - **Gluteus maximus gait** (Fig. 5.22): Injury to the inferior gluteal nerve due to posterior hip dislocation or a surgical complication leads to **weakness in the gluteus maximus muscle**, the chief extensor and lateral rotator of thigh at the hip. The **trunk extends** to compensate for weak extension of the hip, and the patient may hold the **shoulders backwards** on heel strike to relocate the centre of gravity behind the hip joint.

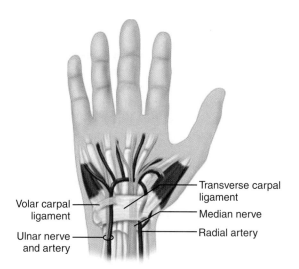

FIGURE 5.16   Hand with carpal tunnel syndrome.
Source: *Gwathmey FW. Anatomy. Miller's review of orthopaedics. p. 148–263.e1, Chapter 2.*

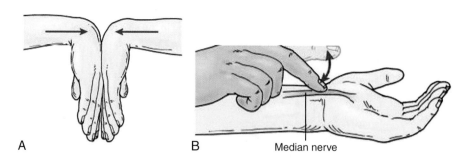

FIGURE 5.17   (A) Diagram of Phalen's test; (B) diagram of Tinel's test.
Source: *Redrawn from Brotzman SB. Hand and wrist injuries: nerve compression syndromes. In Brotzman SB, Manske RC, editors. Clinical orthopaedic rehabilitation, 3rd ed. Philadelphia: Elsevier; 2011, Fig. 1–24AB.*

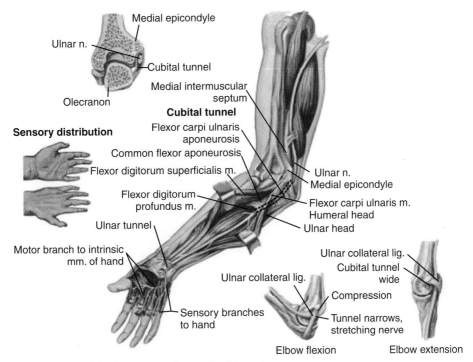

FIGURE 5.18 The anatomy of the ulnar nerve and areas of entrapment.
Source: *Carter GT, MD, MS. Diagnosis and treatment of work-related ulnar neuropathy at the elbow. Phys Med Rehabil Clin North Am 26(3):513–22.*

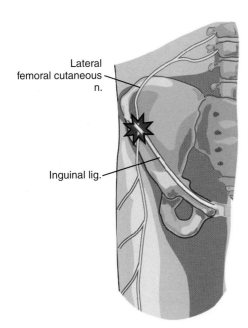

FIGURE 5.19 Burning pain in the lateral thigh is indicative of meralgia paraesthetica.
Source: *From Waldman SD. Physical diagnosis of pain: an atlas of signs and symptoms, Philadelphia: Saunders; 2006. p. 279.*

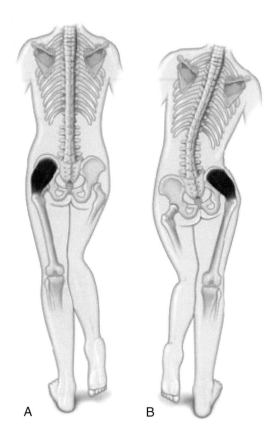

FIGURE 5.20 Trendelenburg gait. The Trendelenburg test is positive on the right side – the location of the weak gluteus medius and minimus muscles. (A) As the patient stands with the weight on the normal side, the pelvis is maintained in the horizontal position by the contraction and tension of the normal hip abductor muscles. (B) As the patient shifts weight to the affected side, the pelvis on the opposite and normal side drops as a result of the weakness of the hip abductor muscles. The sideways lean of the body towards the affected side is known as the Trendelenburg sign.

Source: *Herring JA. Developmental dysplasia of the hip. Tachdjian's pediatric orthopaedics. p. 483–579, Chapter 16.*

A   B

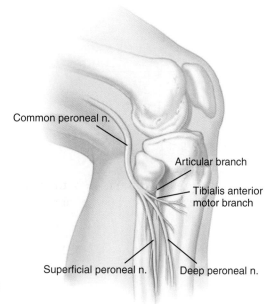

FIGURE 5.21 Peroneal nerve anatomy.
Source: *Prince MR, DO. Peroneal nerve injuries: repair, grafting, and nerve transfers. Operative techniques in sports medicine 23(4): 357–61.*

Weak gluteus maximus gait

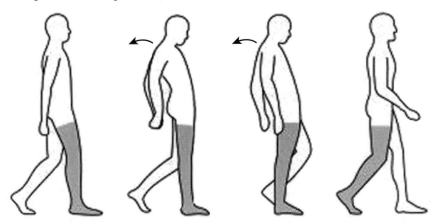

FIGURE 5.22 Gluteus maximus gait. The shading indicates the limb with the weak muscle, and the black arrows indicate the diagnostic movements. Because the gluteus maximus muscles are extensor muscles, abnormalities of these muscles produce characteristic findings during the stance phase. In the weak gluteus maximus gait, there is an abnormal backward lean during stance.
Source: *McGee S, MD. Stance and gait. Evidence-based physical diagnosis. p. 48–62, Chapter 6.*

SOMATIC REFLEXES

In general, a **reflex** has the following characteristics:

- **Rapid**: The paucity or even absence of interneurons in a reflex arc permits minimal synaptic delay compared to other nervous system processes.
- **Provoked**: The presence of sensory inputs is essential to initiate a reflex.
- **Involuntary**: Awareness of a reflex occurs only after its initiation or ending. Conscious, voluntary suppression of a reflex is possible but usually hard to achieve.
- **Predictable**: A reflex occurs in the same way in response to similar stimuli.

A **reflex arc** is the structural pathway upon which a somatic reflex takes place. It is composed of:

- **Receptors**: Somatic receptors that are located in muscles, tendons or skin.
- **Afferent fibres**: Sensory fibres that relay information collected at the receptors to the dorsal horn of the spinal cord.
- **Interneurons**: Interneurons are located in the grey matter of spinal cord and process the incoming information. They are absent from some reflex arcs.
- **Efferent fibres**: Motor fibres that carry motor information to the concerned muscles.
- **Effector organs**: In the case of somatic reflexes, skeletal muscles perform the final motor response of the reflex.

Types of Somatic Reflexes
Muscle Spindle (Fig. 5.23)

Before discussing the physiology of the stretch reflex, it is important to learn about one of its key components: the muscle spindle.

Muscle spindles are **sensory receptors** scattered within the bulk of skeletal muscles and respond to **stretch stimuli**.

- Fine-control muscles, such as intrinsic hand muscles, are richer in muscle spindles than large muscles responsible for rough movements.
- **Intrafusal fibres** refer to the **modified muscle fibres** located inside the capsule of muscle spindles, whereas **extrafusal fibres** constitute the bulk of **skeletal muscle fibres**. Two types of intrafusal fibres exist:
  - **Nuclear chain fibres**: Have a **single straight chain of nuclei** organized in the middle of the fibre, which is the noncontractile part (only the fibre endings are able to contract).

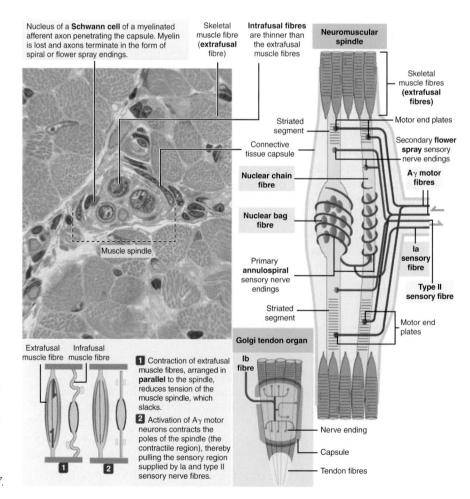

FIGURE 5.23 Neuromuscular (muscle) spindle and Golgi tendon organ. Source: *Kierszenbaum AL, MD, PhD. Muscle tissue. Histology and cell biology: an introduction to pathology. p. 217–38, Chapter 7.*

Nucleus of a **Schwann cell** of a myelinated afferent axon penetrating the capsule. Myelin is lost and axons terminate in the form of spiral or flower spray endings.

Skeletal muscle fibre (**extrafusal** fibre)

Intrafusal fibres are thinner than the extrafusal muscle fibres

Neuromuscular spindle

Skeletal muscle fibres (**extrafusal fibres**)

Striated segment

Motor end plates

Connective tissue capsule

Secondary **flower spray** sensory nerve endings

Nuclear chain fibre

Aγ **motor fibres**

Nuclear bag fibre

Primary **annulospiral** sensory nerve endings

Ia **sensory fibre**

Type II sensory fibre

Striated segment

Motor end plates

Muscle spindle

Golgi tendon organ

Extrafusal muscle fibre   Infrafusal muscle fibre

Ib fibre

1 Contraction of extrafusal muscle fibres, arranged in **parallel** to the spindle, reduces tension of the muscle spindle, which slacks.

2 Activation of Aγ motor neurons contracts the poles of the spindle (the contractile region), thereby pulling the sensory region supplied by Ia and type II sensory nerve fibres.

Nerve ending

Capsule

Tendon fibres

- Nuclear bag fibres: Are **longer** and **thicker** – especially at the middle – than the nuclear chain fibres, and their **nuclei are concentrated in the middle region**.
- Three types of nerve fibres innervate a muscle spindle:
  - **Primary sensory fibres**: Have **annulospiral endings** that wrap around the midregion of intrafusal fibres and are activated during the **initiation of a muscle stretch**.
  - **Secondary sensory fibres**: Have **flower-spray endings** distributed over the tails of intrafusal fibres and react to **prolonged stretch stimuli**.
  - **Axons of gamma motor neurons**:
    - Similar to alpha motor neurons that supply extrafusal fibres, cell bodies of gamma motor neurons are located in the ventral horn of the spinal cord and their axons innervate **intrafusal fibres**.
    - Around **one-third** of fibres in a spinal nerve originate from gamma motor neurons.
    - The intended effect is to guarantee the response of intrafusal fibres by keeping them **tense** all the time.

Stretch Reflex *(Fig. 5.24)*

A **stretch reflex** initiates when a muscle is stretched, an inherently **protective** mechanism against tearing of muscle fibres. Stretch reflexes are also responsible for **maintaining posture** and **equilibrium**.

- A simple stretch reflex utilizes the following pathway:
  - Stretching of a muscle activates muscle spindles by contraction of intrafusal fibres.
  - Sensory information is carried out by the primary and secondary fibres from muscle spindles to the spinal cord, brain stem and finally to the cerebellum.
  - After processing the incoming information, the cerebellum projects it to the cerebral cortex.
  - The cortex further integrates the cerebellar information and relays motor stimuli to the concerned muscle. The latter would contract, with the contraction force being proportional to that of the initial stretching.
- More commonly, a stretch reflex involves a **set of flexor** and **extensor muscles**. Contraction of flexors around a joint extends the extensors and initiates a stretch reflex. Similarly, extension triggers a stretch reflex in the flexors.
- In particular, sudden, strong stimuli are processed in a shorter pathway that does not involve the brain, but only the spinal cord.
- **Tendon reflexes** (knee-jerk or patellar, biceps, triceps, brachioradialis, Achilles reflexes) are typical examples of a **rapid stretch reflex** integrated **solely** at the spinal cord level (Fig. 5.25). These reflexes form a **monosynaptic reflex arc** as described herein:
  - Tapping the tendon pulls the muscle and stimulates the primary sensory fibres connected to the intrafusal fibres.

FIGURE 5.24   Knee-jerk (myotatic) reflex. Tapping the patellar tendon with a percussion hammer elicits a reflexive knee jerk caused by contraction of the quadriceps muscle: the stretch reflex. Stretching the tendon pulls on the muscle spindle, exciting the primary sensory afferents, which convey their information via group Ia axons. These axons make monosynaptic connections to the α motor neurons that innervate the quadriceps, resulting in the contraction of this muscle. The Ia axons also excite inhibitory interneurons that reciprocally innervate the motor neurons of the antagonist muscle of the quadriceps (the flexor), resulting in relaxation of the semitendinosus muscle. Thus, the reflex relaxation of the antagonistic muscle is polysynaptic.
Source: *Connors BW. Circuits of the central nervous system. Medical physiology. p. 390–407.e1, Chapter 16.*

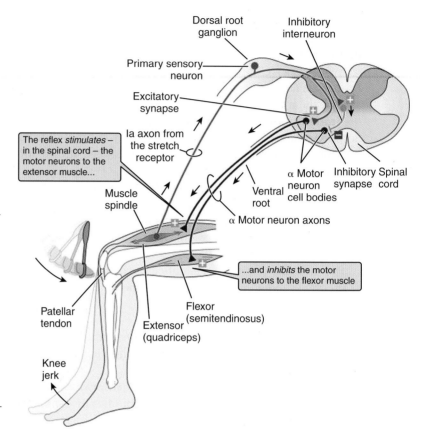

The reflex *stimulates* – in the spinal cord – the motor neurons to the extensor muscle...

...and *inhibits* the motor neurons to the flexor muscle

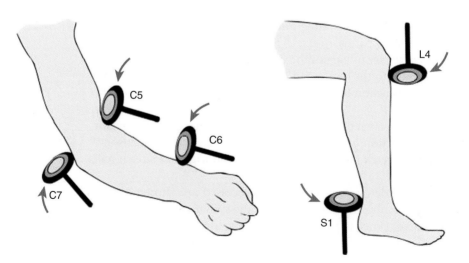

FIGURE 5.25   Upper and lower extremity muscle stretch reflexes and the responsible nerve roots.
Source: *Ju KL. Initial evaluation of the spine in trauma patients. Skeletal trauma: basic science, management, and reconstruction. p. 303–14.e2, Chapter 10.*

- Primary sensory fibres synapse and relay impulses directly onto the cell bodies of alpha motor neurons in the grey matter of the spinal cord.
- Alpha motor neurons convey the stimulus to the concerned muscle leading to contraction.
- **Reciprocal inhibition**, which is closely associated with the reflex arc, ensures the **prevention of contraction of antagonist muscles** that may interfere with the contraction of the concerned muscle. It occurs as the following:
  - Primary sensory fibres supply the same excitatory impulses to interneurons, which in turn inhibit alpha motor neurons innervating antagonist muscles.
  - Thus, while excitatory impulses activate the concerned muscle, the antagonist muscles are not able to contract due to central (spinal cord) inhibition of their motor neurons.

CLINICAL INSIGHT

- **Hyporeflexia versus hyperreflexia**
  - **Hyporeflexia** and **areflexia** are **diminished** and **absent** stretch responses to tendon tapping, respectively. These usually indicate the presence of a **lower motor neuron** disease, i.e. pathology involving alpha motor neurons, nerve roots or peripheral nerves.
  - **Hyperreflexia** is an enhanced response to tendon tapping. It indicates the presence of an **upper motor neuron** disease, i.e. brain or spinal cord injury.
  - **Clonus** is the **involuntary**, **rhythmic contractions** and **relaxations** of muscles. In severe **upper motor neuron** disease, hyperreflexia may be associated with clonus.
  - Table 5.3 depicts the interpretation of the grading system of muscle stretch reflexes.

Table 5.3 Interpretation of the grading system of muscle stretch reflexes	
Grade	**Interpretation**
0	Absent reflex
1+	Diminished reflex
2+	Normal reflex
3+	Enhanced reflex
4+	Enhanced reflex + nonsustained clonus
5+	Enhanced reflex + sustained clonus

Golgi Tendon Reflex (Fig. 5.23)

The **Golgi tendon reflex** utilizes **Golgi tendon organs**, which are **encapsulated nerve endings**. They are spread between collagen fibres near the **tendon–muscle junction** and are responsive to **pressure forces**.

- Golgi tendon organs relay information about muscle–joint tension to the CNS.
- The reflex regulates the tension by inhibiting alpha motor neurons to prevent excessive force that may tear the tendon or pull off the muscle from the bone.
- The reflex also distributes the tension force on all muscle fibres evenly by inhibiting over-tensed muscle segments and allowing for the recruitment of less contracted fibres.

Flexor and Crossed Extensor Reflexes (Fig. 5.26)

The **flexor reflex**, also known as **withdrawal reflex**, occurs in response to pain and functions to protect the body against damage from the external environment. Depending on the body part involved and the stimulus strength, a **crossed extensor reflex** may accompany the flexor reflex.

- The flexor reflex utilizes an **ipsilateral reflex arc**, where pain fibres **stimulate** and **inhibit ipsilateral** alpha motor neurons of **flexor** and

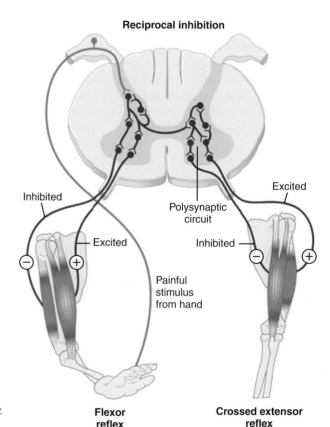

FIGURE 5.26   Flexor reflex, crossed extensor reflex and reciprocal inhibition.
Source: *Hall JE, PhD. Motor functions of the spinal cord; the cord reflexes. Guyton and Hall textbook of medical physiology. p. 695–706, Chapter 55.*

extensor muscles, respectively. Thus, they allow rapid withdrawal of the body part from the stimulus.

- The crossed extensor reflex is activated by the same pain fibres **inhibiting** and **stimulating contralateral** alpha motor neurons of **flexor** and **extensor** muscles, respectively. This reflex employs a **contralateral reflex arc** and is essential to **relocate the centre of gravity** and **retain equilibrium** during rapid withdrawal from pain.
- Occasionally, the reflex requires involvement of myotomes from different levels of the spinal cord, and thus utilizes an **intersegmental reflex arc** with more input from the cerebrum and cerebellum compared to the aforementioned less complicated reflexes.

CASE STUDY DISCUSSION

GBS is an **acute inflammatory demyelinating disorder** presenting as **multiple peripheral nerve dysfunctions**. Classically, GBS patients present with acute-onset, **ascending sensory deficits** that progress to **diminished reflexes and muscle weakness**, which could be **fatal** when **respiratory muscles** are involved.

Clinical Features

The presentation and progression of the disease may include any combination of the following signs/symptoms:

- **Sensory**: Dysaesthesia, numbness, and paraesthesia. Usually, these symptoms appear distally (toes; fingertips) and progressively ascend to involve proximal sites (ankles followed by legs, thighs and abdomen; wrists followed by forearms, elbows, arms).
- **Motor**: Weakness and areflexia. Weakness starts at the **proximal** muscles of lower extremities, then **progresses** to involve the truncal muscles, arms, CNs and respiratory muscles.
- **Autonomic**: Facial flushing, anhidrosis/diaphoresis, tachycardia/bradycardia, paroxysmal/orthostatic hypertension and urinary retention.
- Symptoms/signs secondary to **CNs dysfunction**: Ophthalmoplegia, diplopia, facial weakness, dysarthria and dysphagia.
- **Pain**: Throbbing and aching in nature. It mostly involves the back, shoulder girdle, buttocks and thighs.

Several GBS variants have been extensively described in the literature, the most important of which are summarized herein:

- **Acute inflammatory demyelinating polyneuropathy (AIDP)**: Sensory and CNs more involved than motor nerves.
- **Acute motor axonal neuropathy (AMAN)**: Motor nerves affected without sensory involvement.

- **Acute motor and sensory axonal neuropathy (AMSAN)**: Sensory and motor deficits with rapid progression and paralysis; pain more prevalent and prolonged recovery period.
- **Miller Fisher syndrome**: Triad of ophthalmoplegia, ataxia and areflexia; rare variant.
- **Pure panautonomic neuropathy**: Sympathetic and parasympathetic systems involvement; slow and incomplete recovery; high morbidity and mortality; very rare variant.

Pathophysiology

GBS is an **autoimmune** disease that is usually triggered by an infectious process.

- GBS may start at any time from **few days to few weeks** after a **respiratory** or **gastrointestinal infection**.
- The most commonly identified organisms are *Campylobacter jejuni* and **Cytomegalovirus**.
- **Molecular mimicry**, the presence of specific antigens shared by the organism and human nerves, is the initial step in the pathogenesis of GBS.
- Antibodies produced by the body against these antigens attack not only the organism but also certain **gangliosides** and **glycolipids** present in the human **myelin sheath**.
- This is followed by lymphocytic infiltration of spinal nerve roots, peripheral and/or CNs, and phagocytic attack of myelin by macrophages.

Management

- Any GBS patient showing signs of cardiac or respiratory compromise or rapid progression of the disease should be admitted to the ICU for close monitoring.
- IVIG and plasmapheresis are equally effective in clearing autoantibodies from the circulation and minimizing the recovery time.

- Physical rehabilitation to strengthen weak muscles and speech therapy to ensure safe swallowing skills and improve speech are highly advised.

Prognosis

The disease **outcomes are highly variable** between GBS patients; neurologic sequelae range from a mild weakness that causes difficulty in ambulation, to diffuse and profound weakness that could lead to tetraplegia and even death from respiratory compromise.

- Walk independently at 6 months: 80% of GBS patients.
- Full recovery of motor strength at 1 year: 60% of GBS patients.
- Very delayed/incomplete recovery and prolonged ventilator dependency for several months: 10–15% of GBS patients.
- Mortality rate: up to 12% of GBS patients.
- Recurrence rate: up to 5% of GBS patients.

CHAPTER 6

Spinal Cord

Nour Estaitieh, Mohammad Shehade

CASE STUDY

Presentation and Physical Examination: A 46-year-old woman, previously healthy, presented for worsening pain in the shoulders with associated paraesthesia in the hands and fingers, more so on the right side. She reported dropping objects from her hands. She denies lower extremity paraesthesias/weakness or gait disturbance.

Neurological examination showed normal motor power in her four extremities, hyperreflexia (3+) all over with a positive Hoffman sign, and decreased pinprick and temperature sensation in the upper extremities. Vibration was intact.

Diagnosis, Management and Follow-Up: Given the history of sensory deficit involving the upper extremity in a cape-like distribution while sparing the lower extremities, the lesion is consistent with a **central cord syndrome** in the cervical region.

The patient underwent magnetic resonance imaging (MRI) of the cervical spine, which revealed Arnold–Chiari malformation type-I with associated cervical **syringomyelia** (accumulation of fluid in the central canal) (Fig. 6.1). She was referred for surgical management (suboccipital craniotomy). Follow-up after 2 weeks showed complete resolution of symptoms.

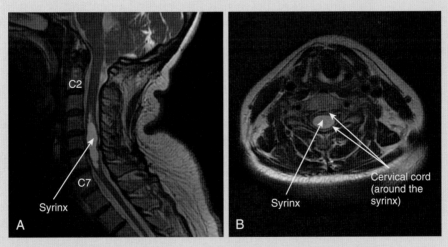

FIGURE 6.1 Sagittal (A) and axial (B) T2-weighted MRI showing a syrinx extending from C4 to C7 with thinning of the cervical cord.
Source: *Courtesy of Mohammad Shehade, MD. Lebanese American University Medical Center.*

BRIEF INTRODUCTION

The spinal cord, the second component of the central nervous system (CNS) after the brain, plays an important role in the control of body movements and sensations.

- The spinal cord has grey and white matter constituents that are arranged in a cylindrical shape, with nerve roots extending from the lateral foramina of the vertebral column, the protective cage in which the spinal cord lies.
- Several descending and ascending tracts utilize the spinal cord as a highway with multiple relay stations, each serving a specific physiological function.
- The spinal cord's blood supply is segmental and originates from multiple independent arteries.
- Any type of damage (compression, ischaemia, inflammation, metabolic) to the spinal cord will lead to devastating neurological consequences, which may be irreversible if not managed promptly.

This chapter introduces the gross and microanatomy of the spinal cord and discusses the ascending, descending and autonomic pathways passing through it.

SPINAL CORD STRUCTURE

The **spinal cord** lies inside the vertebral canal and is well protected by the strong vertebral bones, ligaments and paravertebral musculature (Fig. 6.2).

- It occupies the upper two-thirds of the vertebral column in adults.
- It extends from the upper border of the foramen magnum to the level of the disc between the **first and second lumbar vertebrae**. In newborns, it stretches to the level of the third lumbar vertebra.
- It consists of **31 spinal segments**: 8 cervical, 12 thoracic, 5 lumbar, 5 sacral and 1 coccygeal.
- Each spinal segment gives a ventral motor and a dorsal sensory root.
- The ventral and dorsal roots unite to give rise to **31 pairs of spinal nerves**, which exit through the intervertebral foramina.
- The spinal cord has two enlargements, a **cervical enlargement**, which gives rise to the roots of the brachial plexus supplying the upper extremities, and a **lumbosacral enlargement**, which gives rise to the roots of the lumbosacral plexus supplying the lower extremities.
- The spinal cord tapers off into the conus medullaris at the apex, from which extends the filum terminale, a pia mater extension that anchors the cord to the posterior surface of the coccyx.

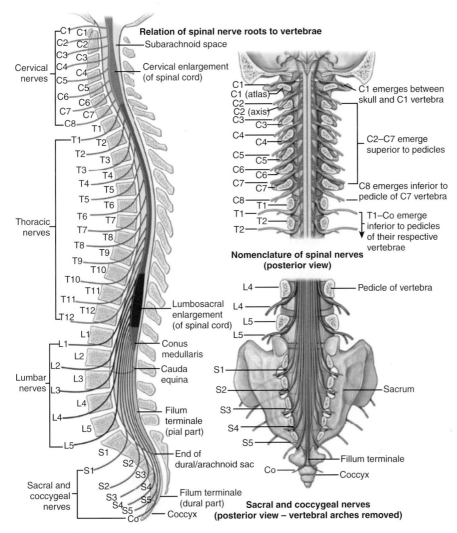

FIGURE 6.2 Relation of spinal cord and nerve roots to vertebrae.
Source: *From Drake RL et al. editors. Gray's atlas of anatomy, 2nd ed., Philadelphia: Churchill Livingstone; 2015.*

CLINICAL INSIGHT

- **Tethered cord syndrome**
  - Is the result of a **short filum terminale with reduced viscoelasticity**; this causes dysfunction of the spinal cord due to excessive stretching
  - Typically occurs in children and less commonly in adults
    - In children: usually associated with meningoceles, myelomeningoceles, split cord malformations, dermal and lipomatous tumours and/or skin stigmata (e.g. tufts of hair and dermal sinus tract) (Fig. 6.3)

- In adults: usually associated with thickened filum, an intradural lipoma and/or fibrous adhesions
■ Clinical features include:
  - Early: burning, nondermatomal pain
  - Late: nonmyotomal weakness, urologic dysfunction, muscle atrophy
■ Aggravated by growth spurts in children and stretching manoeuvres, disc herniation and trauma in adults
■ Surgery is the treatment of choice in all age groups
  - To relieve the tension on the spinal cord and prevent further neurological deterioration

Similar to the brain, three meningeal membranes surround the spinal cord: dura mater, arachnoid mater and pia mater. These are in continuity with the cranial meninges and provide protection and suspension of this CNS structure within the vertebral canal (Fig. 6.4).
- **Twenty-one pairs of dentate ligaments** anchor the spinal cord to the dura mater. These are pial extensions from the lateral surface of the spinal cord between the sensory and motor roots.
- The cerebrospinal fluid (CSF) protects the spinal cord in the subarachnoid space.

The spinal cord has a **cylindrical shape** (Fig. 6.5).
- It consists of a central butterfly-shaped grey matter and a peripheral white matter.

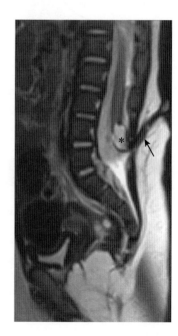

FIGURE 6.3 Tethered cord syndrome with an intradural lipoma and a dermal sinus tract. Tethered cord terminating at L4–L5 disc space level with an intradural lipoma. See the downward oblique orientation of the dermal sinus tract (arrow) extending from the skin surface to the lipoma (asterik).
Source: *Nadgir R, MD. Congenital anomalies of the central nervous system. Neuroradiology: the requisites. p. 263–310, Chapter 8.*

- The grey matter primarily contains the **cell bodies of neurons and glia**. The white matter contains the **fibre tracts**.
- The anterior median fissure and the posterior median septum divide it into right and left halves.

A **central canal** pierces the grey commissure of the spinal cord and is continuous with the fourth ventricle.

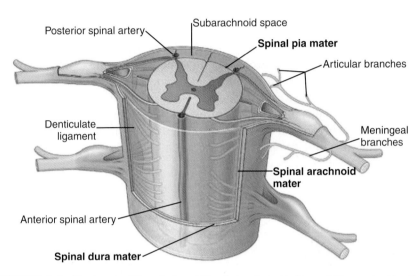

FIGURE 6.4 Membranes of the spinal cord. The pia is adherent to the cord. The arachnoid encloses the cerebrospinal fluid. The denticulate ligaments anchor the cord to the dura. The dura is continuous with the nerve sheaths. The denticulate ligaments are lateral extensions of the spinal pia mater to the spinal arachnoid and dura mater along both sides of the spinal cord. They serve to attach the spinal cord in the centre of the subarachnoid space.
Source: *Paulsen F. Brain and spinal cord. Sobotta atlas of human anatomy. vol. 3, p. 211–342, Chapter 12.*

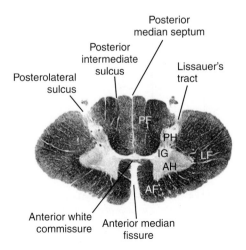

FIGURE 6.5 Axial cut at the level of C8. AF, anterior funiculus; LF, lateral funiculus; PF, posterior funiculus; AH, anterior horn; IG, intermediate grey matter; PH, posterior horn.
Source: *Vanderah TW, PhD. Spinal cord. Nolte's the human brain. p. 233–71, Chapter 10.*

Grey Matter

The **grey matter** of the spinal cord features an H-shaped appearance (Fig. 6.5).

- It has **posterior** and **anterior horns** on each side.
- An additional **intermediolateral horn** exists in the thoracic and the upper two levels of the lumbar segments.
- The right and left parts are connected by anterior and posterior **grey commissures** around the central canal.

Bror Rexed divided the spinal grey matter into **ten laminae or nuclei** with variable functions. The dorsal horn laminae (I to VI) significantly overlap and contain small-sized sensory neurons. The nuclei of the ventral horns contain the largest cells, the motor neurons. The intermediate lamina (VII) is located between the dorsal and the ventral horns and contains medium-sized neurons (Fig. 6.6).

- **Lamina I** contains the **marginal zone nuclei**. It consists of neurons that display horizontal dendrites in order to maximize their contact with the incoming fibres of the dorsal root.

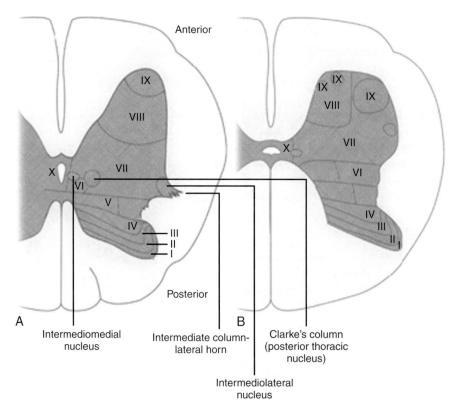

FIGURE 6.6   Rexed laminae of the 2nd thoracic (A) and the 4th lumbar (B) spinal cord.
Source: *Redrawn from Williams PL, editor. Gray's anatomy: the anatomical basis of clinical practice, 38th ed. Edinburgh: Churchill Livingstone; 1999.*

- **Lamina II (substantia gelatinosa)** is composed of **Golgi type II neurons** and receives afferent fibres that convey pain, temperature and touch sensations.
- **Laminae III and IV** contain the **nucleus proprius** and occupy a large region of the dorsal horn. They receive fibres related to the senses of position, proprioception and vibration from the posterior white column.
- **Lamina V** occupies the neck of the posterior horn and establishes synapses with the corticospinal and rubrospinal tracts. The lateral part of this nucleus is known as the **reticular nucleus**.
- **Lamina VI** is present in the spinal cord enlargements (cervical and lumbosacral) and particularly **absent in the fourth thoracic through the second lumbar segments.**
- **Lamina VII** forms the **intermediate zone** and contains Clarke's column (posterior thoracic nucleus, nucleus dorsalis), intermediolateral and intermediomedial nuclei.
  - **Clarke's column** extends from the **first thoracic to the second or third lumbar spinal segments** and gives rise to the dorsal spinocerebellar tract.
  - The **intermediolateral nucleus** occupies the lateral horns between the **first thoracic and the second or third lumbar spinal segments**, providing preganglionic sympathetic axons. At the second, third and fourth sacral spinal segments, this nucleus provides preganglionic parasympathetic fibres *(see chapter 16)*.
  - The **intermediomedial nucleus** extends through the entire length of the spinal cord and receives visceral afferents.
- **Lamina VIII** occupies the medial aspect of the anterior horn in the spinal cord enlargements and contains **commissural neurons.**
- **Lamina IX** contains **motor neurons** that are arranged somatotopically, meaning that:
  - In the cervical segments, neurons supplying the neck muscles lie medially, neuronal cell bodies of the accessory nucleus (C1–5) and phrenic nucleus (C3–5) occupy the central portion and neurons supplying the upper limb muscles lie laterally.
  - In the thoracic segments, the medial group of cells innervate trunk muscles.
  - In the lumbosacral segments, the medial group of cells mainly supply muscles of the lower limbs and perineum.
- **Lamina X (or area X)** consists of small neurons that form the **grey commissures around the central canal**. It receives some afferents from the dorsal root fibres and contains neurological cells in its ventral part that send cytoplasmic extensions to the adjacent pia mater.

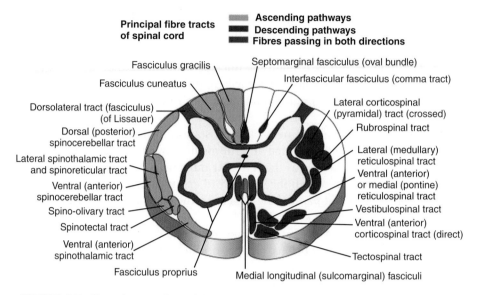

Principal fibre tracts of spinal cord

Ascending pathways
Descending pathways
Fibres passing in both directions

Fasciculus gracilis
Fasciculus cuneatus
Dorsolateral tract (fasciculus) (of Lissauer)
Dorsal (posterior) spinocerebellar tract
Lateral spinothalamic tract and spinoreticular tract
Ventral (anterior) spinocerebellar tract
Spino-olivary tract
Spinotectal tract
Ventral (anterior) spinothalamic tract
Fasciculus proprius

Septomarginal fasciculus (oval bundle)
Interfascicular fasciculus (comma tract)
Lateral corticospinal (pyramidal) tract (crossed)
Rubrospinal tract
Lateral (medullary) reticulospinal tract
Ventral (anterior) or medial (pontine) reticulospinal tract
Vestibulospinal tract
Ventral (anterior) corticospinal tract (direct)
Tectospinal tract
Medial longitudinal (sulcomarginal) fasciculi

FIGURE 6.7   The major ascending and descending tracts of the spinal cord.
Source: *Rosenow JM. Anatomy of the nervous system. Neuromodulation. p. 95–107, Chapter 10.*

White Matter

The **white matter** of the spinal cord surrounds the grey matter. It is divided into anterior, lateral and posterior columns or funiculi (Figs. 6.5 and 6.7).

- The **posterior columns**, also known as the posterior funiculus, are located between the posterolateral sulci, where fibres from the dorsal roots enter the grey matter.
- The **lateral columns**, i.e. the lateral funiculus, are located between the dorsal and ventral roots on each side and contain the lateral corticospinal, rubrospinal and spinothalamic tracts.
- The **anterior column**, i.e. the anterior funiculus, is located between the emerging ventral roots and contains the ventral spinothalamic, tectospinal and reticulospinal tracts as well as the medial longitudinal fasciculus.

SPINAL CORD PATHWAYS

Descending Pathways

The origins of the descending upper motor neuron fibres are the cerebral cortex (the motor area, supplementary motor area, prefrontal area and a portion of the postcentral gyrus) and the brainstem. These descending motor tracts are divided into the lateral and the anterior motor tracts according to their locations in the spinal columns and their synapses in the grey matter at the lateral and medial horn cells, respectively.

The two lateral descending motor tracts are composed of the lateral corticospinal tract and the rubrospinal tract.

- The function of the lateral corticospinal tract is to control voluntary and skilled movements of the limbs, especially rapid and dexterous movements of individual digits.
- The rubrospinal tract's main function is to regulate the flexor muscle movements. It originates in the red nucleus. Fibres decussate in the midbrain, descend to reach the lateral funiculus just anterior to the corticospinal tract and end in the same laminae as the corticospinal tract.
- While the corticospinal tract initiates movement, the rubrospinal tract refines this movement and controls errors.

The four anterior descending tracts are the ventral corticospinal, vestibulospinal, reticulospinal and tectospinal tracts.

- The **vestibulospinal tract** facilitates the activity of extensor muscles and inhibits the activity of flexor muscles, and therefore, controls postural balance.
- The **reticulospinal tract** is mainly responsible for the modulation of the alpha or gamma motor neurons in the anterior grey columns, and therefore, facilitates or inhibits voluntary movement or reflex activity.
- The **tectospinal tract** arises from the superior colliculus and is concerned with reflex postural movement in response to visual stimuli.

Lateral and Ventral Corticospinal Tracts (Figs. 6.7 and 6.8)

A major pathway, the **corticospinal tract** is derived from the precentral gyrus, the premotor and supplementary motor areas, and the postcentral gyrus (Fig. 6.9).

- The largest fibres originate from the **giant pyramidal cells of Betz** in the fifth cortical layer.
- Layer V pyramidal cell projections relay directly to the ventral horn of the spinal cord as well as to spinal interneurons.

Axons from the cerebral cortex join together to enter the upper portion of the cerebral white matter, the corona radiata, in a fan-shaped pattern and descend downwards through the **posterior limb of the internal capsule**.

- The cerebral white matter conveys information to other cerebral areas and to subcortical structures such as the thalamus, basal ganglia and brainstem.
- In the internal capsule, the **somatotopic organization** is well preserved. The motor fibres for the face are in the anterior portion and those for the arm and leg lie progressively posterior.
- Fibres from the internal capsule continue travelling down to the brainstem to reach the ventral part of the midbrain at the cerebral peduncles, the so-called 'feet of the brain'. Somatotopic arrangement for the face, arm and leg is from the medial to lateral, respectively.
- These fibres descend downwards to reach the ventral pons and medulla to form the medullary pyramids.

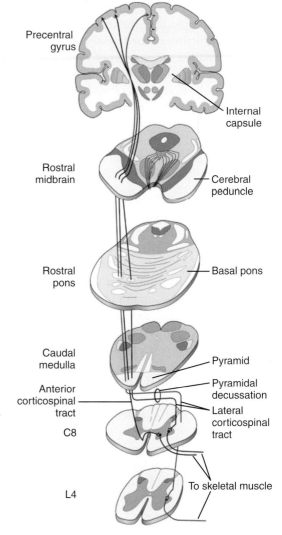

Precentral gyrus

Internal capsule

Rostral midbrain

Cerebral peduncle

Rostral pons

Basal pons

Caudal medulla

Pyramid

Pyramidal decussation

Anterior corticospinal tract

Lateral corticospinal tract

C8

L4

To skeletal muscle

FIGURE 6.8 Corticospinal tracts. Fibres from the precentral gyrus and other nearby cortical areas descend through the cerebral peduncles, pons and medullary pyramids; most cross in the pyramidal decussation to form the lateral corticospinal tract. Those that do not cross in the pyramidal decussation form the anterior corticospinal tract; most of these fibres cross in the anterior white commissure before ending in the spinal grey matter. Most corticospinal fibres do not synapse directly on the motor neurons. They are drawn that way here for simplicity. Source: *A from Nolte J. The human brain: an introduction to its functional anatomy. 4th ed. St. Louis: Mosby; 1999. p. 249.*

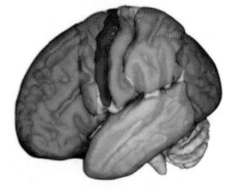

FIGURE 6.9 Brain cortices. Prefrontal (blue); premotor/supplementary motor (orange); primary motor (red); primary sensory (green); posterior parietal (yellow); temporal (pink) and occipital (copper) cortices.
Source: *Bohanna I. Connectivity-based segmentation of the striatum in Huntington's disease: vulnerability of motor pathways. Neurobiol Dis 42(3):475–481.*

- The cervicomedullary junction is located at the level of the foramen magnum, where 85% of the pyramidal tracts decussate to enter the lateral white column of the spinal cord forming the **lateral corticospinal tract**.
- The somatotopic map of fibres representing the upper limbs is medial while fibres representing the lower limbs are located laterally.
- Finally, the axons of the lateral corticospinal tract relay to the anterior horn cells of the spinal cord.
- The remaining 15% of the corticospinal tract continue ipsilaterally without decussation to form the **ventral (anterior) corticospinal tract,** which is located in the anterior white matter column of the spinal cord.
- Fibres of the lateral corticospinal tract, which terminate in the upper spinal cord segments, are medial to fibres that terminate in the lower spinal segments.
- The lateral corticospinal tract controls distal musculature through excitatory multisynaptic interneurons, except for the innervation of the digits, which occurs through direct monosynaptic connections.

Most of ventral corticospinal tract fibres cross midline in the spinal cord at the level of their termination. These fibres:

- Are bilaterally excitatory to the axial and proximal appendicular musculatures.
- Do not extend caudal to upper thoracic levels.

Descending tracts other than the lateral and ventral corticospinal tracts include the **rubrospinal,** reticulospinal, vestibulospinal and tectospinal tracts, the pathways of which are depicted in Figs. 6.7, 6.10–6.12.

Ascending Pathways
Somatosensory Pathways
Somatosensation essentially means the perception of pain, temperature, fine touch, vibration and joint position (proprioception) as well as stereognosis (ability to recognize the form of objects using touch only) and two-point tactile discrimination.

The main somatosensory pathways are as follows:

- **Dorsal column-medial lemniscal pathway**, which conveys proprioception, vibration, fine touch, pressure and two-point discrimination of touch sensations.
- **Anterolateral pathway,** which includes the spinothalamic tract and conveys crude touch, pain and temperature sensations.

Four main types (I through IV) of sensory fibres exist. Each fibre conducts impulses from a specific type of receptor and at a specific speed; large myelinated fibres conduct faster than small unmyelinated fibres (*see Table 1.2 of chapter 1*).

Rubrospinal and reticulospinal tracts

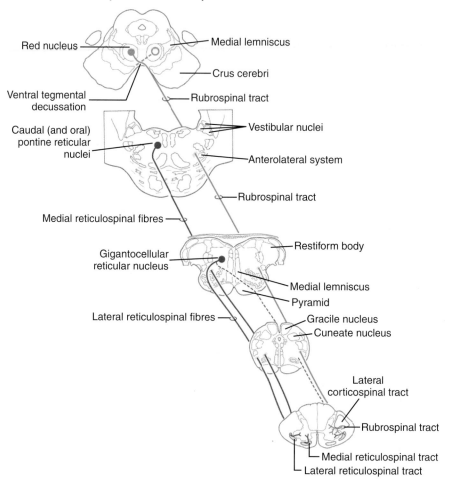

FIGURE 6.10 Rubrospinal and reticulospinal tracts.
Source: *Mihailoff GA. Motor system I: peripheral sensory, brainstem, and spinal influence on anterior horn neurons. Fundamental neuroscience for basic and clinical applications. p. 324–37.e1, Chapter 24.*

Dorsal root ganglia contain cell bodies of sensory neurons. The sensory axon from the dorsal root ganglion bifurcates into a:

- Long process conveying sensory information from a specific dermatome (peripheral process).
- Short process that relays sensory information to the grey matter of the spinal cord (central process).

Posterior Column-Medial Lemniscal Pathway

Proprioception, vibration, light pressure and fine touch information are carried via large myelinated nerve fibres.

Vestibulospinal fibres

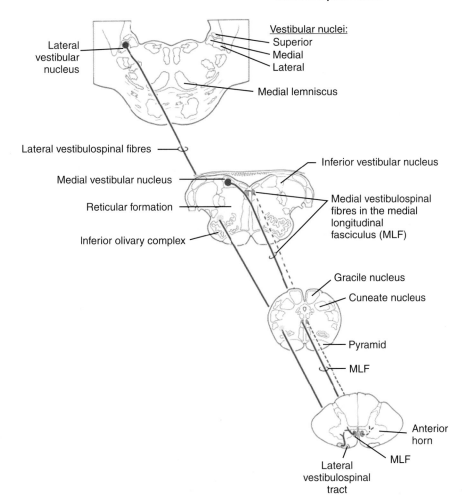

FIGURE 6.11   Medial and lateral vestibulospinal tracts.
Source: *Mihailoff GA. Motor system I: peripheral sensory, brainstem, and spinal influence on anterior horn neurons. Fundamental neuroscience for basic and clinical applications. p. 324–37.e1, Chapter 24.*

- These fibres (first-order neurons) enter the spinal cord through the medial entry zone of the dorsal root ipsilaterally and form the **posterior column tract.**
- Fibres of the posterior column tract ascend to relay the information to the posterior column nuclei, **nucleus gracilis** and **nucleus cuneatus** in the medulla, which house cell bodies of the second-order neurons.
- Some collaterals of the first-order neurons enter the grey matter of the spinal cord to relay to interneurons and ventral (alpha) motor neurons.

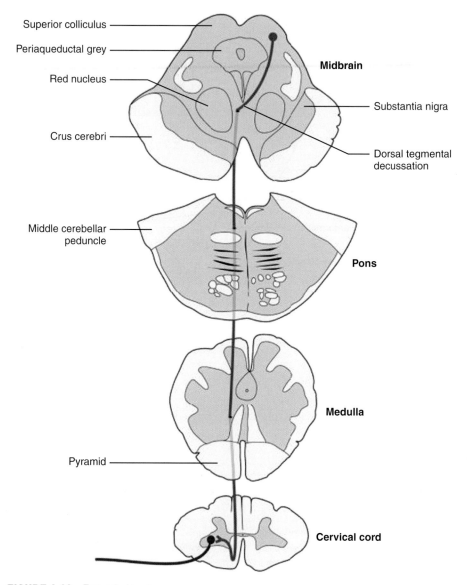

FIGURE 6.12 Tectospinal tract.

Source: *Crossman AR, PhD DSc, Spinal cord. Neuroanatomy: an illustrated colour text. p. 69–90, Chapter 8.*

The somatotopic organization is important to recognize. The dorsal column is formed by two major tracts (Figs. 6.5, 6.7 and 6.13):

- The **gracile fasciculus**, which transmits information from the lower limbs and lower trunk below T6.
- The **cuneate fasciculus**, which carries information for the upper limb and upper trunk above T6. The cuneate fasciculus is absent below T6.

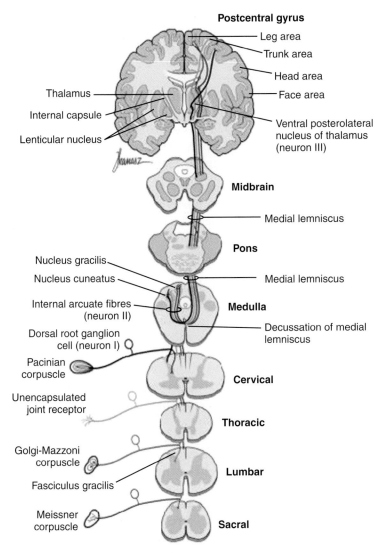

FIGURE 6.13 Posterior column–medial lemniscal pathway.
Source: *Copyright Cleveland Clinic Foundation.*

- Above T6, the **gracile tract is medial** in the dorsal funiculus, whereas the **cuneate tract is lateral**. They are separated by the posterior intermediate septum.
- Fibres conveying information from the sacrococcygeal segments are most medial, while those supplying information from the cervical segments are most lateral.
- The gracile and cuneate tracts project onto the gracile and cuneate nuclei, respectively.

Axons of the second-order neurons decussate in the medulla as the **internal arcuate fibres** to form the medial lemniscal pathway.

- The **medial lemniscal pathway** lies medial at the level of the medulla and progressively becomes more inclined and occupies a lateral position at the level of midbrain.
- At first, the feet are represented ventrally ('little man stands up'), and then it becomes represented laterally as the tract ascends ('little man lies down'), while the arms lie more medially.
- Of note, the legs are always represented laterally, except in the sensory motor cortices and the posterior columns (Fig. 6.13).

When fibres of the medial lemniscus reach the thalamus, they synapse on third-order neurons in the **ventral posterior lateral (VPL) nucleus** of the thalamus. Neuronal axons from the VPL nucleus then travel to the posterior limb of the internal capsule via the thalamic somatosensory radiation to reach the **postcentral gyrus** of the somatosensory cortex.

Anterolateral Pathways

Small unmyelinated nerve fibres convey sensory information from the periphery as first-order neurons to reach the dorsal root entry zone.

- Some collaterals ascend and descend for few segments in **Lissauer's (posterolateral) tract** before entering the grey matter of the spinal cord.
- In **laminae I and V**, fibres relay to second-order neurons.
- Fibres of second-order neurons cross midline in the anterior commissure to ascend in the anterolateral white matter.
- The decussating fibres travel through **two-to-three spinal segments** to reach the opposite side. Therefore, pain and temperature sensation will be affected two-to-three levels below the site of injury on the contralateral side.
- The somatotopic map of the anterolateral pathways preserves the rule emphasizing that legs are represented laterally and arms medially.
- When the anterolateral pathway reaches the medulla, it passes through a groove between the olives and the inferior cerebellar peduncles. Then, it travels in the pontine and midbrain tegmentum just **lateral to the medial lemniscus**.

The anterolateral pathway includes three tracts: spinothalamic, spinoreticular and spinomesencephalic (Figs. 6.7 and 6.14).

The **spinothalamic tract** is responsible for localization as well as recognition of intensity of pain and temperature (Figs. 6.7 and 6.15).

- Second-order neurons relay to the **VPL nucleus** of the thalamus.
- Fibres of third-order neurons travel via the thalamic somatosensory radiation to reach the **postcentral gyrus** of the somatosensory cortex.
- There are additional projections to other thalamic nuclei, including the intralaminar and mediodorsal nuclei.

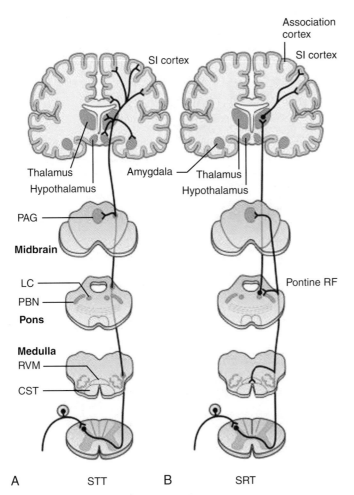

FIGURE 6.14   Pathways for transmission of pain, temperature and crude touch sensations.
(A) Spinothalamic tract (STT); (B) spinoreticular tract (SRT). CST, corticospinal tract; RVM, rostral ventromedial medulla; LC, locus coeruleus; PAG, periaqueductal grey; PBN, parabrachial nucleus; RF, reticular formation. Source: *Redrawn from Michael-Titus A, Revest P, Shortland P. The nervous system. Edinburgh: Churchill Livingstone; 2006, with permission.*

- These projections, along with the spinoreticular tract, participate in conveying the emotional and arousal aspects of pain.
- Fibres of the **spinoreticular tract** end in the pontine and medullary **reticular formation** and send fibres to the thalamic nuclei, which in turn propagate the information to the entire cortex and thus initiate the behavioural reaction to painful stimuli.

The **spinomesencephalic fibres** project to the midbrain periaqueductal grey matter and superior colliculi for the central modulation of pain.

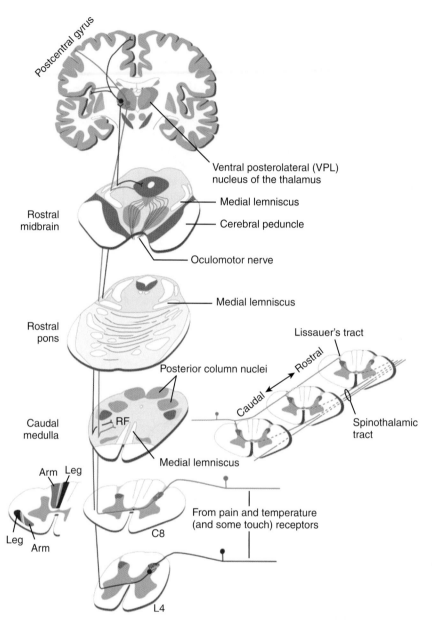

FIGURE 6.15 Spinothalamic tract. Pain, temperature and some touch and pressure afferents end in the posterior horn. Second- or higher-order fibres cross the midline, form the spinothalamic tract and ascend to the ventral posterolateral (VPL) nucleus of the thalamus. Thalamic cells then project to the somatosensory cortex of the postcentral gyrus, to the insula, and to other cortical areas. Along their course through the brainstem, spinothalamic fibres give off many collaterals to the reticular formation (RF). The inset to the left shows the lamination of fibres in the posterior columns and the spinothalamic tract in a leg–lower trunk–upper trunk–arm sequence. The inset to the right shows the longitudinal formation of the spinothalamic tract. Primary afferents ascend several segments in Lissauer's tract before all their branches terminate; fibres crossing to join the spinothalamic tract do so with a rostral inclination. Source: *Vanderah TW, PhD. Spinal cord. Nolte's the human brain. p. 233–71, Chapter 10.*

The spinothalamic and spinomesencephalic tracts arise from laminae I and V, whereas the spinoreticular tract arises from the intermediate and ventral horn laminae (VI through VIII).

The anterolateral pathway also conveys crude touch information; thus, touch sensation is not lost when the posterior column is damaged.

Spinocerebellar Pathway (Fig. 6.16)
The **spinocerebellar pathway** consists of the following tracts:
- **Dorsal (posterior) spinocerebellar tract**, which is associated with the **cuneocerebellar tract**.

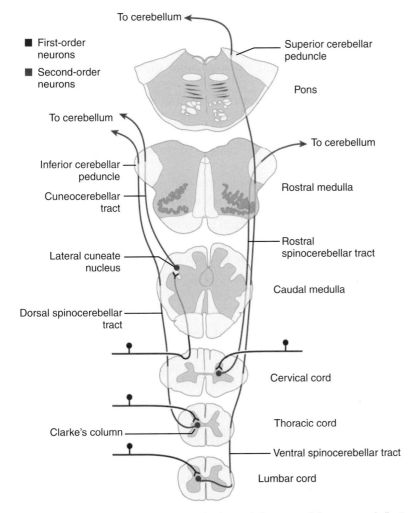

FIGURE 6.16 Spinocerebellar tracts. The dorsal spinocerebellar tract and the cuneocerebellar tract are shown on the left side. The ventral spinocerebellar tract and the rostral spinocerebellar tract are shown on the right side.

Source: *Crossman AR, PhD DSc. Spinal cord. Neuroanatomy: an illustrated colour text. p. 69–90, Chapter 8.*

- **Ventral (anterior) spinocerebellar tract**, which is associated with the **rostral spinocerebellar tract**.

The dorsal and ventral spinocerebellar tracts convey information from the lower limbs, while the cuneocerebellar and rostral spinocerebellar tracts convey information from the upper limbs.

- The dorsal spinocerebellar and cuneocerebellar tracts transmit information about limb movement (i.e. proprioceptive information from muscle spindles).
- The ventral and rostral spinocerebellar tracts project to the cerebellum and relay information related to the activity of interneurons and the effectiveness of descending regulatory pathways (i.e. proprioceptive information from Golgi tendon organs).

First-order neurons with large myelinated nerve fibres carry information of proprioception, pressure and vibration from the lower limbs and enter the dorsal root entry zone.

- Instead of entering the posterior column, these fibres relay to neurons residing in Clarke's column.
- Second-order neuron fibres ascend as the dorsal spinocerebellar tract, which is located in the dorsolateral funiculus, lateral to the lateral corticospinal tract.
- This tract gives rise to **mossy fibres** that travel via the **ipsilateral inferior cerebellar peduncle** to reach the **ipsilateral** cerebellum.

Sensory movement information from upper limbs is conveyed via large myelinated fibres that travel to reach the cuneate fasciculus in the posterior column.

- Fibres ascend to the **cuneate nucleus** in the medulla ipsilaterally and relay to second-order neurons that give rise to the cuneocerebellar tract.
- The cuneocerebellar tract travels to the **ipsilateral** cerebellar hemisphere via the **inferior cerebellar peduncle**.

Fibres from the **lateral border spinal neurons** of the grey matter and the **intermediate lamina** give rise to the ventral spinocerebellar tract.

- The ventral spinocerebellar tract is located lateral to the anterolateral pathway near the surface of the spinal cord.
- It **crosses midline** at the anterior white commissure and ascends to the pons, where it crosses again to enter the **superior cerebellar peduncle**. Thus, the ventral spinocerebellar tract crosses twice: once in the cord and once in the pons.
- Finally, it enters to the cerebellar hemisphere **ipsilateral** to the limb of origin.

The rostral spinocerebellar tract is similar to the ventral spinocerebellar tract. However, there are two main differences:

- The rostral spinocerebellar tract relays information from the upper limbs.
- It never crosses the midline and remains ipsilateral all the way to the cerebellum.

SPINAL CORD SYNDROMES: CLINICAL CASES

CASE 1

A 65-year-old man presented to the emergency department for 7 months history of progressive difficulty in walking, left leg numbness and urinary problems. The patient, who was previously healthy, gradually developed mid-back pain and left leg stiffness and weakness. The right leg was numb, and he complained of imbalance. Few weeks prior to presentation, he started having urinary frequency, incontinence and constipation.

The neurologic examination revealed left lower extremity (LLE) spasticity, decrease in motor power (3/5) and increase in deep tendon reflexes in the left knee and left ankle (3+ and 4+, respectively) with positive clonus. Sensory exam revealed decreased vibration and position sense in the LLE and decreased pain and temperature sense up to slightly below the mid-belly on the right. Anal tone was decreased. The rest of the neurologic exam was normal.

Discussion

Unilateral weakness and upper motor neuron signs in the left leg associated with contralateral sensory abnormalities up to the horizontal level below the umbilicus and midthoracic pain support the diagnosis of a lesion in the left hemicord at the T8 level leading to **Brown-Sequard syndrome**. Bladder and bowel involvement raises the suspicion of bilateral cord disease.

The progressive course of deficits over several months with local pain is highly suggestive of differential diagnoses such as a tumour compressing the spinal cord, arthritic bony changes or disc disease with myelopathy. The patient turned out to have a tumour compressing the spinal cord (Fig. 6.17).

Brown-Sequard syndrome is caused by a functional or physical **hemicord injury**. Dysfunction of the following spinal cord components leads to a peculiar combination of signs/symptoms.

- **Corticospinal tract:** resulting in **ipsilateral** hemiparesis, spasticity, hyperactive reflexes and clonus below the level of injury as well as a Babinski sign.
- **Dorsal column:** resulting in **ipsilateral** loss of vibration, position, two-point discrimination, pressure and fine touch sense below the level of injury.
- **Spinothalamic tract:** resulting in **contralateral** loss of pain and temperature sensation and numbness as of **two-to-three dermatomes** below the level of injury.
- **Ventral horn injury:** resulting in **ipsilateral** lower motor neurons signs manifesting as muscle paralysis, atrophy and fasciculations.

Brown-Sequard syndrome is rarely complete as in this classical picture.

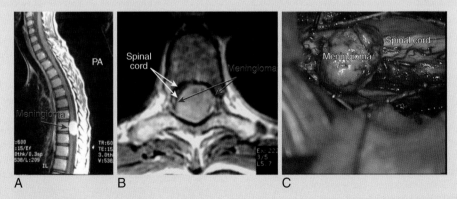

A   B   C

FIGURE 6.17 (A) Intradural extramedullary tumour (meningioma, red arrow) seen on the T1 sagittal MRI at T8-9 compressing the spinal cord. (B) The axial image shows the eccentric tumour on the left (red arrows demarcating the tumour limits) with significant compression of the spinal cord (white arrows demarcating the compressed spinal cord limits), which is displaced to the right. (C) The intraoperative photograph shows the reexpansion of the spinal cord as the tumour is being removed.
Source: *Courtesy of George Jallo, MD. John Hopkins All Children's Hospital.*

CASE 2

A 37-year-old woman presented with tingling and numbness in the trunk and all four limbs of 1-week duration. She also complained of clumsiness upon walking and decreased dexterity in her hands. She had electricity-like sensation in her spine that run downwards to her toes when moving her neck.

Neurologic examination was notable for dysmetria on the finger-to-nose test. Tandem gait was unsteady, and Romberg sign was positive. There was remarkable loss of vibration reaching the knuckles. Position sense was impaired in the toes and, to a lesser extent, in the fingers. While pinprick examination was normal, light touch sensation was impaired.

Discussion

Loss of vibration and proprioception in all four limbs that is associated with unsteady gait and positive Romberg and Lhermitte's signs suggests a diagnosis of **posterior column syndrome** at the level of cervical spine. The patient was found to have posterior column myelitis and was later diagnosed with multiple sclerosis (Fig. 6.18).

Posterior Column Syndrome

- The clinical picture includes **ipsilateral or bilateral** loss of vibration, proprioception, two-point discrimination and deep touch depending on the extent of injury.

- Aetiologies include myelitis (due to multiple sclerosis, postinfectious, etc.), tabes dorsalis and vitamin B12 deficiency.

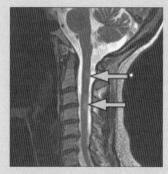

FIGURE 6.18 Spinal cord MRI in multiple sclerosis. Sagittal T2-weighted MRI of the cervical spinal cord shows typical dorsal, short-segment signal abnormalities (arrows) characteristic of multiple sclerosis.
Source: *Wingerchuk DM, MD. The spectrum of neuromyelitis optica. Lancet Neurol 6(9):805–15.*

CASE 3

A 26-year-old woman developed sudden acute neck pain and upper extremities pain and weakness. Shortly afterwards, she started having difficulty in urination and stool incontinence.

Neurological examination revealed motor deficits on elbow extension (3/5), handgrip (0/5), finger extensors (0/5) and lower extremities (0/5) bilaterally with absent triceps and lower extremities reflexes. She also had a C7 sensory level, where pinprick and light touch sensations were diminished. Vibration and proprioception were normal. Rectal tone was absent.

Discussion

The combination of bilateral hand weakness, loss of tone and reflexes, sensory level and bowel and bladder dysfunction suggests an acute anterior spinal lesion at the C7–T1 level. Aetiologies could be spinal cord infarction, myelitis, infectious or trauma.

Anterior Spinal Artery Syndrome

- Due to occlusion of the anterior spinal artery that results in ischaemia affecting the anterior two-thirds of the spinal cord.

- Onset is abrupt and associated with flaccid paralysis below the level of the lesion initially (due to spinal shock) with loss of bowel and bladder function.

- Sensory loss is dissociated, where patients develop loss of pain and temperature sense starting from two-to-three levels below the lesion level (due to loss of spinothalamic tract function) and preservation of vibration and proprioception sense (dorsal column remains intact).

- After the initial phase, upper motor neuron signs predominate due to bilateral loss of corticospinal tracts.

ADDITIONAL SPINAL CORD SYNDROMES

Complete Cord Transection

- Complete paralysis and loss of sensation below the level of injury
- Pain and temperature sensation are lost starting from two-to-three dermatomes below the level of injury
- Aetiologies include trauma, transverse myelitis, infarction, tumour and abscess

Subacute Combined Degeneration (Posterolateral Column) Syndrome

- Bilateral, selective degeneration involving the posterior and lateral funiculi, resulting in loss of vibration and proprioception that is associated with upper motor neuron signs (due to injury to corticospinal tracts).
- Aetiologies include Friedreich's ataxia and pernicious anaemia (vitamin B12 deficiency).

Combined Anterior Horn Cell-Pyramidal Tract Syndrome (Amyotrophic Lateral Sclerosis)

- Progressive, combined upper and lower motor neuron findings due to the degeneration of the motor neurons (Betz cells in layer V of the cerebral cortex and their axons that form the corticospinal tract; motor neurons of the cranial nerves; anterior horn [alpha motor neuron] cells and their axons that form the peripheral nerves).
- Clinical features are variable and include involvement of any of the end organs innervated by the motor nervous system.

Cauda Equina Syndrome (Fig. 6.19)

- Occurs due to compression/damage of the cauda equina (lumbar and sacral nerve roots) by various causes (tumour, disc, abscess, etc.)
- Early onset of radicular and back pain
- Late onset of anal sphincter problems, saddle anaesthesia and bladder, bowel and sexual dysfunction
- Lower motor neuron signs, including paralysis/paresis in the affected roots, hypoactive reflexes and muscle atrophy
- A surgical emergency and requires rapid decompression of the affected roots before the damage becomes irreversible

Conus Medullaris Syndrome (Fig. 6.20)

- Occurs due to compression/damage of the conus medullaris at T12–L2 levels by various causes (tumour, disc, abscess, etc.)
- Early onset of sphincter dysfunction, urinary incontinence, saddle anaesthesia (S2–S4 roots) and erection and ejaculation difficulties
- Late onset of lower extremity motor deficits
- May have a similar presentation to the cauda equina syndrome, but signs of upper motor neuron involvement due to direct spinal cord injury confirm the diagnosis

Table 6.1 lists some of the discriminatory features of cauda equina and conus medullaris syndromes.

Transverse Myelitis

- Acute inflammation of grey and white matter involving one (or more) whole spinal segment(s)
- Clinical features include:
  - Bilateral sensory, motor and/or autonomic dysfunction originating from the spinal cord

- Clearly defined sensory level, usually at a thoracic level, i.e. the most commonly affected location
- Confirmation of spinal cord inflammation by gadolinium-enhanced MRI or CSF studies showing pleocytosis or elevated immunoglobulin G (IgG) index (CSF IgG to CSF albumin ratio compared to serum IgG to serum albumin ratio)
- Idiopathic in up to 36% of cases; could be associated with a variety of diseases such as multiple sclerosis, neuromyelitis optica (Devic diseases), systemic lupus erythematosus and postinfectious

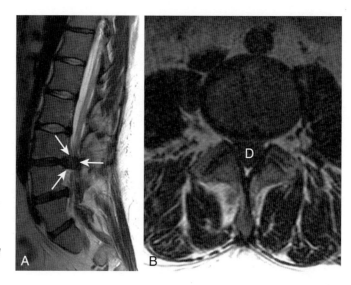

FIGURE 6.19   Cauda equina syndrome. Sagittal T2-weighted MRI (A) and axial T2-weighted MRI (B) at the L3–4 disc level. Large disc herniation (arrows, image A) completely obliterates the thecal sac at L3–4. Axial image (B) demonstrates absence of the normal increased T2-weighted signal intensity of the thecal sac because the disc herniation (D) occupies all the available space.
Source: *Fenton DS, MD. Cauda equina syndrome. Imaging painful spine disorders. p. 102–7, Chapter 14.*

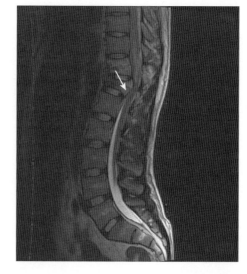

FIGURE 6.20   Conus medullaris syndrome. T2 sagittal magnetic resonance imaging study showing a T12 burst fracture (arrow) resulting in conus medullaris syndrome.
Source: *Snyder LA. Spinal cord trauma. Bradley's neurology in clinical practice. p. 881–2.e3, Chapter 63.*

Table 6.1 Discriminatory features of cauda equina syndrome and conus medullaris syndrome

Feature	Cauda Equina Syndrome	Conus Medullaris Syndrome
Level of injury	T12–L2	Below L2
Symmetry	Asymmetrical motor and sensory impairment	Symmetrical motor and sensory impairment
Level of motor Neuron injury	Lower (nerve root) motor neuron	Upper (spinal cord) and/or lower motor neuron

CASE STUDY DISCUSSION

Central cord syndrome results from injury to the area around the central canal. Aetiologies include syringomyelia and spinal cord hyperextension injury.

■ Caused by compression of the **crossing fibres of spino-thalamic tract** in the anterior white commissure.

■ Results in loss of pain and temperature sensation in affected dermatomes (dermatomes starting from two-to-three levels below the injured decussation) in upper extremities with absence of symptoms in lower extremities at the initial stage.

■ When the injury extends, there will be involvement of other parts of the spinal cord such as anterior, lateral and posterior columns with their associated signs and symptoms.

CHAPTER 7

Brainstem

Rajiv Iyer, George Jallo

CASE STUDY

Presentation and Physical Examination: A 7-year-old boy is brought to the emergency room accompanied by his parents due to frequent vomiting and difficulty ambulating. He has also had trouble swallowing with coughing after meals. Physical examination reveals a well-developed young boy with dysconjugate gaze and trouble with left eye lateral motion, in addition to dysmetria and ataxic gait.

Diagnosis and Management: Magnetic resonance imaging (MRI) of the brain reveals a hyperintense lesion on T2-weighted imaging within the brainstem (Fig. 7.1). He is referred to a neurosurgeon and an oncologist due to concern for an intra-axial brainstem lesion.

What is the most likely diagnosis? Try to answer this question after studying this chapter!

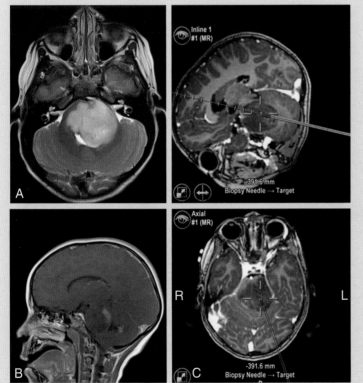

FIGURE 7.1 Magnetic resonance (MR) imaging of a child with a diffuse pontine lesion. Axial T2-weighted (A) and sagittal (B) T1-weighted with contrast MRI demonstrating a T2-hyperintense lesion within the pons, extending into the left and right middle cerebellar peduncles. (C) Intraoperative view of the surgical plan and trajectory utilized to accurately navigate a needle biopsy forceps to the lesion.
Source: *Courtesy of George Jallo, MD. John Hopkins All Children's Hospital.*

BRIEF INTRODUCTION

Much of the basis for human function exists within, or traverses the **brainstem.**

- The human brainstem has three components: the **midbrain,** which is derived embryologically from the **mesencephalon**; the **pons,** which is derived from part of the **metencephalon,** a subcategory of the rhombencephalon and the **medulla,** which is derived from the **myelencephalon,** another subclassification of the rhombencephalon.
- The majority of the structures comprising the brainstem are contained within the posterior fossa of the human calvarium, and it lies between the cerebral cortex and the spinal cord.
- Part of the ventricular system containing cerebrospinal fluid (CSF) is surrounded by the brainstem and includes the **cerebral aqueduct** (of Sylvius) and the **4th ventricle** (Fig. 7.2).

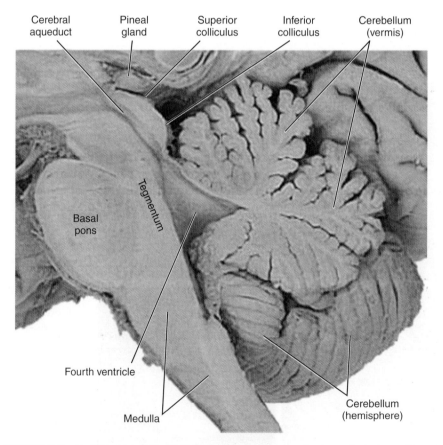

FIGURE 7.2   Medial surface of the right half of a hemisected brain, showing major features of the brainstem and cerebellum.
Source: *Courtesy Grant Dahmer, University of Arizona College of Medicine. Modified from Nolte J, Angevine JB Jr. The human brain in photographs and diagrams, 3rd ed, St. Louis: Mosby; 2007.*

- Some of the delicate structures within the brainstem include cranial nerve nuclei and nerve fibres, as well as critical ascending and descending tracts that allow for motor and sensory innervation to the face, neck and body.
- Other connections, including the brainstem connections to subcortical structures, such as the basal ganglia, as well as the cerebellum, also exist.
- Fundamental subconscious cardiorespiratory mechanisms that are essential to human life, as well as centres involved in sleep-wake cycles and alertness are also governed by structures within the brainstem.
- Given the most basic, yet vast function housed within a relatively small amount of neural real estate, it is not surprising that brainstem injury can cause a significantly detrimental loss of function. Maintaining a thorough working knowledge of the ultrastructural architecture of the brainstem can help a clinician localize neurological lesions with better accuracy.

In this chapter, we discuss the macrostructural organization of the brainstem and cite some common clinical applications that aid in understanding its complex anatomical framework. A more exhaustive discussion of individual cranial nerve function and nuclei is discussed elsewhere. The purpose of this chapter, rather than exhaustively listing each structure and tract located in or passing through the brainstem, is to provide a framework and foundation for understanding brainstem anatomy to aid in clinical diagnosis and interpretation.

BRAINSTEM ORGANIZATION

- Rostral to caudal organization: midbrain, pons, medulla.
  - Cerebellum is attached to the posterior surface of the brainstem.
- Part of the ventricular system is surrounded by the brainstem.
  - Cerebral aqueduct (of Sylvius) is surrounded by the midbrain (mesencephalon) and connects the 3rd and 4th ventricles.

CLINICAL INSIGHT

- **Congenital hydrocephalus**
  - Congenital hydrocephalus, or buildup of CSF in the ventricular system, can occur as a result of obstructive processes such as **aqueductal stenosis,** or the presence of a tectal tumour (Fig. 7.3), which can narrow, occlude or scar the cerebral aqueduct. To treat these obstructive conditions, CSF diversion can be accomplished with an **endoscopic third ventriculostomy** (ETV), in which a fenestration is created in the floor or the third ventricle to allow an alternate route for CSF egress into the subarachnoid cisterns at the base of the skull.

- The 4th ventricle lies at the level of the pons and medulla.
  - Floor made up of the rostral medulla; roof composed of the ventral surface of the cerebellum and tela choroidea.

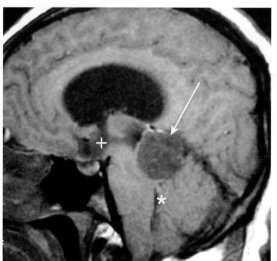

FIGURE 7.3   Tectal tumour causing aqueductal stenosis. T1-weighted sagittal MRI demonstrating a hypointense tectal lesion (arrow) causing effacement of the cerebral aqueduct, which connects the 3rd ventricle (plus sign) and 4th ventricle (asterisk). Due to obstruction of cerebrospinal fluid (CSF) flow, this patient will likely require a CSF-diversionary procedure such as an endoscopic third ventriculostomy, or ventriculoperitoneal shunt placement. Source: *Courtesy of George Jallo, MD. John Hopkins All Children's Hospital.*

- 4th ventricular outlet into the cisternal spaces:
    - Medially – foramen of Magendie.
    - Laterally – **foramina of Luschka** (bilateral).
  - 4th ventricular outlet into the central canal of the spinal cord via the **obex** of the fourth ventricle.
- Cranial nerve function is organized within the brainstem in a rostro-caudal fashion. Some cranial nerve nuclei are elongated structures that extend across components of the brainstem. Some cranial nerve nuclei also receive input from or send input to multiple cranial nerves, especially the sensory nuclei.
  - Cranial nerve nuclei can be considered in general columns consisting of motor and sensory control. The **basal plate** gives rise to **motor nuclei**. The more dorsolateral **alar plate** gives rise to **sensory nuclei**. During development, the alar plate becomes situated more lateral to the basal plate. On the floor of the 4th ventricle, cranial nerve nuclei are also arranged in columns, with the **sulcus limitans** separating the basal and alar plates.
  - Midbrain: contains oculomotor (III) nerve, trochlear (IV) nerve nuclei.
  - Pons: contains most of trigeminal (V) nerve nuclei, abducens (VI) nerve nuclei, facial nerve (VII) nuclei, vestibulocochlear nerve (VIII) nuclei (extends into rostral medulla).
  - Medulla: contains nuclei receiving input/output from the glossopharyngeal (IX) nerve, vagus (X) nerve, spinal accessory (XI) nerve (also extends into cervical spinal cord) and hypoglossal (XII) nerve.
- Cranial nerve function is subdivided by type of innervation and motor/sensory function (general review).

- General somatic efferent fibres
  - Cranial nerves III, IV, VI, XII.
- Special visceral efferent fibres (branchiomotor – innervate muscles derived from branchial arches)
  - Cranial nerves V, VII, IX, X/XI complex.
- General visceral efferent fibres
  - Cranial nerves **III, VII, IX, X**.
- General somatic afferent fibres
  - Cranial nerves **V, VII, IX, X**.
- General visceral afferent fibres
  - Cranial nerves **VII, IX, X**.
- Special visceral afferent fibres
  - Cranial nerves **I, VII, IX, X**.
- Special somatic afferent fibres
  - Cranial nerves **II, VIII**.
- Ascending and descending tracts traverse the brainstem
  - Ascending (afferent)
    - Dorsal column-medial lemniscal (DC-ML) tract
      - This tract conveys joint position sense and **discriminative touch** from the body. First-order neurons lie within the dorsal root ganglia at various levels in the spinal cord. Central processes of these neurons ascend in the **gracile fasciculus** (medial) and **cuneate fasciculus** (lateral), which together comprise the **dorsal column** on either side. In the caudal brainstem, second-order neurons in this pathway are located in the **nucleus gracilis** and **nucleus cuneatus**. After synapsing there, decussation occurs by means of the **internal arcuate** fibres, eventually leading to the **ventral posterolateral (VPL) nucleus** of the thalamus, and subsequently to the postcentral gyrus.
      - Brainstem decussation.
    - Spinothalamic tract (anterolateral system)
      - This tract conveys **pain** and **temperature** as well as **some light touch sensation** from the body. Connection between the first-order and second-order neurons occurs in the dorsal horn of the spinal cord. Following this, fibres decussate in the spinal cord within the **anterior white commissure** and travel in the spinothalamic tract. These fibres ascend to the **VPL nucleus of the thalamus** and from there, to the postcentral gyrus.
      - Spinal cord decussation.
  - Descending (efferent)
    - Corticospinal tract
      - **Motor** function from cerebral cortex to spinal cord.
      - Brainstem (pyramidal) decussation.
    - Corticobulbar tract
      - Fibres projecting from cerebral cortex to brainstem.
      - Symmetric, bilateral input to brainstem nuclei.

MEDULLA

- Caudal medulla – the most caudal aspect of the brainstem prior to the cervicomedullary junction, which is the border between the brainstem and the spinal cord (Figs. 7.4 and 7.5).
  - Similar in appearance to the cervical spinal cord
    - Part of the anterior horn still remains at this level and the lower motor neurons supplying the spinal accessory nerve (XI) arise from this location.
    - Correlating with the dorsal root entry zone, or Lissauer's tract, the **spinal nucleus of the trigeminal nerve** and the **spinal trigeminal**

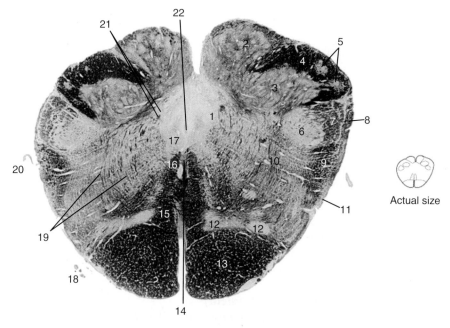

Actual size

FIGURE 7.4   Caudal medulla (close to the level of the obex). 1. Dorsal motor nucleus of the vagus. 2. Nucleus gracilis. 3. Nucleus cuneatus. 4. Fasciculus cuneatus. 5. Lateral cuneate nucleus. Arm equivalent of Clarke's nucleus. Proprioceptive primary afferents travel through fasciculus cuneatus to reach the lateral cuneate nucleus, which then gives rise to uncrossed cuneocerebellar fibres that enter the cerebellum through the inferior cerebellar peduncle. 6. Spinal trigeminal nucleus (caudal nucleus). 7. Spinal trigeminal tract. 8. Posterior spinocerebellar tract. 9. Anterolateral pathway. 10. Location of nucleus ambiguus. 11. Anterior spinocerebellar tract. Crossed fibres from lumbosacral spinal grey matter, carrying proprioceptive and other information from the leg. This tract stays in approximately the same position until the rostral pons, where it moves over the surface of the superior cerebellar peduncle and turns posteriorly into the cerebellum. 12. Inferior olivary nucleus (medial accessory nucleus). Climbing fibres from the accessory nuclei project mainly to the vermis and flocculus, those from the principal inferior olivary nucleus to the cerebellar hemisphere. 13. Pyramid. 14. Raphe nuclei. 15. Medial lemniscus. 16. Medial longitudinal fasciculus (MLF). At this level, the fibres of the medial vestibulospinal tract. 17. Hypoglossal nucleus. 18. Hypoglossal nerve fibres, on their way to the muscles of the ipsilateral half of the tongue. 19. Internal arcuate fibres, crossing from nuclei gracilis and cuneatus to form the medial lemniscus. 20. Fibres of the vagus nerve, on their way to muscles of the ipsilateral half of the larynx and pharynx. 21. Solitary tract and its nucleus. Primary afferents conveying visceral information from cranial nerves VII, IX and X (and some chemosensory information from the trigeminal nerve) travel through the solitary tract to reach the surrounding nucleus of the solitary tract. 22. Central canal.
Source: *Vanderah TW, PhD. Atlas of the human brainstem. Nolte's the human brain. p. 383–93, Chapter 15.*

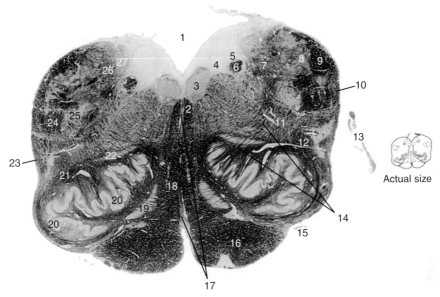

Actual size

FIGURE 7.5 Rostral medulla. 1. Fourth ventricle. 2. Medial longitudinal fasciculus (MLF). 3. Hypoglossal nucleus. 4. Dorsal motor nucleus of the vagus. 5. Nucleus of the solitary tract. 6. Solitary tract. 7. Nucleus cuneatus. 8. Lateral cuneate nucleus. 9. Inferior cerebellar peduncle. By the time it enters the cerebellum, it contains crossed olivocerebellar fibres, the uncrossed posterior spinocerebellar tract, vestibulocerebellar fibres, trigeminocerebellar fibres and other cerebellar afferents. 10. Posterior spinocerebellar tract entering the inferior cerebellar peduncle. 11. Location of nucleus ambiguus. 12. Anterolateral pathway. 13. Vagus nerve. 14. Internal arcuate fibres. 15. Hypoglossal nerve fibres. 16. Pyramid. 17. Raphe nuclei. Serotonergic neurons that at this level are one source of descending pain-control fibres to the spinal cord. 18. Medial lemniscus. 19. Inferior olivary nucleus (medial accessory nucleus). 20. Inferior olivary nucleus (principal nucleus). 21. Fibres of the central tegmental tract reaching the inferior olivary nucleus. 22. Inferior olivary nucleus (dorsal accessory nucleus). 23. Anterior spinocerebellar tract. 24. Spinal trigeminal tract. 25. Spinal trigeminal nucleus (interpolar nucleus). 26. Inferior vestibular nucleus with bundles of vestibular primary afferents running through it. 27. Medial vestibular nucleus. Site of origin of the medial vestibulospinal tract (among other connections). Source: *Vanderah TW, PhD. Atlas of the human brainstem. Nolte's the human brain. p. 383–93, Chapter 15.*

tract lie dorsolaterally in the caudal medulla and receive fibres from the unilateral face to supply **pain** and **temperature** sensation from the **head** and **neck.**

- The more medial gracile fasciculus and lateral cuneate fasciculus enter the brainstem and synapse in the gracile and cuneate nuclei, respectively, located in the caudal brainstem.
  - After synapsing in the gracile and cuneate nuclei, the internal arcuate fibres decussate in the caudal medulla to form the **medial lemniscus.**
  - Somatotopy of the medial lemniscus at this level is such that **cervical** segments are represented **dorsally**, and **lumbar** segments are represented **ventrally** (homunculus standing atop the medullary pyramids).
- **Decussation of the pyramids**
  - The majority of corticospinal tract fibres from motor cortex cross ventrally at the level of the **medullary pyramids** to travel in the spinal cord as the **lateral corticospinal tract.**

- **Hypoglossal nuclei** and **hypoglossal nerve fibres**
  - Nuclei are just ventral to the 4th ventricle and the nerves exit ventrally. Each hypoglossal nerve supplies muscles of the **ipsilateral tongue**; injury causes tongue deviation to the ipsilateral side.

CLINICAL INSIGHT

- Iatrogenic hypoglossal nerve injury
  - In high anterior cervical approaches (e.g. anterior cervical discectomy and fusion, or carotid endarterectomy), the hypoglossal nerve may be encountered and inadvertently injured as it passes over the carotid artery (Fig. 7.6).

- **Spinothalamic tract** remains in an **anterolateral** position at this level of the brainstem.
- **Medial longitudinal fasciculus** sits atop the medial lemniscus just ventral to the ventricular system and relays fibres from the **medial vestibulospinal tract**.
- Rostral medulla
  - Inferior olivary nuclei
    - Paired nuclei that appear grossly as prominent anterior surface swellings, separated from the medullary pyramids by the anterolateral sulci.
    - Receive input from cortex, spinal cord and brainstem and send impulses to the cerebellar hemispheres via **climbing fibres** that cross in the **inferior cerebellar peduncles**.
  - Some specific cranial nerve nuclei
    - Nucleus ambiguus: **Lower motor neurons** that supply the **glossopharyngeal** (IX – stylopharyngeus muscle) nerve and **vagus** (X) nerve fibres that supply the muscles of the pharynx and larynx.

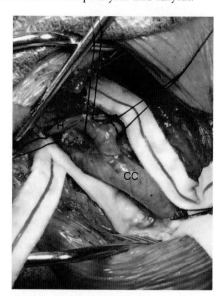

FIGURE 7.6 Hypoglossal nerve in the neck. Intraoperative view during carotid endarterectomy demonstrating common carotid artery (CC) and superiorly, the hypoglossal nerve (H) as it crosses close to the carotid bifurcation.
Source: *Courtesy of George Jallo, MD. John Hopkins All Children's Hospital.*

- Solitary nucleus: Receives **afferent** input regarding **taste** sensation from VII, IX and X nerves.
  - Dorsal motor nucleus of vagus nerve: **Parasympathetic motor** innervation to the thoracoabdominal viscera.
- Vestibular nuclei
  - Medial, lateral and inferior vestibular nuclei contain **primary vestibular afferent** fibres. Immediately underlying these structures is **area postrema**, on the 4th ventricular wall, one of the emesis control centres.

CLINICAL INSIGHT

- Case – Area Postrema
  - A 3-year-old boy presented with vomiting and MRI of the brain revealed a large, cystic posterior fossa lesion that appeared to arise from the 4th ventricle (Fig. 7.7). T2-weighted imaging demonstrated enlarged ventricles with evidence of transependymal flow, indicating the presence of hydrocephalus. Hydrocephalus in combination with compression of area postrema likely resulted in his persistent emesis. Surgical resection was completed via a suboccipital approach and intraoperative view following excision demonstrates a widely patent 4th ventricle with a view of the cerebral aqueduct above.

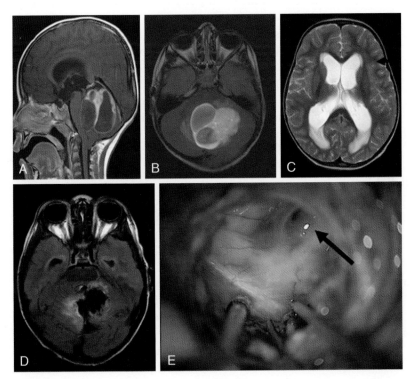

FIGURE 7.7 Child with a juvenile pilocytic astrocytoma and associated hydrocephalus. Sagittal (A) and axial (B) T1-weighted MRI demonstrating a ring-enhancing lesion in the posterior fossa effacing the 4th ventricle and causing downward tonsillar herniation of the cerebellar tonsils due to mass effect, seen on sagittal image. (C) Axial T2-weighted image demonstrating supratentorial ventricular enlargement and transependymal flow of CSF from the ventricular space, consistent with hydrocephalus as a result of the obstructive 4th ventricular tumour. (D) Postoperative axial T2-FLAIR image showing the surgical path and minimal tissue oedema around surgical site. (E) Intraoperative image following suboccipital craniotomy and resection of the brain tumour, with visualization of a patent 4th ventricle and cerebral aqueduct within (arrow). Source: *Courtesy of George Jallo, MD.*

- **Inferior cerebellar peduncle (restiform body)**
  - This **primarily afferent** connection to the cerebellum provides input from the vestibulospinal tracts, dorsal spinocerebellar tracts, olivocerebellar tracts and others.

PONS

The **pons**, the Latin term for 'bridge' given its connectivity to the cerebellum, is composed of a ventrally protuberant base, known as the **basal pons**, and a dorsal **tegmentum**. Located between the medulla and the midbrain, and given its cerebellar connectivity, it is not surprising that the pons contains many traversing, orthogonal tracts. Several of the continuing ascending and descending tracts of the medulla are also found within the pontine tegmentum (Fig. 7.8).

- **Facial colliculus**
  - Part of the caudal pons serves as the floor of the 4th ventricle.
  - The abducens (VI) nucleus lies close to the floor of the 4th ventricle.
  - As the facial nerve runs dorsal to the abducens nucleus (facial nerve genu), it forms a swelling in the 4th ventricle floor, i.e. the facial colliculus.
- **Pontine nuclei**
  - Scattered amongst longitudinally and transversely oriented fibres within the basal pons are several pontine nuclei.
    - Longitudinal fibres in the basal pons are partly composed of the corticospinal tracts.
  - **Corticopontine fibres** entering the brainstem from the cerebral cortex may synapse on pontine nuclei, which subsequently send impulses to the cerebellum via decussation in the **middle cerebellar peduncle** (brachium pontis).
    - Injury to the basal pons can lead to ataxia due to involvement of pontocerebellar tracts and damage to pontine nuclei, such as in a child with a pontine glioma *(see Case Study)*.
    - The middle cerebellar peduncles are the largest of the three cerebellar peduncles.
- **Medial lemniscus**
  - In the medulla, the homunculus of the medial lemniscus is oriented in a rostrocaudal fashion (upright homunculus). In the pons, the homunculus begins to flatten. Its somatotopic organization lies in a mediolateral fashion, with **lumbar** regions being represented **lateral** and **cervical** regions represented **medially.**
- **Lateral lemniscus**
  - Conduct **auditory** impulses from the dorsal cochlear nuclei by connecting to the inferior colliculi within the midbrain.
- **Raphe nuclei**
  - Group of **serotonergic** neurons that project to the cerebral cortex and throughout the brain, as well as caudal projections that help mediate **pain** sensation in the spinal cord.

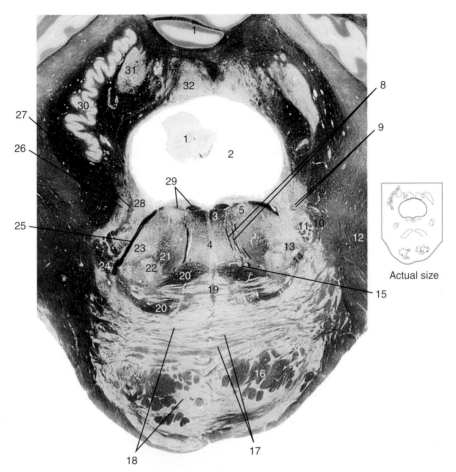

Actual size

FIGURE 7.8 Caudal pons. 1. Vermis of the cerebellum. 2. Fourth ventricle. 3. Medial longitudinal fasciculus (MLF). At this level, fibres from vestibular nuclei and abducens interneurons, active in coordinating eye movements. 4. Raphe nuclei. 5. Abducens nucleus. Contains the lower motor neurons for the ipsilateral lateral rectus and the interneurons that project through the contralateral MLF to medial rectus motor neurons. 6. Superior cerebellar peduncle. Fibres from the deep cerebellar nuclei to the contralateral red nucleus and thalamus (ventral lateral nucleus [VL]). 7. Inferior cerebellar peduncle entering the cerebellum. 8. Abducens nerve fibres. 9. Solitary tract and its nucleus. 10. Spinal trigeminal tract. 11. Spinal trigeminal nucleus (oral nucleus). 12. Middle cerebellar peduncle. Fibres from contralateral pontine nuclei that end as mossy fibres in all areas of cerebellar cortex. 13. Lateral lemniscus. Ascending auditory fibres from the cochlear and superior olivary nuclei, representing both ears. 14. Anterolateral pathway. 15. Errant avian. 16. Corticospinal, corticobulbar and corticopontine fibres, from ipsilateral cerebral cortex. 17. Pontocerebellar fibres, from pontine nuclei of one side to the opposite middle cerebellar peduncle. 18. Pontine nuclei. Source of pontocerebellar fibres that cross the midline and form the middle cerebellar peduncle. 19. Trapezoid body. Crossing auditory fibres, primarily from the ventral cochlear nucleus. 20. Medial lemniscus. 21. Central tegmental tract. Descending fibres from the red nucleus to the inferior olivary nucleus, together with fibres to and from different levels of the reticular formation. 22. Superior olivary nucleus. First site of convergence of fibres representing the two ears and the source of many of the fibres of the lateral lemniscus. 23. Facial motor nucleus. 24. Anterior spinocerebellar tract. 25. Facial nerve fibres. 26. Lateral vestibular nucleus, source of the lateral vestibulospinal tract. 27. Juxtarestiform body. Fibres of the inferior cerebellar peduncle interconnecting the vestibular nuclei and cerebellum. 28. Superior vestibular nucleus. 29. Internal genu of the facial nerve. 30. Dentate nucleus. The deep nucleus connected to lateral parts of the cerebellar hemisphere and the source of most of the fibres in the superior cerebellar peduncle. 31. Interposed nucleus. The deep cerebellar nucleus connected to medial parts of the cerebellar hemisphere. 32. Fastigial nucleus. The deep cerebellar nucleus connected to the vermis and flocculus.

Source: *Vanderah TW, PhD. Atlas of the human brainstem. Nolte's the human brain. p. 383–93, Chapter 15.*

MIDBRAIN

The most rostral component of the brainstem is known as the **midbrain**, and is characterized by the dorsal, paired superior and inferior collicula, all together known as the **tectum** or **corpora quadrigemina**, as well as the ventrally situated **cerebral peduncles**. The structures comprising the midbrain surround the cerebral aqueduct, which connects the 3rd and 4th ventricles (Fig. 7.9).

- **Superior colliculus**
  - Part of the tectum that functions in the **visual** system with involvement in mechanisms for **saccadic eye movements**.

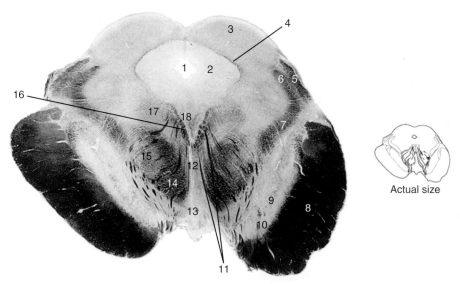

Actual size

FIGURE 7.9 Rostral midbrain. 1. Cerebral aqueduct. 2. Periaqueductal grey. Site of origin of the descending pain-control pathway that relays in the nucleus raphe magnus (among other connections). 3. Superior colliculus. Involved in visual attention and eye movements, and the site of termination of most fibres of the superior brachium. 4. Mesencephalic trigeminal tract. Processes of cell bodies in the adjacent mesencephalic trigeminal nucleus that innervate mechanoreceptors in and around the mouth. 5. Brachium of the inferior colliculus. Ascending auditory fibres on their way from the inferior colliculus to the medial geniculate nucleus. 6. Anterolateral pathway. 7. Medial lemniscus. 8. Cerebral peduncle. Descending corticospinal, corticobulbar and corticopontine fibres from ipsilateral cerebral cortex. 9. Substantia nigra (compact part). Dopaminergic neurons whose axons terminate in the caudate nucleus and putamen. 10. Substantia nigra (reticular part). Site of termination of fibres from the caudate nucleus and putamen and site of origin of fibres to the thalamus, superior colliculus and reticular formation. 11. Oculomotor nerve fibres. Axons of lower motor neurons and preganglionic parasympathetic neurons for the ipsilateral medial, superior and inferior recti; inferior oblique; levator palpebrae; pupillary sphincter; and ciliary muscle. 12. Raphe nuclei. 13. Ventral tegmental area. Dopaminergic neurons whose axons terminate in limbic and frontal cortical sites. 14. Crossed superior cerebellar peduncle entering the red nucleus. Fibres from the contralateral deep cerebellar nuclei, on their way to the red nucleus and thalamus. 15. Red nucleus. Receives inputs from the contralateral deep cerebellar nuclei via the superior cerebellar peduncle and projects primarily to the inferior olivary nucleus via the central tegmental tract. 16. Medial longitudinal fasciculus (MLF). 17. Central tegmental tract. Descending fibres from the red nucleus to the inferior olivary nucleus, together with fibres to and from different levels of the reticular formation. 18. Oculomotor nucleus. Lower motor neurons for the ipsilateral medial and inferior recti and inferior oblique, the contralateral superior rectus and the levator palpebrae of both sides; preganglionic parasympathetic neurons for the pupillary sphincter and the ciliary muscle.

Source: *Vanderah TW, PhD. Atlas of the human brainstem. Nolte's the human brain. p. 383–93, Chapter 15.*

- Descending input from the **frontal eye fields** onto the retinotopically arranged superior colliculus.

- **Inferior colliculus**
  - Part of central **auditory** pathway
    - Receives input from the **superior olivary nucleus** and **lateral lemniscus**.
    - Sends input to the **medial geniculate body** via the brachium of the inferior colliculus.
- **Periaqueductal grey**
  - Surrounds the cerebral aqueduct and is a grey matter structure responsible for partly mediating the descending **pain** control systems.
- **Cerebral peduncles**
  - Most ventral component of the midbrain, containing **corticospinal** and **corticobulbar** fibres.
    - Between the bilateral cerebral peduncles is the **interpeduncular cistern** (or fossa) in which the **oculomotor (III)** nerves travel.

CLINICAL INSIGHT

- **Uncal herniation**
  - In patients with a large subdural or epidural hematoma, mass effect on the temporal lobe can cause shift of its most medial aspect, the uncus, known as **uncal herniation** (Fig. 7.10). Uncal herniation results in compression of the **3rd nerve** and the **cerebral peduncle**, resulting in a dilated unilateral pupil, and contralateral hemiparesis. The **Kernohan's notch** phenomenon occurs when lesions are of such significant size and mass effect that the contralateral cerebral peduncle becomes compressed against the tentorial edge, resulting in **ipsilateral paresis**, a false-localizing sign.

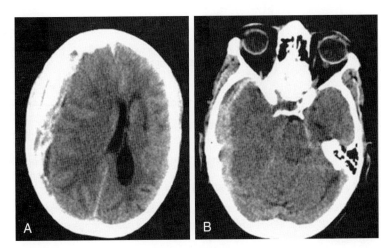

FIGURE 7.10 Axial brain CT scans showing (A) an extensive right hemispheric acute subdural hematoma, causing a 2-cm-midline shift and (B) a right uncal herniation with deformation of both cerebral peduncles and obliteration of the perimesencephalic cisterns. Source: *Carrasco R. Kernohan-Woltman notch phenomenon caused by an acute subdural hematoma. J Clin Neurosci 16(12):1628–31.*

- **Substantia nigra**
  - Immediately dorsal to the cerebral peduncles, and composed of the **pars compacta** and **pars reticulata.**
  - Communicates with the **basal ganglia** and other structures through **dopaminergic** signalling.
    - Reduction in pigmented dopaminergic neurons within the substantia nigra results in **Parkinson disease.**
- **Red nucleus**
  - Immediately dorsal to the substantia nigra in the tegmentum of the midbrain, this nucleus receives **crossed cerebellar input** via the superior cerebellar peduncles as they decussate in the midbrain.
  - Efferent fibres give rise to the **rubrospinal tract**, which conveys impulses that affect **flexor tone** on the contralateral side (ipsilateral to the cerebellar input of red nucleus).

BRAINSTEM RETICULAR FORMATION

A complex network of polysynaptic cells with extensive axonal and dendritic connectivity is known as the **reticular formation** (Fig. 7.11). The reticular formation extends throughout the brainstem and sends input diffusely throughout the cerebral cortex, the diencephalon and caudally into the spinal cord. Its function spans several systems including **motor control, wakefulness,**

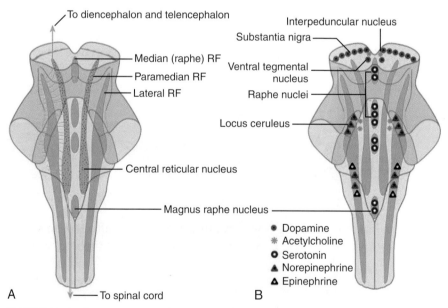

FIGURE 7.11   Reticular formation (RF). (A) Subdivisions; (B) aminergic and cholinergic cell groups. Source: *Mtui E, MD. Reticular formation. Fitzgerald's clinical neuroanatomy and neuroscience. p. 230–42, Chapter 24.*

cardiorespiratory centres and pain sensation. Uniquely, while many functional systems pass through the thalamus as a relay to exert influence on the cerebral cortex, the reticular formation contains outputs that project to the thalamus as well as direct projections to the cerebral cortex.

- **Median** reticular formation
  - **Raphe nuclei**, serotonergic projections
- **Paramedian** reticular formation
  - **Magnocellular neurons** just lateral to midline in the pons and medulla, including **gigantocellular neurons**
  - Gives rise to the **pontine** and **medullary reticulospinal tracts**
- **Lateral** reticular formation
  - **Parvocellular zone** containing small cells receiving primarily afferent input that subsequently send signals to the central nuclei
    - Input to the reticular formation includes **olfactory**, **auditory**, **visual**, **vestibular** and **somatic information**
- Reticular formation function
  - **Motor control**
    - Pontine and medullary reticulospinal tracts
      - **Opposing influence on extensor muscle tone** via alpha and gamma motor neurons
        - **Pontine** reticulospinal tract **facilitates** extensor muscle tone
        - **Medullary** reticulospinal tract **inhibits** extensor muscle tone; cortical input to this tract helps facilitate its function
    - Patients with brainstem injury **caudal to the red nucleus** exhibit **extensor posturing**
      - Unopposed action of the pontine reticulospinal tract if cortical input to medullary reticulospinal tract is affected
  - **Pain modulation**
    - The **gating concept** of regulated transmission from reticular formation via **gamma aminobutyric acid (GABA) projections to the dorsal grey horns** of the spinal cord can affect the perception of pain in different circumstances (i.e. a soldier during battle may experience less pain depending on environmental factors)
  - **Wakefulness**
    - **Ascending reticular activating system** (ARAS) contains **noradrenergic** (originating in **locus ceruleus**), **serotonergic** and **cholinergic** neurons (as well as others) and exerts influence on sleep-wake cycles and arousal through thalamic and cortical influence
  - **Cardiorespiratory function**
    - The **dorsal** and **ventral medullary respiratory centres** and the **pontine pneumotaxic centre**, as well as neurons involving cardiac function, are all held under influence by the reticular formation and reticulospinal tracts; input via the carotid sinus and blood carbon dioxide or pH influence these functions

CASE STUDY DISCUSSION

The child exhibits signs of cranial nerve dysfunction (6th nerve palsy), vomiting and ataxia, signs and symptoms that are concerning for a pontine lesion. A brainstem biopsy was performed to obtain a tissue diagnosis of the lesion, which was found to be a **diffuse intrinsic pontine glioma (DIPG)** *(see Fig. 1.22 of chapter 1).*

CHAPTER 8

Cranial Nerves

Mohammad Shehade, Nour Estaitieh

CASE STUDY

Presentation and Physical Examination: An 18-year-old female patient with a history of recurrent sinusitis presented with the acute onset of fever, headache, diplopia, pain and decreased vision in her left eye.

On physical examination, she had low-grade fever of 38.5°C with stable vital signs. Neck examination showed minimal terminal stiffness. She was found to have left eye ptosis and proptosis, engorged conjunctiva and periorbital oedema. She also had anisocoria (pupils of unequal size) with a right pupil of 3 mm and a left of 5–6 mm. The direct pupillary reflex was normal on the right side, whereas the consensual was sluggish. On the left, both direct and consensual reflexes were sluggish. She was unable to move her left eye in any direction, while her right eye had a full range of motion. She had diminished sensation to all modalities in the left forehead and middle part of the face but normal sensation in the lower face. Funduscopy revealed left papilloedema. There was no bruit heard over the eye.

Try to guess the most probable location and aetiology of this young patient's symptoms after studying this chapter!

BRIEF INTRODUCTION

Twelve pairs of cranial nerves (CNs) exist in humans. Each has a specific name and is also referred to by a **roman number**. CNs are divided into three categories depending on their function.

- **Pure sensory:** olfactory (I), optic (II) and vestibulocochlear (VIII)
- **Pure motor:** oculomotor (III), trochlear (IV), abducens (VI), accessory (XI) and hypoglossal (XII)
- **Mixed motor and sensory:** trigeminal (V), facial (VII), glossopharyngeal (IX) and vagus (X)

The olfactory nerve is the only afferent sensory pathway that does not relay to the cerebral cortex through the thalamus. The vagus nerve is the only nerve that supplies structures outside the head and neck.

Sensory and motor nuclei of CNs are embedded in different parts of the **brainstem** (Figs. 8.1 and 8.2).

- **Somatic motor** (to skeletal muscles via general somatic efferent fibres) and **branchiomotor** (to muscles originating from branchial arches via special visceral efferent fibres) nuclei contain cell bodies of **efferent fibres** of motor CNs.

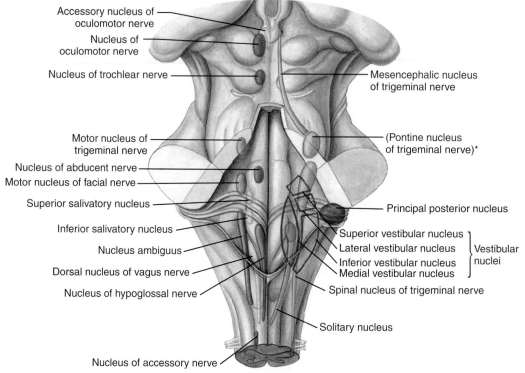

Accessory nucleus of
oculomotor nerve

Nucleus of
oculomotor nerve

Nucleus of trochlear nerve

Mesencephalic nucleus
of trigeminal nerve

Motor nucleus of
trigeminal nerve

(Pontine nucleus
of trigeminal nerve)*

Nucleus of abducent nerve

Motor nucleus of facial nerve

Superior salivatory nucleus

Principal posterior nucleus

Inferior salivatory nucleus

Superior vestibular nucleus
Lateral vestibular nucleus   } Vestibular
Inferior vestibular nucleus   } nuclei
Medial vestibular nucleus

Nucleus ambiguus

Dorsal nucleus of vagus nerve

Nucleus of hypoglossal nerve

Spinal nucleus of trigeminal nerve

Solitary nucleus

Nucleus of accessory nerve

FIGURE 8.1   Cranial nerves nuclei; posterior view. With the exception of the cranial nerves I and II, all cranial nerves (III–XII) have nuclei located in the brainstem. The mesencephalon contains the nuclei of the cranial nerves III and IV, the nuclei of the cranial nerves V to VII lie in the pons, and the medulla oblongata contains the nuclei of the cranial nerves VII to XII. *Clinical term: principal sensory nucleus of trigeminal nerve.

Source: *Paulsen F. Brain and spinal cord. Sobotta atlas of human anatomy. vol. 3, p. 211–342, Chapter 12.*

- These nuclei receive **input** from the inferior part of the precentral gyrus **directly** through **corticobulbar** and **indirectly** through **corticoreticu- lobulbar fibres.**
- The majority of these fibres **cross to the opposite side** before reach- ing their target nuclei.
- All **motor CN nuclei** receive bilateral input from both cerebral hemispheres **except** for the **part of motor facial** nucleus supply- ing the **muscles of facial expression in the lower face** and the **part of hypoglossal** nucleus supplying the **genioglossus muscle**; these exceptions receive input from the **contralateral hemisphere** only.
- **Visceral motor** (to cardiac muscle, smooth muscles and glands via gen- eral visceral efferent fibres) nuclei contain cell bodies of efferent para- sympathetic pathways.
  - These nuclei include:
    - Edinger–Westphal (accessory) nucleus of CN III
    - Superior salivatory and lacrimal nuclei of CN VII

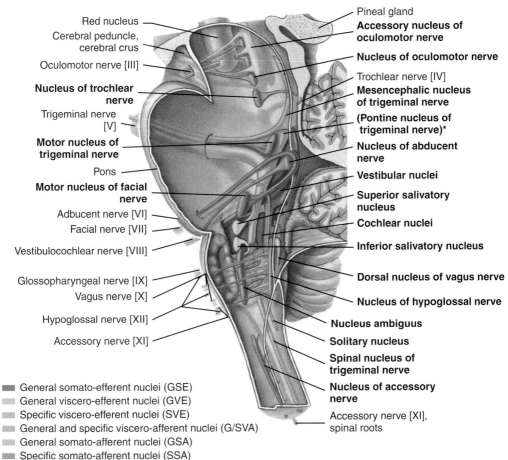

Red nucleus

Cerebral peduncle, cerebral crus

Oculomotor nerve [III]

Nucleus of trochlear nerve

Trigeminal nerve [V]

Motor nucleus of trigeminal nerve

Pons

Motor nucleus of facial nerve

Adbucent nerve [VI]

Facial nerve [VII]

Vestibulocochlear nerve [VIII]

Glossopharyngeal nerve [IX]

Vagus nerve [X]

Hypoglossal nerve [XII]

Accessory nerve [XI]

Pineal gland

Accessory nucleus of oculomotor nerve

Nucleus of oculomotor nerve

Trochlear nerve [IV]

Mesencephalic nucleus of trigeminal nerve

(Pontine nucleus of trigeminal nerve)*

Nucleus of abducent nerve

Vestibular nuclei

Superior salivatory nucleus

Cochlear nuclei

Inferior salivatory nucleus

Dorsal nucleus of vagus nerve

Nucleus of hypoglossal nerve

Nucleus ambiguus

Solitary nucleus

Spinal nucleus of trigeminal nerve

Nucleus of accessory nerve

Accessory nerve [XI], spinal roots

▬ General somato-efferent nuclei (GSE)
▬ General viscero-efferent nuclei (GVE)
▬ Specific viscero-efferent nuclei (SVE)
▬ General and specific viscero-afferent nuclei (G/SVA)
▬ General somato-afferent nuclei (GSA)
▬ Specific somato-afferent nuclei (SSA)

FIGURE 8.2   Cranial nerves; topographic overview of the nuclei of the cranial nerves III to XII in the median plane. Nuclei of origin with perikarya (cell bodies) of the efferent/motor fibres divide into: general somatoefferent nuclei (nuclei of oculomotor nerve [III, extraocular muscles], nucleus of trochlear nerve [IV, superior oblique], nucleus of abducent nerve [VI, lateral rectus], and nucleus of hypoglossal nerve [XII, muscles of the tongue]); general visceroefferent nuclei (accessory nuclei of oculomotor nerve or Edinger–Westphal nuclei [III, sphincter pupillae and ciliary muscle], superior salivatory nucleus [VII, submandibular, sublingual, lacrimal, nasal and palatine glands], inferior salivatory nucleus [IX, parotid gland], dorsal (posterior) nucleus of vagus nerve [X, viscera]); special visceroefferent nuclei (motor nucleus of trigeminal nerve [V, masticatory muscles, muscles of the floor of the mouth], motor nucleus of facial nerve [VII, mimic muscles], nucleus ambiguus [IX, X, cranial root of XI, pharyngeal and laryngeal muscles] and nucleus of accessory nerve [XI, spinal root, shoulder muscles]). Terminal nuclei are targeted by afferent/sensory fibres and divide into: general visceroafferent nuclei (nuclei of solitary tract, inferior part [IX, X, sensory innervation of smooth muscles (viscera)]); special visceroafferent nuclei (nuclei of solitary tract, superior part [VII, IX, X], taste fibres); general somatoafferent nuclei (mesencephalic nucleus of trigeminal nerve [V, proprioception of masticatory muscles], pontine (principal sensory) nucleus of trigeminal nerve [V, touch, vibration, position of temporomandibular joint], spinalis nucleus of trigeminal nerve [V, pain and temperature sensation in the head region]); special somatoafferent nuclei (superior, lateral, medial and inferior vestibular nuclei [VIII, vestibularis part, equilibrium] as well as anterior and posterior cochlear nuclei [VIII, cochlear part, hearing]). *Clinical term: principal sensory nucleus of trigeminal nerve.

Source: *Paulsen F. Brain and spinal cord. Sobotta atlas of human anatomy. vol. 3, p. 211–342, Chapter 12.*

- Inferior salivatory nucleus of CN IX
- Dorsal motor nucleus of vagus nerve
- They receive **input from the hypothalamus** through the descending autonomic pathways.
- **Sensory nuclei** contain cell bodies of **second-order neurons,** which receive axons of **first-order neurons** located in the **nerve ganglia.** These second-order neurons project to the **contralateral thalamic nuclei** and from there, the **third-order neurons** send their axons via the **internal capsule** to the **postcentral gyrus.** Sensory nuclei convey:
  - General sensation and proprioception via **general somatic afferent** fibres.
  - General sensation from visceral organs via **general visceral afferent** fibres.
  - Special sensations (vision and hearing) via **special somatic afferent** fibres.
  - Special sensory input (smell and taste) via **special visceral afferent** fibres.

OLFACTORY NERVE (CN I) (Fig. 8.3)

The **olfactory nerve** is formed by the centripetal unmyelinated axons of **bipolar neurons** in the upper nasal mucosa. The peripheral axons are connected to hair-like structures that react to **chemical odours** in the air. The olfactory nerve enters the anterior cranial fossa through the fenestrated **cribriform plate** to synapse on secondary neurons in an elongated structure attached to the basal surface of the brain known as the **olfactory bulb.**

CLINICAL INSIGHT

- **Cribriform plate fracture**
  - Fracture of the cribriform plate can lead to anosmia (loss of smell) in one or both of the olfactory nerves.

Axons of **mitral** and **tufted neurons,** collectively known as **projection neurons,** in the olfactory bulb form the **olfactory tract.**

- The olfactory tract courses posteriorly in the olfactory sulcus until it reaches the **anterior perforated substance.**
- There, the olfactory tract divides into medial and lateral olfactory striae.
  - The **lateral stria** projects on the **primary olfactory cortex** in the periamygdaloid and peripiriform areas.
  - The **medial stria** crosses through the anterior commissure to project on the **contralateral olfactory bulb.**

The primary olfactory cortex is connected to the **entorhinal cortex** (Brodmann area 28) of the **parahippocampal gyrus,** which is responsible for **appreciation of odours.**

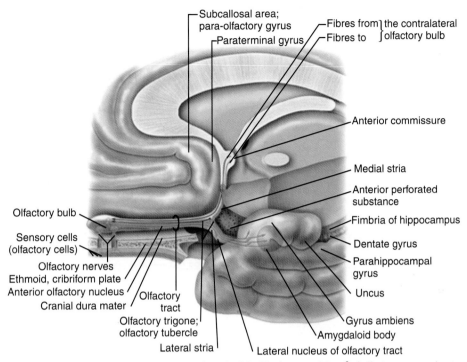

Subcallosal area;
para-olfactory gyrus
Paraterminal gyrus

Fibres from⌉ the contralateral
Fibres to ⌋ olfactory bulb

Anterior commissure

Medial stria

Anterior perforated
substance

Olfactory bulb

Sensory cells
(olfactory cells)

Fimbria of hippocampus

Dentate gyrus

Olfactory nerves
Ethmoid, cribriform plate
Anterior olfactory nucleus
Cranial dura mater

Olfactory
tract

Parahippocampal
gyrus

Uncus

Olfactory trigone;
olfactory tubercle

Gyrus ambiens
Amygdaloid body

Lateral stria

Lateral nucleus of olfactory tract

FIGURE 8.3   Olfactory nerve [I] and olfactory tract; view from the left side. An area of 3 cm^2 of olfactory mucosa locates to both sides at the roof of the nasal cavity. It contains approximately 30 million receptor cells (olfactory sensory cells) which respond to chemical signals. These are bipolar neurons. On one side, they connect with the outer environment, and on the other side, their axons form the olfactory nerves. The olfactory neurons have a short life span of 30–60 days and are replaced by neuronal stem cells throughout life. The olfactory nerves are collectively named olfactory nerve [I]. In each olfactory bulb, they converge onto approximately 1000 glomeruli. From here, the olfactory information reaches different areas at the cranial base and the temporal lobe (primary olfactory cortical area) and, through direct and indirect connections, projects to secondary olfactory cortical areas and other brain regions. That way, the conscious realization of olfactory stimuli and the connection with other sensory perceptions is accomplished.
Source: *Paulsen F. Brain and spinal cord. Sobotta atlas of human anatomy. vol. 3, p. 211–342, Chapter 12.*

OPTIC NERVE (CN II) (Fig. 8.4)

Formed by axons of **multipolar ganglion cells** of the retina, the **optic nerve** originates at the optic disc, travels posteromedially and exits the orbit through the optic canal. Since the retina is embryologically an outward extension of the central nervous system, the optic nerve is ensheathed by an **extension of brain meninges** and floats in the **cerebrospinal fluid (CSF).**

Shortly after leaving the orbit, the optic nerve meets the **contralateral nerve** and forms the **optic chiasm.**

- The optic chiasm is located just **anterior** to the **lamina terminalis below** the **genu of** the **corpus callosum.**
- At the optic chiasm, nerve fibres originating from the **nasal retina** cross to join nerve fibres originating from the **temporal retina** of the second eye (which remain uncrossed) and form the **optic tract.**

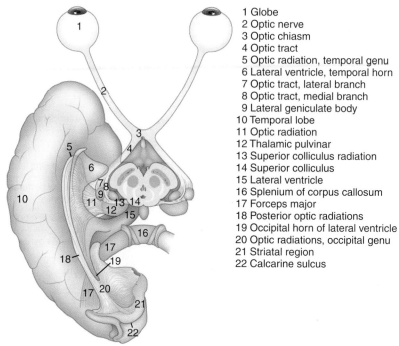

1 Globe
2 Optic nerve
3 Optic chiasm
4 Optic tract
5 Optic radiation, temporal genu
6 Lateral ventricle, temporal horn
7 Optic tract, lateral branch
8 Optic tract, medial branch
9 Lateral geniculate body
10 Temporal lobe
11 Optic radiation
12 Thalamic pulvinar
13 Superior colliculus radiation
14 Superior colliculus
15 Lateral ventricle
16 Splenium of corpus callosum
17 Forceps major
18 Posterior optic radiations
19 Occipital horn of lateral ventricle
20 Optic radiations, occipital genu
21 Striatal region
22 Calcarine sulcus

FIGURE 8.4 Visual system anatomy.

Source: *Nieuwenhuys R, Voogd J, van Huijen C. The human central nervous system: a synopsis and atlas. Rev 3rd ed. Berlin: Springer-Verlag; 1988.*

- Thus, the **optic tract** contains fibres originating from the **temporal retina of the ipsilateral eye** and the **nasal retina of the contralateral eye**.

The optic tract passes posterolaterally in the subarachnoid space around the cerebral peduncles to project on the **lateral geniculate nucleus (LGN) in the thalamus**. Before reaching the LGN, few fibres leave the pathway to project on the **pretectal nucleus** and **superior colliculus**. These fibres are involved in the **visual reflexes**.

Neurons of the lateral geniculate body project by means of the **optic radiation (geniculocalcarine tract)** to the **primary visual cortex (Brodmann area 17)**, which lies on the banks of the calcarine sulcus in the **mesial occipital lobe**.

- Fibres originating from the **upper retina** are directed posteriorly and lateral to the trigone of the lateral ventricle to project on the **upper calcarine bank**.
- Fibres originating from the **lower retina** project anteriorly in the roof of the temporal horn, then loop backward (**Meyer's loop**) to project on the **lower calcarine bank**.
- As a result, the visual cortex in the upper calcarine bank is connected to the upper temporal retina in the ipsilateral eye and the upper nasal retina in the contralateral eye and allows the visualization of the lower quadrant in the contralateral hemifield.
- Similarly, the lower calcarine bank visualizes the upper quadrant of the contralateral hemifield.

- The **macula** projects **posteriorly** whereas the **peripheral retina** projects **anteriorly** along the visual cortex.
- The macular area receives **dual blood supply** from the posterior cerebral (PCA) and the middle cerebral (MCA) arteries. Thus, it is usually spared in PCA strokes.

OCULOMOTOR NERVE (CN III)

Oculomotor nerve fibres arise from two nuclei located in the **midbrain** (Figs. 8.1 and 8.2).

- **Main motor nucleus**
  - Located in the **periaqueductal grey matter** at the level of the superior colliculus.
  - Supplies all **extraocular muscles except** the **superior oblique** and **lateral rectus** muscles.
  - Receives **input** from:
    - Cerebral hemispheres through the **corticobulbar tract**
    - Superior colliculus – and visual cortex indirectly – through the **tectonuclear tract**
  - Interacts with **CNs IV, VI and VIII nuclei** through the **medial longitudinal fasciculus (MLF)**.
- **Edinger–Westphal (accessory parasympathetic) nucleus**
  - Located just **posterior to the motor nucleus**.
  - Receives **corticobulbar** fibres and fibres from the **pretectal nucleus**.
  - Its **preganglionic parasympathetic** fibres accompany **CN III** to the orbit where they project on the **ciliary ganglion** (Fig. 8.5).
  - **Postganglionic** fibres form the **short ciliary nerves**, which supply the **pupillary constrictors** and **other ciliary muscles**.

The oculomotor nerves, together with the parasympathetic fibres, pass directly forward through the **red nuclei** (Fig. 8.2) to emerge from the anterior surface of the midbrain in the **interpeduncular fossa**.

- Along the oculomotor nerve, **parasympathetic** fibres are located at the **periphery** whereas **motor** fibres travel at the **centre**.
- The oculomotor nerve passes between the PCA and the superior cerebellar artery (SCA) before entering the lateral wall of the cavernous sinus.

CLINICAL INSIGHT

- **Diabetic versus vascular lesions of CN III**
  - Posterior communication artery (PCom) aneurysms, basilar artery aneurysms and uncal herniation may compress the oculomotor nerve. Since the parasympathetic fibres are peripherally situated, the patient develops **mydriasis (dilated pupil)** on the **ipsilateral** side **before** the **onset of motor weakness**. Conversely, **vascular lesions** (such as those seen in **diabetes**) preferentially damage the centrally located motor fibres and cause **oculomotor weakness** with relative **sparing** of **pupillary-motor function** (pupillary-sparing CN III palsy).

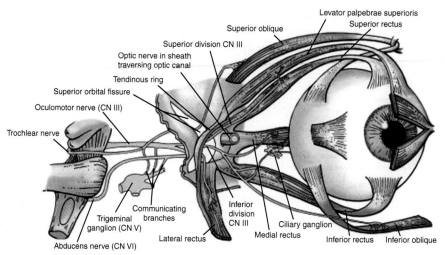

FIGURE 8.5 Anatomic structures subserving eye movements: lateral view of the right eye. The oculomotor nerve (CN III), trochlear nerve (CN IV) and abducens nerve (CN VI) arise from the brainstem. After passing through the subarachnoid space and cavernous sinus, they enter the orbit through the superior orbital fissure. The oculomotor nerve divides into superior and inferior divisions, and ultimately innervates the superior rectus, inferior rectus, medial rectus, inferior oblique (shown cut) and levator palpebrae muscles. In addition, parasympathetic fibres of the third nerve synapse in the ciliary ganglion, then innervate the pupillary constrictor muscle. The trochlear nerve innervates the superior oblique muscle. The abducens nerve innervates the lateral rectus muscle (shown cut).
Source: *Adapted from Agur AMR, Dalley AF. Grant's atlas of anatomy. 12th ed. Philadelphia: Lippincott, Williams & Wilkins; 2009; with permission.*

The oculomotor nerve passes in the lateral wall of the **cavernous sinus** (Fig. 8.6), where it divides into **superior** and **inferior rami**.

- These rami enter the orbit through the **superior orbital fissure**.
- The **motor** component supplies the **levator palpebrae**, the **superior, medial** and **inferior recti,** which are responsible for lifting the eyelid, turning the eye upwards, inwards and downwards, respectively (Fig. 8.5). It also supplies the **inferior oblique**, which is an ocular external rotator, elevator and abductor.

Through the short ciliary branches, the oculomotor nerve constricts the pupil and controls the lens thickness during accommodation.

Visual Body Reflex

Several types of the **visual body reflex** exist. These include:
- Involuntary movement of the eyes, head and neck towards a visual stimulus
- Involuntary movements of the eyes and head while reading
- Involuntary raising the hand and closing the eyes (as a protective mechanism) in response to a visual stimulus

Visual impulses are carried by the optic nerve, chiasm and tract to the **superior colliculus**, from which the following tracts arise:
- **Tectobulbar tract**, which projects on CNs III, IV, VI, VII and XI

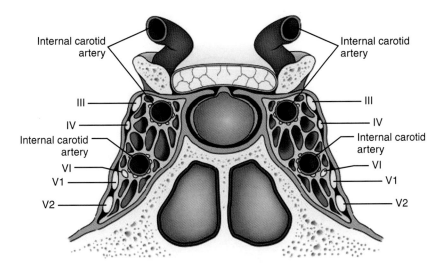

FIGURE 8.6 The cavernous sinus, harbouring cranial nerves III, IV, V and VI, as well as the internal carotid artery, cradle the two sides of the pituitary gland.
Source: *(Image modified from Nelson Oyesiku). Bi WL. Pituitary surgery. Endocrinology: adult and pediatric. p. 275–90.e4, Chapter 16.*

- **Tectospinal tract**, which projects on alpha motor neurons in the anterior horn of the spinal cord

Commands from these tracts eventually reach muscles responsible for appropriate eyes, head and neck movements.

TROCHLEAR NERVE (CN IV)

The **trochlear nerve** is the only CN that emerges from the posterior surface of the brainstem (Fig. 8.7). The **trochlear nucleus** is located in the **anterior** part of the **periaqueductal grey matter** at the level of the inferior colliculus (Figs. 8.1, 8.2 and 8.7).

- Receives **corticobulbar input** from both cerebral hemispheres
- Receives **tectobulbar input** from the **superior colliculus**
- Connected to CNs III, VI and VIII via the **MLF**

When the trochlear nerve leaves the nucleus, it **turns backwards** around the cerebral aqueduct to emerge from the **posterior surface** of the brainstem. Then, it **decussates** to the opposite side and passes forward to enter the **lateral wall of the cavernous sinus** (Fig. 8.6). It enters the orbit through the **superior orbital fissure** to supply one muscle, the **superior oblique muscle**, which is responsible for turning the eye globe downwards and lateral with internal rotation (Fig. 8.5).

CLINICAL INSIGHT

- **Trochlear nerve injury**
  - Patients with injury to the trochlear nerve develop **double vision when looking downwards**. Consequently, they typically report difficulty when going down the stairs.

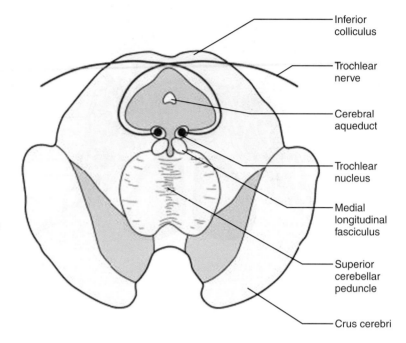

Inferior colliculus

Trochlear nerve

Cerebral aqueduct

Trochlear nucleus

Medial longitudinal fasciculus

Superior cerebellar peduncle

Crus cerebri

FIGURE 8.7 Transverse section through the midbrain at the level of the inferior colliculus. The diagram shows the location of the trochlear nucleus and the course of trochlear nerve fibres.
Source: *Crossman AR, PhD DSc. Cranial nerves and cranial nerve nuclei. Neuro-anatomy: an illustrated colour text.* p. 102–16, Chapter 10.

TRIGEMINAL NERVE (CN V)

The **trigeminal nerve** is the **largest** CN. It has **major sensory** and **minor motor** components. The trigeminal nerve has **three sensory nuclei** and **one motor nucleus** (Figs. 8.1 and 8.2):

- **Mesencephalic nucleus:**
  - Located in the **lateral periaqueductal grey matter** in the caudal mesencephalon at the level of the inferior colliculus.
  - Reaches down to the main sensory nucleus.
  - Conveys **kinaesthesia** (proprioceptive sensation) from the **muscles of mastication** (masseter, temporalis, medial and lateral pterygoids).
- **Main sensory (pontine) nucleus:**
  - Located in the **posterior pons**.
  - Receives fibres that mediate **tactile** and **pressure sensation** from almost the **whole face**.
  - Is continuous with the spinal nucleus caudally.
- **Spinal nucleus:**
  - Extends from **C2 level** in the upper cervical cord and crosses the whole medulla to reach the **caudal pons** where it is continuous with the main sensory nucleus.
  - Receives fibres that mediate **pain** and **temperature sensation** from different parts of the face; these fibres follow what is referred to as **'onion skin distribution'** (Fig. 8.8).
    - Fibres from the **most anterior part** of the face (nose, cheeks and lips) synapse with cells of the **most cranial part** (at caudal pons) of the spinal nucleus.

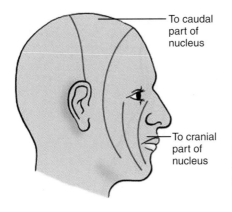

To caudal part of nucleus

To cranial part of nucleus

FIGURE 8.8 'Onion-skin' representation of the facial areas in the spinal nucleus of the trigeminal nerve. Fibres from the most anterior part of the face synapse with cells of the most cranial part of the nucleus.
Source: *Sinnatamby CS, FRCS. Head and neck and spine. Last's anatomy. p. 329–454, Chapter 6.*

- Fibres with the **peripheral face** (scalp, ears and chin) synapse with cells of the **most caudal part** (at upper cervical cord and lower medulla) of the spinal nucleus.
- **Motor nucleus:**
  - Located **medial to the main sensory nucleus in the pons**.
  - Receives **corticobulbar** and **corticoreticulobulbar** fibres from both cerebral hemispheres, and fibres from the MLF, tectum and mesencephalic nucleus.
  - Supplies muscles of mastication, tensor tympani, tensor veli palatini, mylohyoid muscle and anterior belly of the digastric muscle.

The trigeminal nerve emerges from the **anterolateral surface** of the mid-pons as a **large sensory** root and a **small motor** root. Both roots travel anteriorly until they reach the upper border of the petrous apex where the sensory root enlarges into the **semilunar (Gasserian) ganglion**. The Gasserian ganglion sits inside a dural pouch, **Meckel's cave,** and gives rise to three nerves (Fig. 8.9).
- **Ophthalmic nerve (V1)** (Figs. 8.9 and 8.10):
  - Travels in the **lateral wall of the cavernous sinus** (Fig. 8.6) and gives rise to three branches: nasociliary, lacrimal and frontal. All three branches enter the orbit through the **superior orbital fissure.**
  - Supplies the conjunctiva, skin over the forehead, upper eyelids and much of the external surface of the nose.
  - The supraorbital division of the frontal branch supplies the scalp posteriorly as far as the lambdoid suture.
- **Maxillary nerve (V2)** (Figs. 8.9 and 8.10):
  - Exits the cranium through the **foramen rotundum** to enter the **pterygopalatine fossa**, where it gives rise to the infraorbital and the zygomatic nerves as well as other smaller branches.
    - The **infraorbital nerve** emerges from the orbit through the **inferior orbital foramen** to supply the skin extending from the lower eyelid to the upper lip.

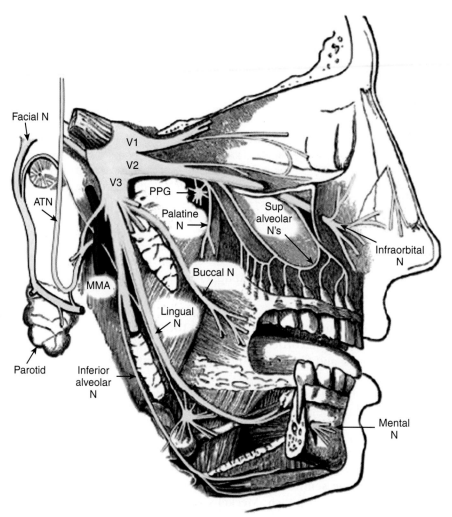

FIGURE 8.9   Cranial nerve V anatomy. Cranial nerve V divides into the ophthalmic (V1), maxillary (V2) and mandibular (V3) branches in the Meckel cave. V1 passes through the cavernous sinus lateral wall and enters the orbit via the superior orbital fissure. V2 passes through the cavernous sinus and exits the skull via foramen rotundum. V3 exits the skull via foramen ovale and enters the masticator space, where it gives off sensory and muscular branches. The auriculotemporal nerve arises from V3 via two roots that encircle the middle meningeal artery and then form a single root, which enters the parotid gland and intermingles with branches of cranial nerve VII. ATN, auriculotemporal nerve; MMA, middle meningeal artery; N, nerve; PPG, pterygopalatine ganglion.

Source: *Moonis G, MD. Patterns of perineural tumor spread in head and neck cancer. Mag Reson Imaging Clin North Am 20(3):435–46.*

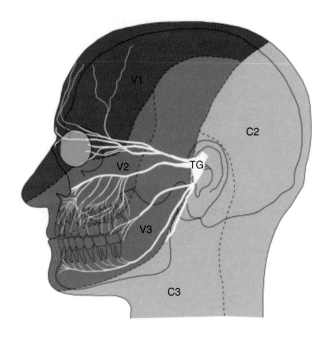

FIGURE 8.10 Innervation of cranio- and orofacial tissues by the three branches of the trigeminal nerve (TG): the ophthalmic (V1), maxillary (V2) and mandibular (V3) divisions. Some parts of the head receive their sensory innervation from branches of the upper cervical nerves (C2 and C3). Each division supplies one of the three different dermatomes of the face and the underlying deeper mucosal, vascular, muscular and meningeal tissues. TG, trigeminal ganglion.

Source: *Villanueva L. Trigeminal mechanisms of nociception. Wall & Melzack's textbook of pain. p. 793–802, Chapter 56.*

- The **zygomatic nerve** passes through the **lateral orbital wall** to supply the prominence over the cheek and the skin over the temple.
- The small branches supply the nose, palate and pharynx.
■ **Mandibular nerve (V3)** (Figs. 8.9 and 8.10):
  ■ Exits the skull through the **foramen ovale** and takes a downward direction to enter the **infratemporal fossa**.
  ■ Is a mixed motor and sensory nerve.
  ■ The **motor** component travels alone from the brainstem and is located medial to the ganglion.
    - Passes through and joins the mandibular nerve just distal to the foramen ovale.
    - Supplies the muscles of mastication, tensor tympani, tensor veli palatini, mylohyoid and anterior belly of the digastric muscle.
  ■ The **sensory** component transmits somatic sensory sensation from the mandibular gum and teeth, external meatus and tympanic membrane, lower lip and lower face, anterior two-thirds of the tongue and floor of the oral cavity.

Afferent axons of **second-order neurons** in the trigeminal sensory (spinal, main sensory and mesencephalic) nuclei cross to the opposite side and ascend through the **trigeminal lemniscus,** which travels with the **medial lemniscus** and is sometimes referred to as its cephalic division, to project on the **ventral posteromedial (VPM) nucleus** of the **thalamus. Third-order thalamic neurons** then travel through the internal capsule and project onto the **postcentral gyrus** (Fig. 8.11).

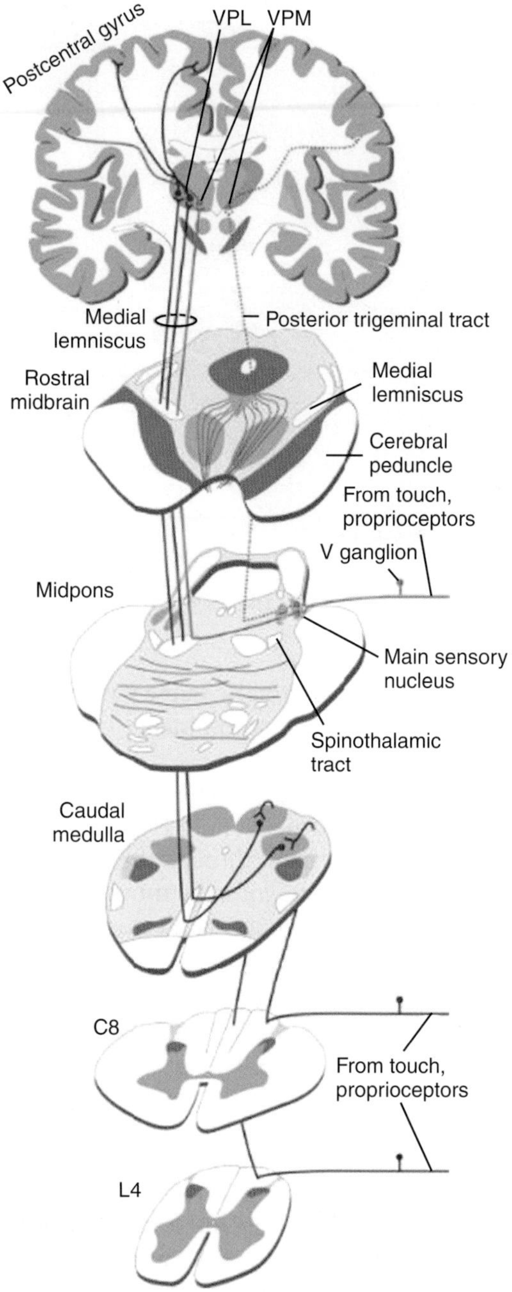

FIGURE 8.11 Ascending trigeminal pathways from the main sensory nucleus. VPL, ventral posterolateral nucleus; VPM, ventral posteromedial nucleus.
Source: *Vanderah TW, PhD. Cranial nerves and their nuclei. Nolte's the human brain. p. 301–28, Chapter 12.*

ABDUCENS NERVE (CN VI)

The **nucleus for the abducens nerve** is located in the **lower pons** and lies **beneath the upper half of the fourth ventricular floor** (Figs. 8.1 and 8.2). The abducens nerve is **purely motor** and innervates only one muscle, the **lateral rectus**, which is responsible for moving the eye laterally.

- The abducens nucleus is connected to CNs III, IV and VIII by means of the **MLF**. It receives input from:
  - Both cerebral hemispheres
  - Superior colliculus
- Fibres travel directly forward from the nucleus, and the nerve emerges from the **anterior surface** of the brainstem at the junction between the pons and medulla oblongata.
- The abducens nerve then travels through the **cavernous sinus** (Fig. 8.6) and enters the orbit through the **superior orbital fissure** where it supplies the lateral rectus muscle (Fig. 8.5.)

CLINICAL INSIGHT

- **Abducens nerve injury**
  - The abducens nerve has the **longest trajectory in the cranium**. Therefore, it is vulnerable to injury in patients with **increased intracranial pressure (ICP)**. Unilateral or bilateral CN VI palsy (inability to move the eye laterally) is frequently associated with increased ICP due to hydrocephalus or head trauma.

FACIAL NERVE (CN VII) (Figs. 8.1, 8.2 and 8.12)

The **facial nerve** contains fibres originating from the following nuclei:
- **Main motor nucleus**: supplies the facial, stapedius and posterior belly of the digastric muscles
- **Parasympathetic nuclei**, i.e. **superior salivary nucleus** and **lacrimal nucleus**
- **Sensory nucleus:**
  - Occupies the **upper part** of the **nucleus solitarius**
  - Is mainly responsible for **taste sensation** in the **anterior two-thirds** of the tongue

Sensory Component

Sensory information is carried by the **nervus intermedius**, whose cell bodies are located in the **geniculate ganglion** (Fig. 8.12). It transmits two types of sensory information:
- **Somatic sensation from the external ear:**
  - Projects onto the **spinal trigeminal nucleus**
  - Afferent fibres project on the contralateral **VPM nucleus of the thalamus** and from there to the somatosensory cortex in the **postcentral gyrus**
- **Specialized sensation (taste)** from taste buds in the **anterior two-thirds** of the tongue that projects onto the **gustatory part** of the **upper nucleus solitarius** (Fig. 8.12).

Motor Component

- The facial nerve has two types of motor fibres:
  - **Somatic motor** component composed of fibres that form the **motor root.**

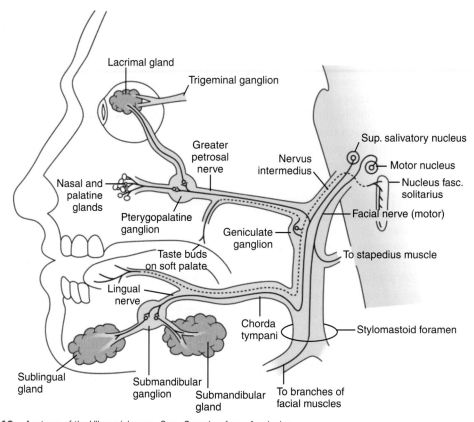

FIGURE 8.12   Anatomy of the VII cranial nerve. Sup., Superior; fasc., fasciculus.
Source: *Bertorini TE, MD. A woman with unilateral facial weakness. Neuromuscular case studies, CASE 29, p. 218–21.*

- **Visceral motor** component composed of **parasympathetic preganglionic** fibres that travel with the **nervus intermedius.**
- The **somatic motor** fibres supply muscles of facial expression, stapedius muscle that controls the quality of hearing, as well as the stylohyoid and the posterior belly of the digastric muscles (Fig. 8.12).
  - These fibres arise from the **main motor nucleus** at the level of the lower pons.
  - Initially, they course posteromedially and **bend around the abducens nucleus** beneath the upper part of the floor of the fourth ventricle forming the **facial colliculus** (Fig. 8.2).
  - Then, they course ventrolaterally to emerge off the **lateral surface** of the pons into the cerebellopontine angle.
  - Neurons in the facial motor nucleus are somatotopically distributed into the following divisions:
    - **Dorsal** division: neurons supplying **upper facial muscles.**
    - **Lateral** division: neurons supplying **lower facial muscles.**
    - **Medial** division: neurons supplying the **platysma** and **auricular muscles.**

- The facial motor nucleus receives several inputs:
  - **Cerebral cortex:**
    - Through the **corticobulbar tract** and to a lesser extent through the **corticoreticulobulbar** pathways.
    - The **dorsal** division of the nucleus, supplying the **upper** facial muscles, receives input from **both cerebral hemispheres.**
    - The **lateral** division, supplying the **lower** facial muscles, receives input from the **contralateral hemisphere only.**

CLINICAL INSIGHT

- **Central versus peripheral facial paresis**
  - In the **peripheral** type, the injury is **at or distal to the motor nucleus. All muscles** of facial expression are affected in the **ipsilateral** face.
  - In the **central** type, the injury is **above the nucleus** resulting in paralysis of the **lower facial muscles contralateral** to the site of injury (since upper facial muscles also receive input from the intact corticobulbar tract).

  - **Basal ganglia**
  - **Superior colliculus** (via the **tectobulbar tract**): Part of the **visual reflex arc**, this pathway is responsible for blinking when an object approaches the eye
  - **Sensory nucleus of the trigeminal nucleus**
  - **Superior olive:** Responsible for **reflex grimacing** in response to **loud noise**

CLINICAL INSIGHT

- **Corneal reflex**
  - It is the closure of **both** eyelids upon touching the cornea on **either side**. The afferent component travels through the **ophthalmic division of the trigeminal nerve** to the main sensory nucleus. The latter sends fibres through the **MLF** to **both motor facial nuclei**, which in turn stimulate the contraction of both orbicularis oculi, thus closing both eyelids.

- The **visceral motor** fibres arise from the **parasympathetic nuclei.** These are located in the **pontine tegmentum** posterolateral to the motor nucleus and include the superior salivatory nucleus and the lacrimal nucleus.
  - The **superior salivatory nucleus** receives input from the **hypothalamus** and **taste information** from the **solitary nucleus.**
  - The **lacrimal nucleus** receives input from the **hypothalamus** for **emotional lacrimation** and from the **sensory nucleus of the trigeminal nerve** for **reflex lacrimation.**
  - The **preganglionic fibres do not form a genu** inside the brainstem (Fig. 8.2) and join the **nervus intermedius** along with the sensory fibres. Distal to the geniculate ganglion, they join the motor root.

- Lacrimal fibres join the greater petrosal nerve distally and synapse on the pterygopalatine ganglion before supplying the lacrimal glands (Fig. 8.12).
- Salivary fibres join the chorda tympani and the lingual nerve distally and synapse on the submandibular ganglion, which supplies the submandibular and sublingual glands (Fig. 8.12).

CLINICAL INSIGHT

- **Crocodile tears**
  - **Crocodile tears** occur with injury to the facial nerve **proximal** to the **geniculate ganglion**. **Aberrant regrowth** of salivation fibres towards the lacrimal gland leads to lacrimation **upon eating**.

Course of the Facial Nerve (Fig. 8.12)

The two roots of the facial nerve emerge from the **anterolateral surface** of the pons at the **junction between the pons and medulla**.

- They accompany the vestibulocochlear nerve laterally through the **cerebellopontine angle** to enter the **internal acoustic meatus** in the petrous part of the temporal bone.
- Then, the facial nerve courses in the **facial canal** laterally. Upon reaching the medial border of the tympanic membrane, it expands to give rise to the **geniculate ganglion**.
  - At the geniculate ganglion, **lacrimal fibres** leave through the greater petrosal branch to synapse on the **pterygopalatine ganglion**.
- The nerve, then, turns sharply backwards and downwards. At the posterior wall of the tympanic cavity, it turns downwards on the medial side of the mastoid antrum to emerge from the **stylomastoid foramen**.
- During this downwards course, it gives rise to the **stapedius branch** and then the **chorda tympani** before reaching the stylomastoid foramen.
  - The chorda tympani contains **peripheral afferents** of the sensory neurons in the geniculate ganglion, which supply **taste buds** in the **anterior two-thirds** of the tongue, in addition to **parasympathetic efferents** to the **submandibular** ganglion, which in turn supplies the submandibular and sublingual salivary glands.
- After emerging from the stylomastoid foramen, the facial nerve gives rise to **five main branches** at the angle of the mandible to supply **muscles of facial expression**. From **superior to inferior**, these branches are as follows (Fig. 8.13):
  - Temporal
  - Zygomatic
  - Buccal
  - Marginal mandibular
  - Cervical

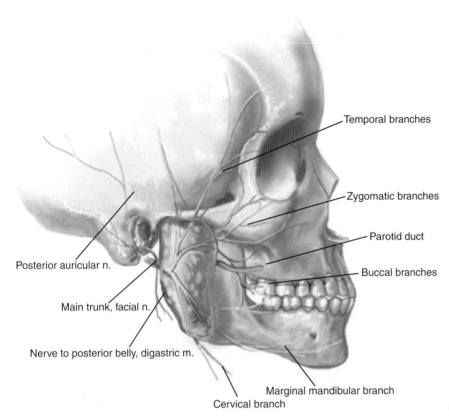

Temporal branches

Zygomatic branches

Parotid duct

Posterior auricular n.

Buccal branches

Main trunk, facial n.

Nerve to posterior belly, digastric m.

Marginal mandibular branch

Cervical branch

FIGURE 8.13 Anatomy of facial nerve branches innervating the facial muscles.
Source: *Herford A. Soft Tissue injuries. Oral and maxillofacial surgery. p. 283–300, Chapter 17.*

CLINICAL INSIGHT

- **Facial nerve lesions**
    - Facial nerve injury (Bell palsy) can be anatomically divided into three levels:
        - **Proximal to the geniculate ganglion**
        - **Distal to the geniculate ganglion**
        - **Stylomastoid foramen**
    - Each level presents with different signs and symptoms.
        - Proximal to the geniculate ganglion, i.e. from the facial nucleus until the geniculate ganglion). This leads to:
            - Paralysis of all muscles of facial expression (upper and lower face)
            - Loss of taste in the anterior two-thirds of the ipsilateral half of the tongue
            - Impaired lacrimation in the ipsilateral eye
            - Hyperacusis (increased sensitivity to sounds) in the ipsilateral ear due to paralysis of the ipsilateral stapedius muscle
            - Impaired salivary secretion by the ipsilateral submandibular and sublingual glands

- Crocodile tears (may occur at a later stage)
- Distal to the geniculate ganglion, i.e. from the geniculate ganglion until before the branching of chorda tympani. **Lacrimation** is **preserved**, but patients will suffer from:
  - Paralysis of all the muscles of facial expression in the ipsilateral face (upper and lower face)
  - Loss of taste in the anterior two-thirds of the ipsilateral half of the tongue
  - Hyperacusis in the ipsilateral ear
  - Impaired salivation in the ipsilateral submandibular and sublingual glands
- Stylomastoid foramen, i.e. from the branching point of chorda tympani until the mastoid foramen. **Parasympathetic preganglionic** and **taste fibres** as well as **fibres innervating the stapedius muscle** are preserved. Injury at this level leads to:
  - Isolated pure motor paralysis involving all muscles of facial expression in the ipsilateral face; both voluntary and involuntary pathways are affected.

VESTIBULOCOCHLEAR NERVE (VIII) (see chapter 14)

The **vestibulocochlear nerve** is **purely sensory**. It is composed of two separate nerves:

- The **vestibular nerve** responsible for **balance**
- The **cochlear nerve** responsible for **hearing**

They accompany the facial nerve from the internal acoustic meatus to the brainstem and enter the brainstem at the **pontomedullary junction** lateral to the facial nerve.

Vestibular Nerve

The **vestibular nerve** is composed of the axons of neurons originating from the **vestibular ganglion,** which extend to the internal acoustic meatus. They conduct impulses related to **static position of the head** from the **utricle** and **saccule** and **kinetic movement** of the head from the **semicircular canals.**

In the medulla, the vestibular nerve relays to the **vestibular nuclear complex** (composed of four nuclei: superior, lateral, medial and inferior) (Figs. 8.1 and 8.2). Few fibres **bypass** the nuclei to project on the cerebellum through the **inferior cerebellar peduncle**. Efferents from vestibular nuclei project to different areas:

- To the **cerebellum** through the **inferior cerebellar peduncle**
- To the **spinal cord** through the **vestibulospinal tract**
  - These two help to maintain posture and balance by regulating muscle tone in the limbs.
- To **CNs III, IV** and **VI nuclei** through the **MLF**
  - This is the pathway for the oculocephalic reflex, which helps to maintain fixation of eyes on a steady object despite the turning of the head
- Ascending fibres to the ventral posterior (VP) nucleus and then to the **cerebral cortex**, which allows for awareness of posture in the space

Cochlear Nerve (Fig. 8.14)

The **cochlear nerve** is formed by axons of neurons originating from the **spiral ganglion**, which extend to the internal auditory meatus.

- These neurons transmit hearing impulses from the organ of Corti located in the cochlea.
- Cochlear fibres project onto the **anterior (ventral)** and **posterior (dorsal) cochlear nuclei** located on the surface of **inferior cerebellar peduncle**.
  - The **ventral** nucleus mediates **low frequency** sounds.
  - The **dorsal** nucleus mediates **high frequency** sounds.

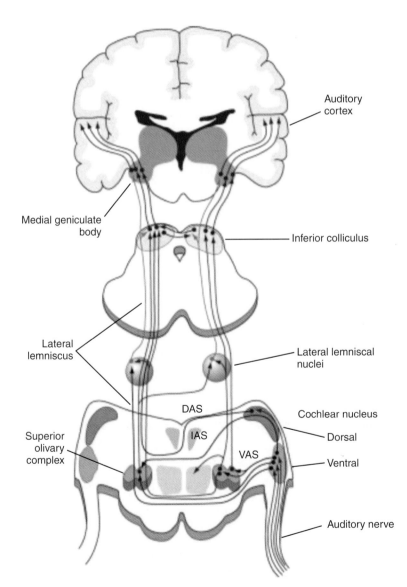

Auditory cortex

Medial geniculate body

Inferior colliculus

Lateral lemniscus

Lateral lemniscal nuclei

DAS

IAS

Cochlear nucleus

Dorsal

Superior olivary complex

VAS

Ventral

Auditory nerve

FIGURE 8.14 Illustration of the major central ascending auditory pathways for sound entering via the right cochlea. DAS, dorsal acoustic stria; IAS, intermediate acoustic stria; VAS, ventral acoustic stria. Source: *Runge CL. Anatomy of the auditory system. Cummings otolaryngology. p. 1987–1993.e2, Chapter 128.*

- Axons of the second-order neurons of the cochlear nerve form **three acoustic striae** (dorsal, intermediate and ventral), which proceed medially through the pontine tegmentum:
  - The **ventral stria (trapezoid body)** is the **largest**.
    - It contains fibres from the **ventral** nucleus.
    - Fibres in this stria project onto the **nucleus** of the **ipsilateral** and **contralateral trapezoid bodies** and the **superior olivary nucleus**.
    - **Third-order neurons** ascend forming the **lateral lemniscus** on both sides, but mostly on the **contralateral** side.
  - Fibres from the dorsal nucleus (**dorsal stria**) and fibres from the **intermediate stria** bypass the trapezoid and superior olivary nuclei and join the **lateral lemniscus** on the **opposite** side.
  - Lateral lemniscus fibres project to the **inferior colliculus** and from there to the **medial geniculate body**. The latter gives rise to the **auditory radiation** that reaches the **primary auditory cortex (Heschl's gyrus)** through the **sublenticular portion of the internal capsule**.

The auditory pathways decussate at least four times before reaching the auditory cortex; this explains why restricted lesions **above** the cochlear nuclei do not lead to hearing loss.

GLOSSOPHARYNGEAL NERVE (IX) (Fig. 8.15)

The **glossopharyngeal nerve** is a **mixed sensory** and **motor** nerve.

Efferent Pathway

The efferent pathway originates from two nuclei (Figs. 8.1, 8.2 and 8.15):
- **Motor nucleus** of the glossopharyngeal nerve

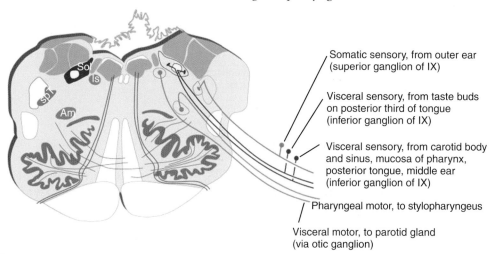

Somatic sensory, from outer ear
(superior ganglion of IX)

Visceral sensory, from taste buds
on posterior third of tongue
(inferior ganglion of IX)

Visceral sensory, from carotid body
and sinus, mucosa of pharynx,
posterior tongue, middle ear
(inferior ganglion of IX)

Pharyngeal motor, to stylopharyngeus

Visceral motor, to parotid gland
(via otic ganglion)

FIGURE 8.15   Fibre types in the glossopharyngeal nerve and their peripheral destinations. Am, nucleus ambiguus; Is, inferior salivary nucleus; Sol, nucleus of the solitary tract; spT, spinal trigeminal nucleus.

Source: *Vanderah TW, PhD. Cranial nerves and their nuclei. Nolte's the human brain. p. 301–28, Chapter 12.*

- Located in the **rostral part** of the **nucleus ambiguus** in the medulla
- Receives **corticobulbar input** from both cerebral hemispheres
- Supplies one muscle, the **stylopharyngeus muscle**
- **Inferior salivatory nucleus**
  - Located in the **dorsal medulla** in close association with the reticular formation
  - Receives **input** from:
    - Hypothalamus
    - **Taste information** from the **nucleus of the solitary tract**
    - **Olfactory information** through the **reticular formation**
  - Sends **preganglionic parasympathetic** fibres to the **otic ganglion**
  - Postganglionic fibres supply the **parotid gland**

Afferent Pathway

The afferent pathway is relayed to the brain by means of two nuclei (Figs. 8.1, 8.2 and 8.15):

- **Spinal trigeminal nucleus:**
  - Mediates **general somatic sensation** from the retroauricular area.
  - Cell bodies are located in the **superior ganglion** of the glossopharyngeal nerve at the level of the jugular foramen.
- **Nucleus solitarius**, which receives two types of visceral afferents:
  - **General visceral afferents** that convey **pain**, **temperature** and **tactile sensations** from the **posterior third** of the tongue, Eustachian tube and tonsils.
  - **Special visceral afferents** that convey **taste** from the **posterior third** of the tongue.

Efferent fibres from the nucleus solitarius cross midline and synapse on third-order neurons in the **ventral thalamus,** which project through the **internal capsule** to the **postcentral gyrus.**

Course of the Glossopharyngeal Nerve

The glossopharyngeal nerve emerges as **multiple rootlets** from the lateral border of the **medulla** between the olive and the inferior cerebellar peduncle (upper medulla).

- It exits through the jugular foramen (Fig. 8.16).
- At this level, it has two dilatations: the **superior** and **inferior ganglia.**
  - Distal to the ganglia, the **lesser petrosal nerve** carries **preganglionic parasympathetic** fibres to the **otic ganglion.**
  - Postganglionic fibres from the otic ganglion supply the parotid gland.
- In the neck, CN IX travels between the internal carotid artery and internal jugular vein until it reaches the posterior wall of the **stylopharyngeus muscle**. Then, it continues forward between the superior and middle pharyngeal constrictors to supply the **mucous membranes in the pharynx** and the **posterior third** of the tongue.

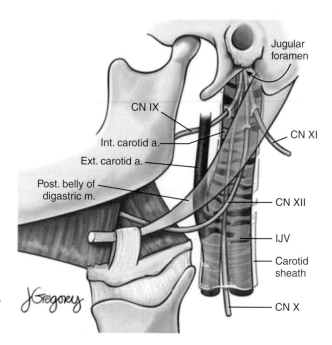

FIGURE 8.16   Lower cranial nerves (IX–XI) emerging through the jugular foramen. IJV, Internal jugular vein; Int., Internal; Ext., External; Post., Posterior; a., artery. Source: *Mourad WF. Oral Oncol 49(9):956–63.*

VAGUS NERVE (CN X)

The **vagus nerve** is a **mixed motor** and **sensory** nerve. It has four nuclei, all of which are located in the medulla (Figs. 8.1 and 8.2):

- **Dorsal motor nucleus of the vagus (parasympathetic)**
- **Ventral motor nucleus of the vagus**
- **Sensory nucleus (nucleus of tractus solitarius)**
- **Spinal nucleus of the trigeminal nerve**

Motor Component

The **motor** component of the vagus nerve is composed of **two nuclei**:

- **Dorsal motor nucleus of the vagus**
  This nucleus is specialized with parasympathetic activity.
  - It is located in the **dorsal** aspect of the lower medulla, beneath the caudal floor of the fourth ventricle and lateral to the hypoglossal nuclei.
  - It receives:
    - **Descending autonomic** fibres from the **hypothalamus**
    - **Collateral branches** from **carotid sinus fibres** of the glossopharyngeal nerve
  - **Preganglionic parasympathetic** fibres emerge from the **anterolateral** surface of the medulla between the olive and inferior cerebellar peduncle.
    - They provide **general visceral efferents** to the viscera of the thorax and abdomen as far down as the proximal two-thirds of the transverse colon.

- **Ventral motor nucleus of the vagus**
  It corresponds to the nucleus ambiguous, which also supplies muscles innervated by CNs IX and XI.
  - It receives **corticonuclear input** from both cerebral hemispheres.
  - Efferent fibres pass dorsomedially, and then turn venterolaterally to emerge from the **anterolateral** surface of the medulla between the inferior olive and the inferior cerebellar peduncle.
    - They supply the **constrictor muscles of the pharynx** and **intrinsic laryngeal muscles**.

Sensory Component

The sensory (afferent) component of the vagus nerve is relayed by two nuclei:
- **Spinal nucleus of the trigeminal nerve**
  - Cell bodies are located in the **superior ganglion of the vagus nerve**.
  - Conveys **tactile sensation** from the external ear.
- **Main sensory nucleus**
  - Corresponds to the **caudal part** of the **nucleus solitarius**.
  - Cell bodies are located in the **inferior ganglion of the vagus**.
  - It receives two types of visceral afferents:
    - **General visceral afferents**, which transmit **pain** and **temperature** from the pharynx, larynx, thoracic and abdominal viscera.
    - **Special visceral afferents**, which convey **taste sensation** from the **epiglottis**.
  - Fibres then cross to the **contralateral** side and ascend to project on the **contralateral thalamus** and from there to the **postcentral gyrus**.

Extramedullary Course of the Vagus Nerve

Upon leaving the medulla, the vagus nerve courses laterally to exit the skull through the jugular foramen (Fig. 8.16).
- At this level, it has two enlargements: the **superior** and **inferior ganglia**.
- In the neck, it travels in the **carotid sheath**, between the internal jugular vein and the internal and common carotid arteries to supply the pharynx and larynx.
- As it enters the thorax, the vagal nerve splits into **right** and **left branches** (Fig. 8.17).
  - The **left vagus nerve** passes **posterior** to the **left lung root**, and then **anterior to the oesophagus** contributing to the pulmonary, cardiac and oesophageal plexuses. It enters the abdomen through the **oesophageal hiatus** as the **anterior vagal trunk**, which supplies the anterior surface of the stomach, liver, pancreas and part of the duodenum.
  - The **right vagus nerve** descends on the right side **posterior** to the **right lung root** and the **oesophagus**. It contributes to the pulmonary, cardiac and oesophageal plexuses and enters the abdomen through the **oesophageal hiatus** as the **posterior vagal trunk**, which

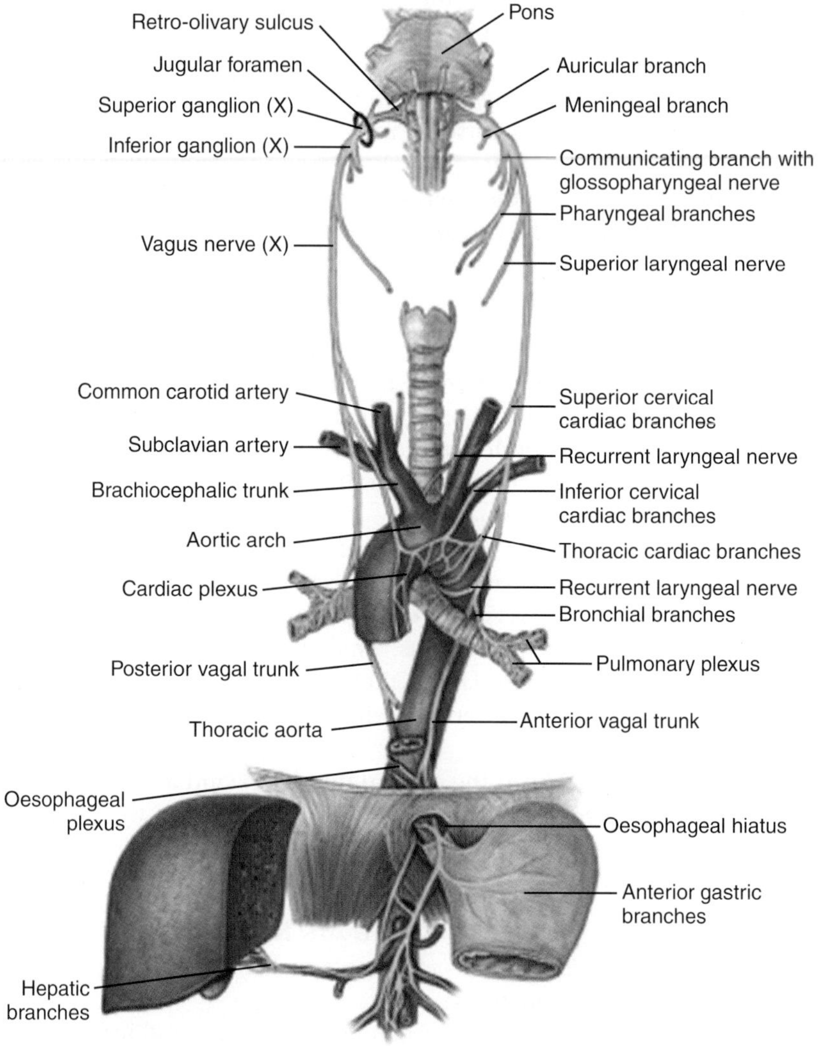

FIGURE 8.17   Vagus nerve [X]; anterior view. The image emphasizes the slightly different course of the right and left vagus nerves and the course of their branches until the anterior and posterior vagal trunks enter the abdominal cavity. Source: *Paulsen F. Brain and spinal cord. Sobotta atlas of human anatomy. vol. 3, p. 211–342, Chapter 12.*

supplies the posterior surface of the stomach. The **large celiac branch** supplies the liver, kidneys and intestines as far distal as the anterior **two-thirds** of the large colon.

CLINICAL INSIGHT

■ **Gag reflex**
   ■ The **gag reflex** is the contraction of the back of throat due to stimulation of the area surrounding the back of the tongue.
   ■ The **afferent limb** of the reflex arc is the **glossopharyngeal nerve**, whereas the **efferent limb** is the **glossopharyngeal** (stylopharyngeus muscle) and **vagus** (pharyngeal constrictors) **nerves**.

ACCESSORY NERVE (CN XI)

The **accessory nerve** has **two** roots: cranial and spinal (Fig. 8.18).

- **Cranial root**
  - Cell bodies are in the **caudal part** of the **nucleus ambiguus**.
  - They receive **bilateral corticonuclear** fibres.
  - Efferent fibres emerge from the **anterolateral** surface of the medulla between the inferior olive and the inferior cerebellar peduncle.

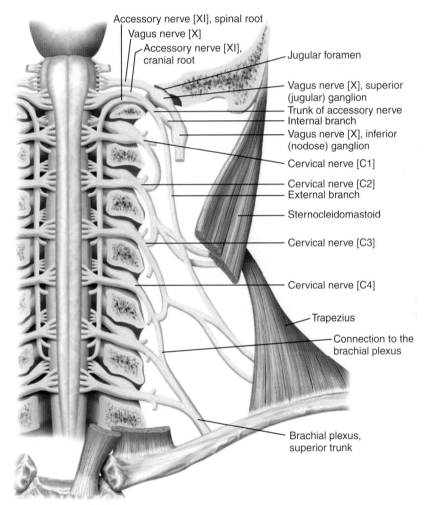

Accessory nerve [XI], spinal root
Vagus nerve [X]
Accessory nerve [XI], cranial root

Jugular foramen

Vagus nerve [X], superior (jugular) ganglion
Trunk of accessory nerve
Internal branch
Vagus nerve [X], inferior (nodose) ganglion

Cervical nerve [C1]

Cervical nerve [C2]
External branch

Sternocleidomastoid

Cervical nerve [C3]

Cervical nerve [C4]

Trapezius

Connection to the brachial plexus

Brachial plexus, superior trunk

FIGURE 8.18   Accessory nerve [XI]; anterior view; vertebral canal and skull have been opened. The accessory nerve [XI] exits the brainstem in the retroolivary sulcus together with the glossopharyngeal nerve [IX] and the vagus nerve [X] and all three cranial nerves traverse the cranial base through the jugular foramen. The accessory nerve [XI] has two different roots. The cranial root of the accessory nerve [XI] originates from the nucleus ambiguus in the medulla oblongata. At the level of the jugular foramen, it joins the spinal root of the accessory nerve [XI] which consists of fibres derived from the anterior and posterior segmental roots in the cervical spinal cord. The fibres of the cranial root form the internal branch and converge on the vagus nerve [X] inferior to the jugular foramen. The cranial root participates in the innervation of the pharyngeal and laryngeal muscles. The fibres of the spinal root project caudally to the sterno-cleidomastoid, course through the lateral cervical triangle to the anterior margin of the trapezius and innervate both muscles.
Source: *Paulsen F. Brain and spinal cord. Sobotta atlas of human anatomy. vol. 3, p. 211–342, Chapter 12.*

- Spinal root
  - Cell bodies are in the **spinal accessory nucleus**, which is situated in the anterior horn of the cervical cord reaching down to the C6 level
  - The **spinal rootlets** emerge from the **lateral** edge of the **cervical cord** between the motor and sensory roots.

Course of the Accessory Nerve

- The spinal root enters the posterior fossa through the **foramen magnum** and joins the cranial root.
- Both roots emerge together through the **jugular foramen** and separate thereafter.
- The spinal root:
  - Runs downwards and laterally
  - Enters the deep surface and innervates the **sternocleidomastoid muscle**
  - Travels through the **posterior triangle** to supply the **trapezius muscle**
- The cranial root:
  - Runs with the **vagus nerve** and joins its **recurrent laryngeal branch** and **pharyngeal branches**
  - Supplies the **intrinsic muscles** of the larynx, pharynx and soft palate

---

CLINICAL INSIGHT

- **Spinal root of accessory nerve injury**
  - Damage to the spinal root of the accessory nerve leads to:
    - Loss of ipsilateral trapezius function, manifesting as winging (downward and outward rotation) of the ipsilateral scapula and mild drop in the ipsilateral shoulder.
    - Loss of ipsilateral sternocleidomastoid function, manifesting as weakness while turning the head to the opposite side.

HYPOGLOSSAL NERVE (CN XII)

The **hypoglossal nerve** is **mainly motor**. It supplies the **intrinsic muscles of the tongue** in addition to the **genioglossus, styloglossus** and **hyoglossus muscles** (Fig. 8.19).

- Cell bodies are found in the hypoglossal nuclei in the **dorsal aspect** of the medulla, beneath the floor of the fourth ventricle and at the level of the inferior olive (Fig. 8.1 and 8.2).
- Each nucleus receives **crossed** and **uncrossed input** from the cerebral hemispheres through the **corticonuclear tracts**.
- Neurons supplying the genioglossus muscle receive input **only from the contralateral side**.
- The efferent axons course anteriorly and exit from **anterolateral** aspect of the medulla in the groove between the pyramids and the inferior olive.

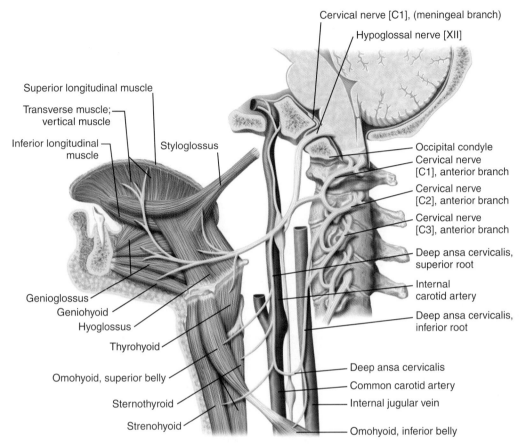

Cervical nerve [C1], (meningeal branch)

Hypoglossal nerve [XII]

Superior longitudinal muscle

Transverse muscle;
vertical muscle

Inferior longitudinal
muscle

Styloglossus

Occipital condyle

Cervical nerve
[C1], anterior branch

Cervical nerve
[C2], anterior branch

Cervical nerve
[C3], anterior branch

Deep ansa cervicalis,
superior root

Internal
carotid artery

Deep ansa cervicalis,
inferior root

Genioglossus

Geniohyoid

Hyoglossus

Thyrohyoid

Omohyoid, superior belly

Sternothyroid

Strenohyoid

Deep ansa cervicalis

Common carotid artery

Internal jugular vein

Omohyoid, inferior belly

FIGURE 8.19   Hypoglossal nerve [XII]; schematic median section; view from the left side. The nucleus of hypoglossal nerve in the medulla oblongata provides the fibres for the hypoglossal nerve [XII]. The fibres exit the brainstem as multiple small bundles between the pyramid and olive in the anterolateral sulcus. They join to form the hypoglossal nerve [XII] which passes through the hypoglossal canal. Inferior to the cranial base, fibres of the spinal nerves C1 and C2 accompany the hypoglossal nerve for a short distance and part again, first as superior root (limb) of the deep ansa cervicalis and then as a branch to the geniohyoid. Together with fibres from C2 and C3, these fibres form the deep ansa cervicalis and, in addition, innervate the geniohyoid. Posterior to the vagus nerve [X] in the neurovascular bundle behind the pharynx, the hypoglossal nerve [XII] passes caudally and, in an arch-shaped bend of 90°, turns rostrally and medially. It runs at the upper margin of the carotid triangle, crosses the external carotid artery at the branching point of the lingual artery and reaches the tongue between the hyoglossus and mylohyoid. The hypoglossal nerve [XII] innervates all internal muscles of the tongue and the styloglossus, hyoglossus and genioglossus.
Source: *Paulsen F. Brain and spinal cord. Sobotta atlas of human anatomy. vol. 3, p. 211–342, Chapter 12.*

- The nerve exits the skull through the **hypoglossal canal** located in the occipital condyle and descends in the neck between the internal carotid artery and internal jugular vein, where it is joined by C1 fibres (Fig. 8.19).
- At the level of inferior edge of the posterior digastric belly, it turns anteriorly and crosses deep to the mylohyoid muscle and lateral to the hypoglossus muscle to reach the oral cavity. At this level, it supplies the muscles with multiple branches (Fig. 8.19).

CLINICAL INSIGHT

- **Hypoglossal nerve injury**
  - Damage to the hypoglossal nerve results in loss of hypoglossal function on the ipsilateral side, manifesting as:
    - Paralysis of the ipsilateral half of the tongue
    - Atrophy and fasciculation of muscles in the ipsilateral aspect of the tongue
    - Deviation of the tongue to the atrophic side when protruded (due to normal function of the opposite genioglossus muscle)

CASE STUDY DISCUSSION

The patient has CN III and VI palsy with dysfunction of the first and second branches of CN V. Involvement of CN V2 and the presence of left papilloedema, most likely due to increased venous pressure, suggest that the problem is at the level of the **cavernous sinus**. Conversely, a superior orbital fissure lesion would spare CN V2. The history of sinusitis and the presence of fever are in favour of an infectious process that has extended into the sinus causing **cavernous sinus thrombosis**. Fig. 8.20 summarizes the clinical sequelae of CNs III, IV and VI palsies.

Nerve Palsy	Muscle(s) "OFF"	Symptoms	Exam Findings
Normal	N/A	N/A	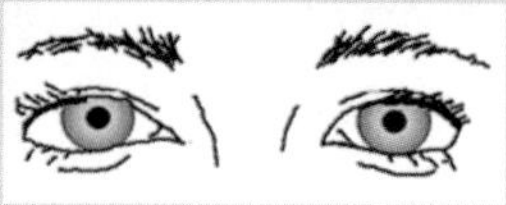
Oculomotor (CN III)	Medial, inferior and superior rectii muscles ■ Inferior oblique muscle ■ Levator palpebrae (eyelid) ■ Ciliary and con-strictor pulillae muscles (pupil)	Multidirectional horizontal and vertical diplopia, except on lateral gaze to the affected side. Eyelid droop.	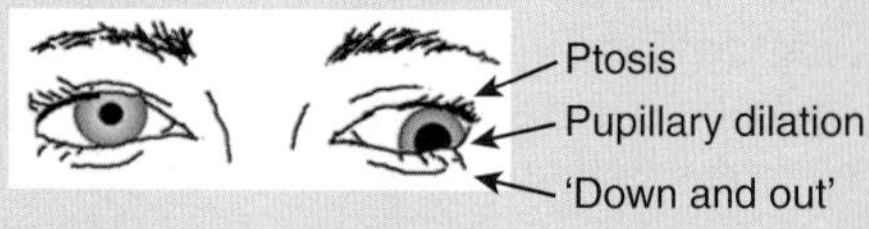 Ptosis — Pupillary dilation — 'Down and out'
Trochlear (CN IV)	Superior oblique muscle	Rotational diplopia that worsens on looking down and towards the nose	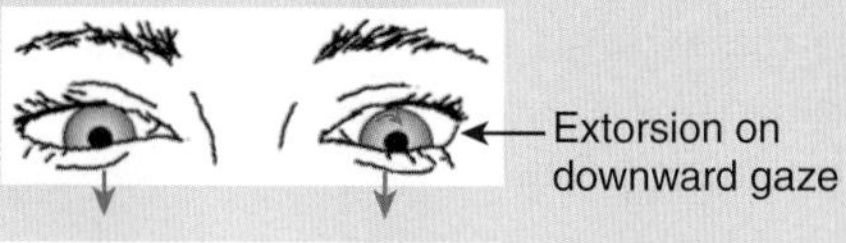 Extorsion on downward gaze
Abducens (CN VI)	Lateral rectus muscle	Horizontal diplopia on gaze towards the affected side	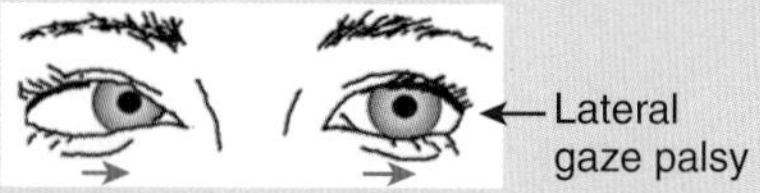 Lateral gaze palsy

FIGURE 8.20   Corresponding muscle dysfunction, symptoms and examination findings for cranial nerves III, IV and VI palsies. CN, cranial nerve.

Source: *Guluma K. Diplopia. Rosen's emergency medicine. p. 176–83.e1, Chapter 21.*

CHAPTER 9

Cerebellum

Samar S. Ayache

CASE STUDY

Presentation and Physical Examination: A 12-year-old right-handed girl, previously healthy, sought medical attention because of headache, vomiting and weird sensation of unsteadiness. Her symptoms started insidiously 2–3 years before consultation and continued to progress steadily to become incapacitating in daily life activities. At first, the patient felt unstable while walking on rough surfaces. This gradually evolved to the point that she became unable to make any step without assistance and felt as if she had completely lost control over her legs. In addition, the family noticed that she had difficulty in using her right hand, describing her movements as 'inelegant' and 'awkward' with a real struggle when picking up objects and inability to execute accurate actions. The family also reported changes in her speech, which became slurred and incomprehensible at times. Ten months prior to presentation, she started having a headache that was described as a frontal tension pain, more severe in the morning and upon awakening. The pain awakened her from sleep. In addition, she had several episodes of vomiting that were sudden and forceful, not preceded by nor associated with nausea. On examination, the patient was wheelchair-bound, unable to stand by herself without her mother's help. In the upright position, she kept on swaying back and forth or side to side, and had a wide-based gait. When asked to walk, she almost fell down upon attempting the first step. She made many errors on finger-to-nose and heel-to-shin tests and had difficulty performing rapid alternating movements. Deficits were seen bilaterally, with the right side being more severely affected than the left one. Remarkably, she had normal motor and sensory examination in all four limbs and intact cranial nerves.

Diagnosis and Management: A brain magnetic resonance imaging (MRI) was done revealing a cystic formation that involved the right cerebellar hemisphere and the cerebellar vermis. Contrast injection highlighted the presence of a mural formation within the cyst (Fig. 9.1).

The preliminary diagnosis was **cystic cerebellar astrocytoma.** A complete surgical excision was done. Pathological examination confirmed the preliminary diagnosis.

Try to guess the significance of our patient's symptoms and their anatomical correlations. How could we explain each clinical finding in the light of neuroanatomy?

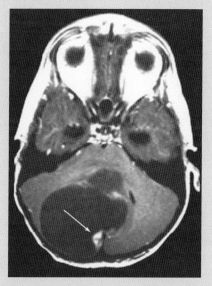

FIGURE 9.1 Contrast-enhanced T1-weighted magnetic resonance imaging showing a cystic cerebellar astrocytoma with a small mural nodule (arrow). This could easily be confused with a simple arachnoid cyst.

Source: *Sutton LN. Cerebellar astrocytomas. Youmans neurological surgery. p. 2105–13.e1, Chapter 202.*

BRIEF INTRODUCTION

The cerebellum is an important structure of the central nervous system (CNS), playing a crucial role in numerous brain functions.

- It is located in the posterior cranial fossa, beneath the cerebral hemispheres, from which it is separated by the **tentorium cerebelli** or the cerebellar tentorium, a dura mater extension.
- Pons and medulla, two parts of the brainstem, are situated ventral to the cerebellum and are connected to it by several thick nerve bundles, known as **cerebellar peduncles.**

The goal of this chapter is to introduce the neuroanatomy and the main functions of the cerebellum and its pathways and highlight important clinical aspects.

CEREBELLAR ANATOMY: MAJOR STRUCTURES

At a macroscopic level, the **cerebellum**, which name means 'little brain', consists of two hemispheres attached by a small midline part known as the vermis (*a Latin word meaning worm*), the latter being clearly demarcated by two longitudinally oriented fissures, called paramedian fissures (Fig. 9.2).

- Similar to the cerebrum, the outside of the cerebellum is folded, with the folds being narrower than those seen on the cerebral surface and almost parallel to each other, giving the cerebellum a banded appearance.

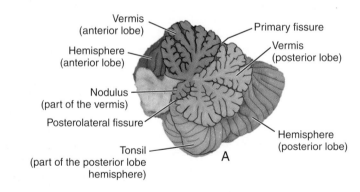

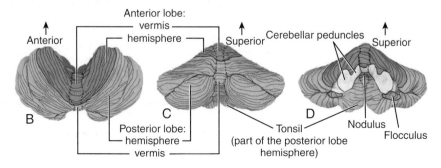

FIGURE 9.2 Gross anatomy of the cerebellum; shown here is the medial surface of a hemisected cerebellum (A), and the same cerebellum before hemisection seen from superior (B), posterior (C) and anterior (D) viewpoints.
Source: *Nolte J, PhD. Functional systems. The human brain in photographs and diagrams.* p. 125–86, Chapter 8.

■ Several fissures and sulci could be distinguished on the cerebellar surface and are best discerned on a sagittal section (Fig. 9.2).

Anatomical Division of the Cerebellum

Among the transversally oriented fissures, **primary** and **posterolateral fissures** are the deepest and by far the most easily identified.

■ They divide the cerebellum into three lobes: anterior, posterior and flocculonodular lobes (Figs. 9.2 and 9.3).

■ The **anterior lobe** is bordered anteriorly by the cerebellar peduncles and posteriorly by the primary fissure.

■ The **posterior lobe** extends between the primary and the posterolateral fissures.

■ The **flocculonodular lobe** lies between the posterolateral fissure and the cerebellar peduncles.

■ Other shallower and transversally oriented fissures subdivide the anterior and posterior lobes into **ten lobules** (Fig. 9.3).

■ To designate these lobules, we should keep in mind that their nomenclature has changed over time.

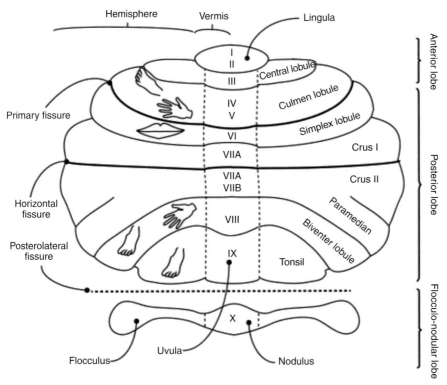

FIGURE 9.3 Unfolded view of the cerebellar cortex showing lobes, fissures and lobules, along with cerebellar somatotopy (left cerebellum only).

Source: *Roostaei T, MD, MPH. The human cerebellum. Neurol Clin 32(4):859–69.*

- In fact, in the eighteenth and nineteenth centuries, the classical nomenclature was adopted, and the choice of lobule names was mainly based on their aspect or their resemblance to particular anatomical structures.
- However, in the twentieth century, anatomical investigations of Lodewijk Bolk and Olof Larsell have introduced another nomenclature, according to which cerebellar lobules were indicated using Roman numerals (Fig. 9.3).

Apart from the above-mentioned anatomical division, the cerebellum could be separated into three different zones.

- On a sagittal plane, we can distinguish the **vermis**, the **intermediate zone** and the **lateral hemispheres**.
- The vermis occupies the midsagittal plane; intermediate zones lie laterally on the right and left sides of the vermis.
- The lateral hemispheres are located lateral to the intermediate zones, with no clear demarcation that is visible on gross anatomy between both zones.

Functional Division of the Cerebellum

Phylogenetically speaking, three cerebellar parts could be distinguished: the archicerebellum, the paleocerebellum and the neocerebellum.

- The **archicerebellum** is made of the flocculonodular lobe (the **flocculus** and the **nodulus**).
- The **paleocerebellum** consists of the vermis, the intermediate zone and its corresponding nuclei (the fastigial and the interposed nuclei) *(see Internal Structure subsection)*.
- The **neocerebellum** is formed by the lateral hemispheres and the dentate nuclei *(see Internal Structure subsection)*.

In fact, based on phylogenetics – the study of organisms' evolution – the flocculonodular lobe was found to be the oldest cerebellar structure, present in various vertebrate species. We, therefore, refer to it as the archicerebellum (*arche means beginning*).

- In other vertebrate species, like birds, the cerebellum is a bit more developed and characterized by the presence of a single median lobe: the paleocerebellum (*paleo means ancient*).
- In mammals, particularly in primates, and lately in humans, the cerebellum has shown a remarkable growth with the extension of two lateral lobes, permitting those species to have more sophisticated and advanced gestures. This new cerebellar part is called the neocerebellum (*neo means new*).

Interestingly, the cerebellar organization is consistent at a functional level.

- The archicerebellum, also known as the **vestibulocerebellum**, is in intimate connection with the vestibular system, thus handling **head and eyes movements**.

- The paleocerebellum, or the **spinocerebellum**, receives proprioceptive sensory inputs from the spinal cord and controls **gait** and **stance** by coordinating **trunk and legs movements**.
- As for the neocerebellum, also known as **cerebrocerebellum** or **ponto-cerebellum**, it is in close interaction with the contralateral cerebral cortex and responsible for the **fine and rapid limb movements**, namely upper limb movements.

Afferent and efferent pathways are explained further in a dedicated section *(see Major Cerebellar Pathways section)*.

CLINICAL INSIGHT

- **Vermian lesions**
  - The cerebellar vermis could be affected by various diseases, including degenerative disorders, toxins and tumours, among others.
  - In particular, chronic and severe alcohol abuse causes **cerebellar atrophy** (loss of volume), which is usually more prominent in the **superior part of the vermis** (Fig. 9.4).
  - Vermian lesions result in abnormal stance and gait (*see Clinical Insights box, p. 250*).

Internal Structure

A folded grey matter covers the cerebellar surface. The centre of the cerebellum is made up of white matter, which has a characteristic tree-like appearance resembling an arbor vitae (*Latin, tree of life*). At the centre of the cerebellar

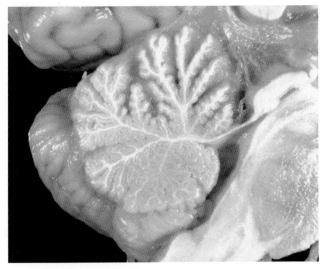

FIGURE 9.4 Alcoholic cerebellar degeneration. The anterior portion of the vermis (upper portion of figure) is atrophic with widened spaces between the folia.
Source: *Frosch MP. The central nervous system. Robbins and Cotran pathologic basis of disease. p. 1251–318, Chapter 28.*

white matter, we can distinguish three pairs of grey matter formations: the **cerebellar nuclei**. These nuclei receive inputs from specific parts of the cerebellar cortex and constitute the **exclusive output structures** of the cerebellum. It is important to point out that the anatomical position of the cerebellar nuclei corresponds to parts of the cerebellar cortex with which they interact.

- The **fastigial nucleus** is the most medially located nucleus.
    - It projects to the **vestibular nuclei** and **reticular formation**.
    - Its inputs majorly come from the **vermis**.
- The **interposed nucleus**, composed of the **globose** and the **emboliform** nuclei, is located lateral to the fastigial nucleus.
    - It receives information from the **intermediate (paravermal) zone** and sends impulses to the **contralateral red nucleus**.
- The **dentate nucleus**, the largest and the most lateral one, has an undulated form, and receives inputs from the **cerebellar hemispheres** and sends impulses to the **contralateral red nucleus and thalamus**.

CLINICAL INSIGHT

- **Guillain–Mollaret triangle (Fig. 9.5)**
    - Three corners define the Guillain–Mollaret triangle, as described by Georges Guillain and Pierre Mollaret in 1931:
        - **Red nucleus** in the midbrain
        - **Inferior olivary nucleus** in the medulla oblongata
        - **Contralateral cerebellar dentate nucleus**
    - The **dentatorubral** fibres, via the superior cerebellar peduncle, link the dentate and the red nuclei. The **olivodentate fibres**, via the inferior cerebellar peduncle, connect the dentate nucleus with the inferior olivary nucleus. The **central tegmental tract** links the inferior olivary nucleus with the red nucleus.
    - Lesions within the Guillain–Mollaret triangle may occur secondary to several aetiologies such as demyelination, cavernoma and vertebrobasilar stroke, among others.
    - Such an injury can lead to **hypertrophic degeneration of the inferior olivary nucleus** and may cause, in some patients, a tremor involving the eyes and palate known as the **oculopalatal tremor**.
    - Brain MRI could help confirm the diagnosis in the majority of cases. It usually unveils the underlying cause and highlights the inferior olivary nucleus hypertrophy; the latter appears as a T2 hyperintensity along with an asymmetry of the anterior rim of the medulla oblongata.
    - In the vast majority of cases, the oculopalatal tremor remains refractory to all medications.
- **Fahr disease**
    - In 1930, a German pathologist, Karl Theodor Fahr, described for the first time an abnormal bilateral and symmetrical **calcification** of the **pallidum, striatum** and **dentate nucleus** (Fig. 9.6). Since then, this entity is known as Fahr disease, Fahr syndrome or **bilateral striatopallidodentate calcinosis**.
    - Fahr disease is a rare neurodegenerative disorder, affecting individuals in their thirties or forties. It may occur sporadically or be transmitted as an autosomal dominant or autosomal recessive trait.

- Although Fahr disease remains idiopathic in the majority of cases, various causes of symmetrical basal ganglia and dentate nuclei calcifications should be excluded. Hence, thorough investigations should be undertaken to rule out calcium metabolism disorders (hypoparathyroidism and pseudohypoparathyroidism), copper metabolism disorders (Wilson disease), infectious processes (neurobrucellosis) and autoimmune disorders (especially systemic lupus erythematosus). In specific clinical contexts, other aetiologies should be eliminated as well; these include mitochondrial encephalopathies and Down syndrome.
- Clinically speaking, movement disorders (Parkinsonism, tremor, dystonia, and dyskinesia) are common manifestations of Fahr disease. Patients may also present with cerebellar disturbances, dementia and other neuropsychiatric symptoms.
- Brain computed tomography (CT) scan helps in establishing the diagnosis by showing bilateral and symmetrical calcium deposits in typical regions (basal ganglia and cerebellum). These deposits, appearing as hyperdense lesions, may also be found in the thalami, the hippocampi and the semioval centres (central areas of white matter located underneath the cerebral cortex).
- To date, the management of Fahr disease is supportive, limited to correcting the underlying cause if possible, and providing symptomatic treatments. Remission or disease stabilization has been the primary purpose of several research protocols. Unfortunately, the aim is yet to be met, and trials resulted in limited clinical benefit. Future studies are highly needed and should focus on the pathophysiology of the disease and the development of new therapeutic options.
- Prognosis of Fahr disease significantly varies among individuals. While some patients stay asymptomatic over a long period, others become disabled within few years.

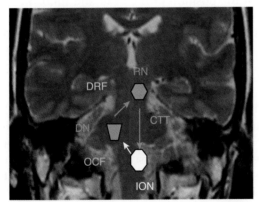

FIGURE 9.5   Coronal T2-weighted MRI with schematic of the Guillain–Mollaret triangle. DRF, dentatorubral fibres; OCF, olivocerebellar fibres; DN, dentate nucleus; ION, inferior olivary nucleus; RN, red nucleus; CTT, central tegmental tract.

Source: *Sánchez HJ. Hypertrophic olivary degeneration secondary to a Guillain–Mollaret triangle lesion. Neurology (Neurología, English ed) 28(1):59–61.*

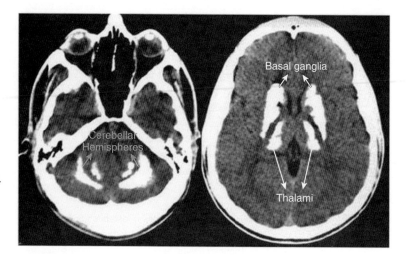

FIGURE 9.6 Brain CT revealed bilateral symmetric calcifications in basal ganglia, thalamus and cerebellar hemispheres. Source: *Alemdar M. Fahr's disease presenting with paroxysmal non-kinesigenic dyskinesia: a case report. Parkinsonism Relat Disorders 14(1):69–71.*

Cerebellar Peduncles

Three pairs of peduncles connect the cerebellum to the brainstem (Fig. 9.7):

- **Superior** peduncles (or **brachium conjunctivum**)
- **Middle** peduncles (or **brachium pontis**)
- **Inferior** peduncles (or **restiform body**)

While superior peduncles mainly convey output fibres, middle and inferior peduncles bring information from the cortex, brainstem and spinal cord into the cerebellum.

MAJOR CEREBELLAR PATHWAYS

In order to control movements, the cerebellum should firstly receive accurate information about the position of the head and limbs in space. Secondly, it should closely interact with the motor cortex before the initiation of any action. In this context, afferent cerebellar pathways convey all the needed information to the cerebellum (Fig. 9.8), while cerebellar outputs are transferred via the efferent pathways to the concerned cerebral regions.

Afferent Pathways

- Afferent pathways within the middle cerebellar peduncles
    - **Pontocerebellar tract**: The major inputs of the cerebellum come from the **cortex**. They are first interposed in the **pontine nuclei**, then, transmitted via the pontocerebellar fibres to the cerebellum to provide information about any intended motion.
- Afferent pathways within the inferior cerebellar peduncles
    Try to imagine the following discussion between the cerebellum, the spine and the brainstem.
    - *Cerebellum: 'Where are the limbs and head in space? How can I advise the motor cortex?'*

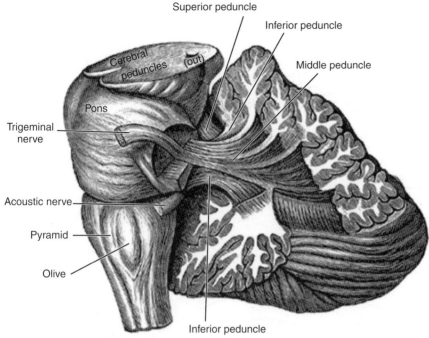

Superior peduncle

Inferior peduncle

Middle peduncle

Cerebral peduncles (out)

Pons

Trigeminal nerve

Acoustic nerve

Pyramid

Olive

Inferior peduncle

FIGURE 9.7   Superior, medial and inferior cerebellar peduncles.

Source: *From: Moses, after Lewis Gray's anatomy (1918), freely available [28]. Van Baarsen KM. The anatomical substrate of cerebellar mutism. Med Hypotheses 82(6):774–80.*

- *Spine and medulla: 'We know where the limbs are. In fact, we convey proprioceptive sensory inputs, which inform about the limb positions and movements'.*
- *Vestibular nuclei: 'I can tell where the head is…'*

Now try to guess what the afferent tracts are, and how the cerebellum can accurately control our various activities.

■ **Spinocerebellar tracts**
- **Dorsal (or posterior) spinocerebellar** tract: It carries **proprioceptive** inputs from the **ipsilateral lower limb** and **lower trunk**.
- **Cuneocerebellar** tract: It brings **proprioceptive** inputs from the **ipsilateral upper limb** and **upper trunk**.
- Both tracts update the cerebellum on the current movement.
- **Ventral (or anterior) spinocerebellar** tract: It runs through the **superior cerebellar peduncle** (not the inferior one), and provides **proprioceptive** information of the **contralateral lower limb**. It primarily deals with the upcoming action of that limb. In fact, the main function of this tract is to monitor the state of activity of the spinal cord interneurons. The latter participate in spinal reflexes and control the firing of motor neurons within the cord. Having access to this information would help the cerebellum in preparing the strategy of future movements.

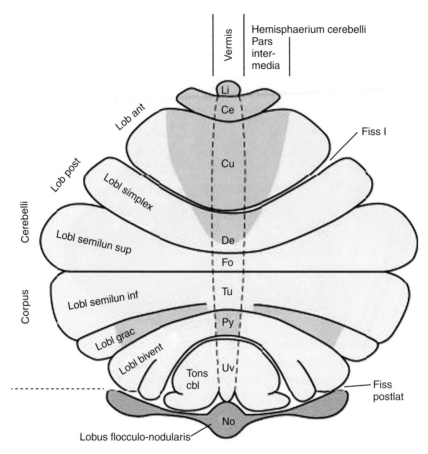

FIGURE 9.8 The cerebellar cortex, unfolded into one plane, showing the fields of termination of cerebellar afferent projections (= mossy fibre system): pontocerebellar fibres (light orange), spinocerebellar fibres (orange) and vestibulocerebellar fibres (dark orange). Ce, central lobe; Cu, culmen; De, declive; Fiss I, primary fissure; Fiss postlat, posterolateral fissure; Fo, folium vermis; Li, lingula; Lob ant, anterior lobe; Lob post, posterior lobe; Lobl bivent, biventer lobule; Lobl grac, gracile lobule; Lobl semilun inf, inferior semilunar lobule; Lobl semilun sup, superior semilunar lobule; Lobl simplex, lobulus simplex; No, nodulus; Py, pyramis; Tons cbl, cerebellar tonsil; Tu, tuber vermis; Uv, uvula.

Source: *Reproduced with permission from Nieuwenhuys R, Voogd J, van Huijzen C. The human central nervous system. A synopsis and atlas. Berlin: Springer; 1988. p. 162.*

- **Rostral spinocerebellar** tract: It enters the cerebellum partly through the **inferior cerebellar peduncle** and partly through the **middle one**. It is responsible for the same function as the ventral spinocerebellar pathway but for the **upper limb**.
- **Trigeminocerebellar** tract
  - Transmits **proprioceptive** inputs from the **face**.
- **Vestibulocerebellar** tract
  - Transfers messages about the **position** and **movement** of the **head**.
- **Olivocerebellar** tract
  - Originates in the **inferior olivary nucleus**.

- Enters the **inferior cerebellar peduncle**, then the cerebellar cortex, and projects onto **Purkinje cells** as the **climbing fibres.**
- Several theories of cerebellar function suggest that information coming from the inferior olive updates the cerebellum about **errors in movement execution.**
- **Reticulocerebellar** tract
  - Originates in the **reticular nuclei** (i.e. lateral reticular, reticulotegmental and paramedian reticular nuclei).
  - Transmits data received by the reticular formation from various structures such as the spinal cord and vestibular system, and participates in the **fine adjustment** of any ongoing action.

Efferent Pathways

Axons of the deep cerebellar nuclei form the main channels through which the cerebellum sends its outputs to the brainstem and cerebral cortex. These axons exit the cerebellum, are mostly conveyed through the superior cerebellar peduncles and form the following tracts:

- **Cerebellothalamic** tract
  - Carries important information to the **contralateral thalamus (ventrolateral nucleus)**, from which inputs are sent to the **motor cortex.**
  - These signals permit **adjustment, correction and readjustment** of any planned movement.
- **Cerebelloreticular** (from the **globose** and **emboliform nuclei**), **cerebelloolivary** and **cerebellorubral** fibres
  - Terminate in the reticular formation, inferior olivary complex and contralateral red nucleus, respectively.
- Two other efferent tracts, the cerebelloreticular (from the **fastigial nucleus**) and the **cerebellovestibular** tracts, which exit the cerebellum via the **inferior cerebellar peduncles** (not the superior peduncles).
  - Transfer signals to the **brainstem** and the **vestibular nuclei**, respectively.

CEREBELLAR FUNCTIONS

When we watch a dance performance, we are rapidly captivated by the complexity, speed and precision of the dancers' steps and moves. In the same way, observing a musician playing piano makes us wonder how it is possible to hit the keys in such an elegant and tactful manner. Amazingly, human beings are the sole creatures to have the capacity to perform accurate, fine and delicate movements, and thus they can execute complex activities such as playing music, writing books, riding bikes and driving cars, to cite a few.

Motor Control

The highly advanced skills of human beings would not be possible if the cerebellum was not present and developed to that extent. In fact, each action puts several muscles into play and requires perfect coordination between them.

For example, to drink some water, we need to pick up the cup and bring it to our mouth; this action requires excellent coordination between hand, forearm and arm muscles. Notably, forearm and arm flexors should be activated, while extensors should be inhibited. In this perspective, the cerebellum is the maestro that offers impeccable motor control.

In addition, the distance between the cup and the mouth, as well as the movement speed should be precisely estimated ahead. Here, the cerebellum intervenes to provide us with these valuable data and permits continuous control of the timing, velocity and power of the movement in question.

As mentioned in the functional division part, we should remember that each cerebellar part is in charge of coordinating specific muscle groups, where the archicerebellum coordinates eyes, head and neck movements, the paleocerebellum supervises gait and stance and the neocerebellum controls limb movements.

Motor Learning

In early childhood, we start to make our first steps, handle objects, use tools and utensils such as cups, forks and spoons. Few years later, we learn to ride tricycles and bicycles, play football or basketball, write and so on. At the beginning, we are clumsy in doing any new action, and then, with practice and through a trial-and-error process, we acquire dexterity and accuracy and become skilful in performing it. This process is known as motor learning, in which the cerebellum plays a crucial role by adapting motor plans and fine-tuning motor strategies.

CLINICAL INSIGHTS

- **Ataxia**
    - Dysfunction of the cerebellum results in loss of the main cerebellar function: motor coordination.
    - **Movement incoordination** could affect any muscle group including eyes, limbs and axial muscles, among others.
    - Ataxia, form Greek meaning 'lack of order', is the term used to indicate motor incoordination and is a key feature of cerebellar disorders.
- **Ataxic gait**
    - Involvement of axial muscles, i.e. neck, and trunk muscles leads to **abnormal stance** and **unsteady gait**.
    - Therefore, a wide-base gait would be adopted to compensate for disequilibrium.
    - **Tandem gait test**: The patient is asked to walk in a straight line, and touch the heel of one foot with the toes of the other on each step. Damage to the **cerebellar vermis** makes this task particularly difficult.
- **Limb ataxia**
    Involvement of limb muscles results in clumsy movements.
    - **Dysmetria**
        - Literally speaking, dysmetria means a 'wrong length'.

- Dysmetria is a type of ataxia and refers to the **inability to estimate distance and speed of movements**.
- Hence, upon reaching an object, the patient either undershoots or overshoots the goal in question. The action undertakes an erroneous trajectory and requires one or several corrections to attain its aim.
- **Finger-to-nose** and **heel-to-shin tests** are commonly used to detect **upper** and **lower limbs dysmetria**, respectively.

■ **Dysdiadochokinesia**

- Dysdiadochokinesia is another aspect of ataxia and a cardinal sign of cerebellar dysfunction.
- The term 'dysdiadochokinesia' is used to describe the **incapacity to perform rapid alternating movements**.
- To examine upper limb dysdiadochokinesia, the patient is asked to place his/her hand on a surface (a table/the other hand/the thigh) and then turn it back and forth as quickly as possible. Patients with cerebellar disorders usually have difficulty in performing this task, which can result in a slow, awkward or impossible movement.
- To test lower limb dysdiadochokinesia, the patient is asked to firmly hold his/her heel against the floor and then rapidly tap his/her toes on the ground as fast as possible.

■ **Intention tremor**

■ Another important manifestation of cerebellar diseases is the tremor.

■ As the name indicates, intention tremor implies that the limb oscillates while moving to reach a target. In fact, when the upper arm is outstretched in an attempt to touch something (a cup for instance), the movement first produces a linear trajectory, then as the hand gets closer to its goal, a tremor of **increasing amplitude** appears.

■ **Nystagmus**

■ Nystagmus is an **involuntary, repetitive** and **rhythmic movement of the eyes**, also described as 'jerking eyes'.

■ Several types of nystagmus exist, and their characteristics depend on the underlying mechanism. For example, eyes could move back and forth like a pendulum (**pendular** nystagmus); or they could travel at a slow velocity in one direction (**slow drift**) and then rapidly move back in the opposite direction (**corrective jerk**).

■ Eyes movements could be **vertical** (up-and-down), **horizontal** (side-to-side), **torsional** (rotatory) or any combination of these motions.

■ A huge number of diseases could cause nystagmus. The most common are disorders of the vestibular apparatus, vestibular pathways and cerebellum.

■ While **peripheral vestibular nystagmus** is typically **horizontal-rotatory**, **cerebellar disturbances** usually generate a **vertical or multidirectional** nystagmus.

Further description of this condition is beyond the scope of this chapter.

■ **Dysarthria**

■ The term dysarthria indicates **abnormal articulation**. This disorder implies that the language content is normal but the **speech production is impaired**.

■ Indeed, dysarthria results from weakness or abnormal control of the muscles involved in the generation of phonemes. In this context, the speech becomes slurred and unintelligible.

■ Several types of dysarthria exist and depend on the underlying cause. Notably, dysarthria resulting from cerebellar diseases is characterized by a **scanning speech**, or **explosive speech**, a condition also known as **ataxic dysarthria**.

CEREBELLOPONTINE ANGLE

The **cerebellopontine angle** (CPA) is the anatomical space located between the cerebellum and the pons:

- Extends from the petrous bone laterally to the lateral aspect of the brainstem medially.
- Its superior and inferior borders are the middle cerebellar peduncle and the arachnoid tissue of lower cranial nerves, respectively.
- This space is filled with cerebrospinal fluid (CSF) and contains meningeal tissue, cranial nerves, along with blood vessels.
- A quick look at this region provides insight into its clinical relevance. Any lesion arising in the CPA would result in complex and invalidating symptoms.
- Curiously, various masses take place in this interesting anatomical area and are relatively specific for it; **schwannoma**, **meningioma** and **epidermoid cyst** are the most frequently encountered CPA lesions.

CASE STUDY DISCUSSION

Cystic cerebellar astrocytoma or **juvenile pilocytic astrocytoma** is a brain tumour that mostly affects **children** and **adolescents** *(see Fig. 1.22 of chapter 1)*.

Clinical Features

Symptoms and signs depend on the structure affected by the tumour growth. Hence, it usually results in cerebellar dysfunction leading to:

- **Abnormal gait and stance**: Broad-based and ataxic gait secondary to a vermian lesion.
- **Clumsiness and tremor** (secondary to involvement of cerebellar hemispheres)
  - Dysmetria: revealed by a finger-to-nose test
  - Dysdiadochokinesia: unveiled by rapid alternating movement test
  - Intention tremor
- Slurred speech
- Nystagmus

When the tumour is enlarged enough to exert pressure on the brainstem and/or obstruct CSF flow in the fourth ventricle causing hydrocephalus, signs and symptoms of raised intracranial pressure dominate in the clinical scenario and manifest as:

- A headache, which is more often frontal and more severe upon awakening and in the morning.
- 'Projectile' vomiting that is usually not accompanied by nausea.
- Bilateral papilloedema on ophthalmologic examination.

Diagnosis

On CT scan or MRI, cystic cerebellar astrocytoma has a classical appearance in less than 50% of cases. It consists of a **cyst with a small enhancing mural nodule**. If the nodule is too small, the tumour may be mistaken for a benign arachnoid cyst.

Management

Complete surgical excision is usually the treatment of choice.

Prognosis

The 20-year survival rate is estimated at 80%. The risk of recurrence increases with age, and the most significant predictor of long-term prognosis is the extent of tumour resection. Completely excised tumours have a better outcome than incompletely resected ones, whose prognosis remains unpredictable.

Diencephalon

Abeer J. Hani

Presentation and Physical Examination: A 60-year-old right-handed woman presented to the clinic for a chief complaint of 2 days of numbness in her right face, arm and leg. She reported waking up about 2 days earlier with sensation that 'her right face and arm were asleep'. The next day, she had loss of sensation in the right foot. Neurologic review of systems was negative for any motor deficits, language difficulties or vision changes. Past medical history is significant for hypertension, cigarette smoking and depression. Her father had a stroke at the age of 64. Physical examination was significant for decreased pinprick, temperature, vibration and light touch sensation in the right face and right side of the body and decreased two-point discrimination in the right hand.

Diagnosis, Management and Follow-Up: Computed tomography (CT) scan of the head was done and revealed a small hypodensity in the left thalamus. An ischaemic lesion was suspected and confirmed by brain magnetic resonance imaging (MRI), which showed restricted diffusion in the lateral thalamus, consistent with a lacunar infarct (Fig. 10.1).

She was admitted to the stroke unit where the workup done was nonrevealing. The numbness gradually improved over few days.

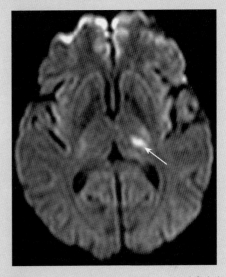

FIGURE 10.1 Diffusion-weighted MRI showing left thalamic infarct (arrow).

Source: *Nentwich LM, MD. Neuroimaging in acute stroke. Emergency Med Clin North Am 30(3):659–80.*

BRIEF INTRODUCTION

The **diencephalon** is the part of the brain lying between the brainstem and cerebral hemispheres.

- It is composed, from dorsal to ventral, of the epithalamus, thalamus, subthalamus and hypothalamus (Fig. 10.2). Some anatomists include the stria medullaris thalami as part of the epithalamus.
- The lateral walls of the diencephalon form the epithalamus most superiorly, the thalamus centrally, and the subthalamus and hypothalamus inferiorly.
- The thalamus is the largest part of the diencephalon.

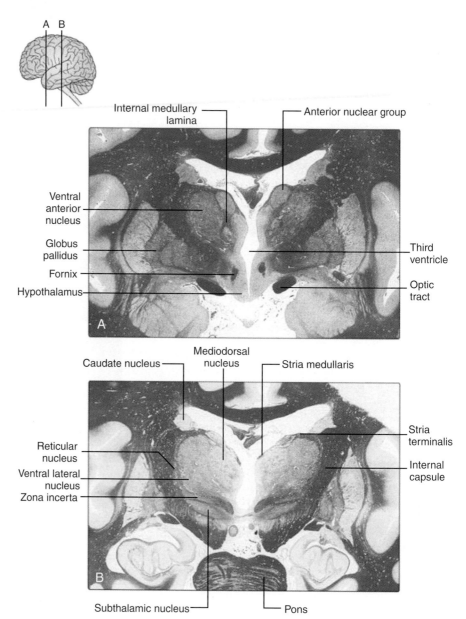

FIGURE 10.2   (A and B) Coronal sections through the diencephalon.
Source: *(A and B) From Crossman AR, PhD DSc. Thalamus. Neuroanatomy: an illustrated colour text. p. 124–30, Chapter 12.*

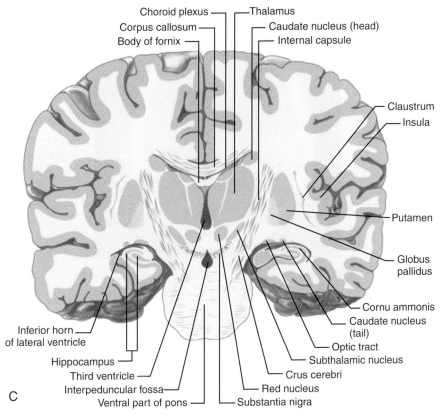

Choroid plexus — Thalamus
Corpus callosum — Caudate nucleus (head)
Body of fornix — Internal capsule
Claustrum
Insula
Putamen
Globus pallidus
Cornu ammonis
Caudate nucleus (tail)
Inferior horn of lateral ventricle
Optic tract
Subthalamic nucleus
Hippocampus
Third ventricle
Crus cerebri
Interpeduncular fossa
Red nucleus
Ventral part of pons
Substantia nigra

C

FIGURE 10.2, cont'd (C) the principal parts of the diencephalon and basal ganglia, coronal section.
Source: (C) From Standring S, MBE, PhD, DSc, FKC, Hon FAS, Hon FRCS. Diencephalon. Gray's anatomy. p. 350–363.e1, Chapter 23.

- The diencephalon is the **main processing centre** for information destined to reach the cerebral cortex from **all ascending sensory pathways** (except those related to olfaction).
- The right and left halves of the diencephalon contain symmetrically distributed cell groups separated by the space of the third ventricle.

The goal of this chapter is to introduce the anatomy of the different structures constituting the diencephalon as well as provide a brief review of their function in normal states and dysfunction in certain pathologic states.

EPITHALAMUS

The **epithalamus** is located in the most dorsal and caudal region of the diencephalon. It consists of the pineal gland and the habenula.

- The **pineal gland** is an endocrine organ that synthesizes **melatonin** and often calcifies in the second decade of life. This gland is involved in controlling the **sleep–wake cycle** (circadian rhythm) and in regulating the **onset of the puberty** (Fig. 10.3).
- The **habenula** or **habenular nucleus** has connections with the limbic system. It receives glutamatergic input from the septal area of the limbic

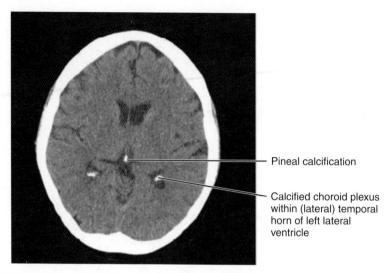

— Pineal calcification

— Calcified choroid plexus within (lateral) temporal horn of left lateral ventricle

FIGURE 10.3 An axial CT image showing calcification of the pineal gland and choroid plexus. Source: *Standring S, MBE, PhD, DSc, FKC, Hon FAS, Hon FRCS. Diencephalon. Gray's anatomy; 2016. p. 350–363.e1, Chapter 23.*

system via the stria medullaris thalami and sends cholinergic tracts to the reticular formation in the midbrain via the habenulointerpeduncular tract. This also helps with the **sleep–wake cycle** (Fig. 10.4).

CLINICAL INSIGHT

■ **Pineal gland shift on imaging**

  ■ A shift of the calcified pineal gland may denote a space-occupying lesion within the skull.

THALAMUS

The **thalamus** (*meaning 'inner chamber' or 'bedroom' in Greek*) is the **largest nuclear mass** in the nervous system. It is also an important processing station in the centre of the brain (Fig. 10.5).

- It forms the lateral wall of the third ventricle along with the hypothalamus.
- The two thalami are joined across the thin slit of the ventricle by the **interthalamic adhesion** also known as **massa intermedia.**
- The thalamus is divided into **three principal nuclear masses** (anterior, medial and lateral) by the internal medullary lamina (Fig. 10.6 and Table 10.1). The nuclei are involved in the following pathways:
  - Nuclei that transmit general and special sensory information to corresponding regions of the sensory cortices.
  - Nuclei that receive impulses from the cerebellum and basal ganglia and interface with motor regions of the frontal lobe.

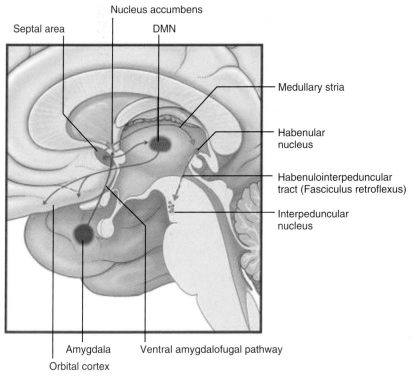

FIGURE 10.4   Connections of the septal area. DMN, dorsal medial nucleus of the thalamus.
Source: *Mtui E, MD. Olfactory and limbic systems. Fitzgerald's clinical neuroanatomy and neuroscience. p. 323–43, Chapter 34.*

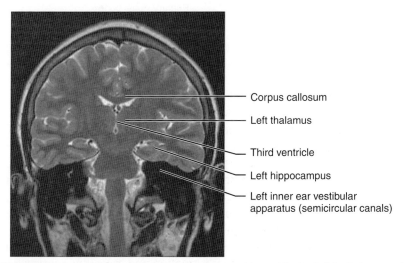

FIGURE 10.5   A coronal T2-weighted magnetic resonance image at the level of the thalamus and third ventricle.
Source: *(Courtesy of Professor Alan Jackson, Wolfson Molecular Imaging Centre, The University of Manchester, Manchester, UK.). Standring S, MBE, PhD, DSc, FKC, Hon FAS, Hon FRCS. Diencephalon. Gray's anatomy; 2016. p. 350–63.e1, Chapter 23.*

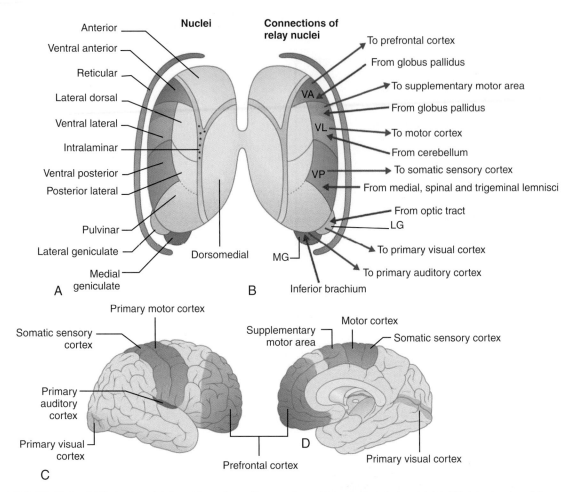

FIGURE 10.6   (A) Thalamic nuclei viewed from above; (B) connections of the specific (relay) nuclei. LG, MG, lateral and medial geniculate nuclei; VA, ventral anterior nucleus; VL, ventral lateral nucleus; VP, ventral posterior nucleus. (C) Lateral and (D) medial surface of the hemisphere showing cortical areas receiving projections from the relay nuclei.
Source: *Mtui E, MD. Thalamus epithalamus. Fitzgerald's clinical neuroanatomy and neuroscience; 2016. p. 260–4, Chapter 27.*

- Nuclei that have connections with associative and limbic areas of the cerebral cortex.
- The **anterior nuclear** group of the thalamus is part of the limbic system. It receives fibres from the mammillary body of the hypothalamus and projects to the cingulate gyrus.
- The **dorsomedial nucleus** in the medial nuclear group has extensive reciprocal connections with the cortex of the frontal lobe.
- The **intralaminar nuclei** located within the internal medullary lamina receive input from the reticular formation and ascending sensory systems and project via other thalamic nuclei to the cerebral cortex and the striatum. They are responsible for activation of the cerebral cortex.
- The **reticular nucleus** receives collaterals of thalamocortical and corticothalamic fibres.

Table 10.1 Thalamic nuclei and their connections

Type	Nucleus	Afferents	Efferents
Specific (or relay)	Anterior	■ Mammillary bodies ■ Hippocampus	■ Cingulate cortex
	Ventral anterior (VA) Ventral lateral (VL)	■ Substantia nigra (pars reticulata)	■ Prefrontal cortex
	VL, anterior part	■ Globus pallidus (internal segment)	■ Supplementary motor area
	VL, posterior part Ventral posterior (VP)	■ Cerebellar nuclei	■ Premotor and motor cortex
	Ventral posterolateral (VPL)	■ Somatic afferents from trunk and limbs	■ Somatic sensory cortex
	Ventral posteromedial (VPM)	■ Somatic afferents from the head region	■ Somatic sensory cortex
	Medial geniculate body	■ Brachium of the inferior colliculus	■ Primary auditory cortex
	Lateral geniculate body	■ Optic tract	■ Primary visual cortex
Association	Lateral dorsal (LD)	■ Hippocampus	■ Cingulate cortex
	Dorsomedial (DM)	■ Prefrontal cortex ■ Olfactory and limbic systems	■ Prefrontal cortex
	Lateral posterior (LP)/Pulvinar	■ Superior colliculus ■ Primary cortices: 　■ Visual 　■ Auditory 　■ Somatosensory	■ Association cortices: 　■ Posterior parietal 　■ Lateral temporal
Nonspecific	Intralaminar (centromedian, parafascicular, others)	■ Reticular formation ■ Basal ganglia ■ Limbic system	■ Cerebral cortex ■ Corpus striatum
	Reticular	■ Thalamus ■ Cortex	■ Thalamus

Source: *Adapted from Fitzgerald's clinical neuroanatomy and neuroscience, 7th ed.; 2016. p. 260–264.*

- The **lateral nuclear** mass includes:
  - **Ventral posterior nucleus:** Receives general sensory afferents from the medial lemniscus, spinothalamic tract and trigeminothalamic tract. It then sends efferents to the primary somatosensory cortex of the parietal lobe.
  - **Lateral geniculate nucleus:** Receives visual afferents from the optic tract and projects to the primary visual cortex of the occipital lobe.
  - **Medial geniculate nucleus:** Receives auditory afferents from the inferior colliculus and sends efferents to the primary auditory cortex of the temporal lobe.
  - **Ventral anterior** and **ventral lateral nuclei:** Receive afferents from the cerebellum and basal ganglia and send efferents to motor cortical areas of the frontal lobe.
- Other 'nonspecific' nuclei connect with wider areas of the cortex, including associative and limbic regions. One such example is the pulvinar that interconnects with associative areas in the parietal, temporal and occipital lobes.

CLINICAL INSIGHT

- **Thalamic lesions**
  - Neurosurgically placed lesions in the region of the ventral lateral nuclei were used to alleviate some of the motor symptoms associated with disorders of the basal ganglia (rigidity, tremor at rest, dyskinesias) seen in Parkinson disease.
  - Strokes and tumours destroying the thalamus lead to loss of sensation in the contralateral face and limbs with a distressing discomfort in the paradoxically anaesthetic areas (thalamic pain also referred to as Dejerine–Roussy syndrome).
  - Thalamic lesions may mimic focal cortical defects because of the richness of thalamocortical connections.

SUBTHALAMUS

The **subthalamus** is a complex region of nuclear groups and fibre tracts.

- It lies beneath the thalamus and dorsolateral to the hypothalamus.
- It contains two main cell groups: the subthalamic nucleus (medial to the internal capsule) and the zona incerta (Fig. 10.7).
- The **subthalamic nucleus** has prominent connections with the globus pallidus (GPi) and the substantia nigra and is important in the **control of movement**.
- The **zona incerta** is a rostral extension of the brainstem reticular formation.

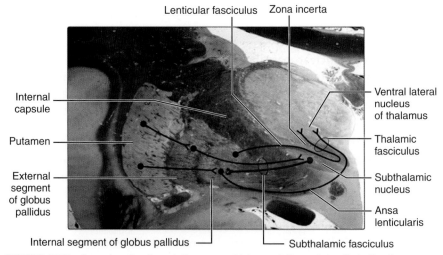

FIGURE 10.7 Coronal section through the corpus striatum and diencephalon illustrating the connections between the globus pallidus and the subthalamic nucleus.

Source: *Crossman AR, PhD DSc. Basal ganglia. Neuroanatomy: an illustrated colour text; 2015. p. 146–54, Chapter 14.*

CLINICAL INSIGHT

■ **Deep brain stimulation**

  ■ In patients with Parkinson disease in whom drug therapy fails, neurosurgical lesioning of the internal segment of the GPi or stimulation of the subthalamic nucleus or GPi through implanted electrodes (deep brain stimulation) may improve or even alleviate the symptoms.

HYPOTHALAMUS

The **hypothalamus** is the most ventral part of the diencephalon, lying beneath the thalamus and ventromedial to the subthalamus. It is connected to the pituitary gland via the pituitary stalk (Fig. 10.8).

- It has **autonomic, neuroendocrine** and **limbic functions** and is involved in the coordination of homeostatic mechanisms. It is referred to as the 'orchestrator of the endocrine system'.
- Activation of the **posterior** hypothalamic domain is associated with **sympathetic** responses, whereas activation of the **anterior** hypothalamus is associated with **parasympathetic** activity.
- The hypothalamus produces **hormones** that are released from the posterior pituitary and also produces releasing factors that control the release of hormones from the anterior pituitary.
- The hypothalamus consists of the following structures and nuclei (Figs. 10.8–10.10; Table 10.2).
  - **Mammillary bodies** that lie between the rostral limits of the two crura cerebri, on either side of the midline and contain the hypothalamic

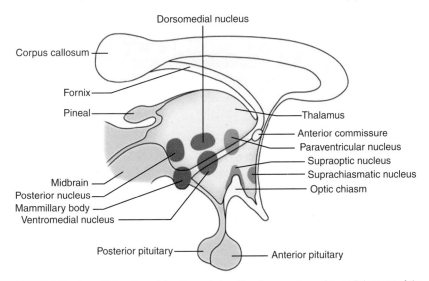

FIGURE 10.8 A sagittal section of the diencephalon. The diagram shows the medial aspect of the hypothalamus. The approximate location of some of the principal hypothalamic nuclei is shown.
Source: *Crossman AR, PhD DSc. Hypothalamus, limbic system and olfactory system. Neuroanatomy: an illustrated colour text; 2015. p. 160–70, Chapter 16.*

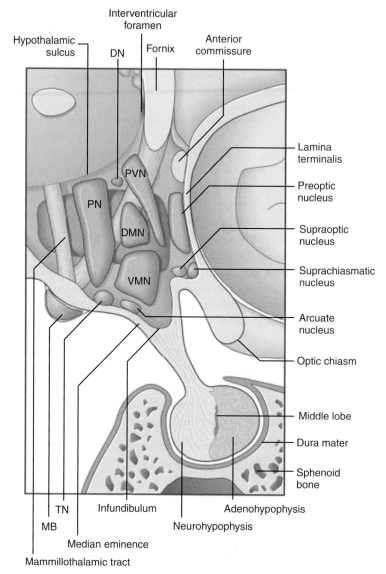

FIGURE 10.9   Hypothalamic nuclei and hypophysis, viewed from the lateral side. DMN, dorsomedial nucleus; DN, dorsal nucleus; MB, mammillary body; PN, posterior nucleus; PVN, paraventricular nucleus; TN, tuberomammillary nucleus; VMN, ventromedial nucleus. The lateral hypothalamic nucleus is shown in pink.

Source: *Mtui E, MD. Hypothalamus. Fitzgerald's clinical neuroanatomy and neuroscience; 2016. p. 253–259, Chapter 26.*

mammillary nuclei. These constitute part of the limbic system, receiving afferents from the hippocampus and projecting to the anterior nuclei of the thalamus and the brainstem.

- **Tuber cinereum** is a small elevated area that lies in the midline, caudal to the optic chiasm. The thin infundibulum or pituitary stalk

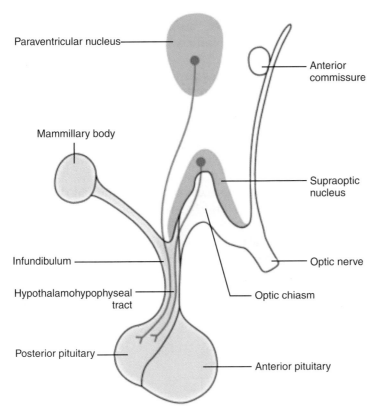

FIGURE 10.10 Supraoptic and paraventricular nuclei projecting to the posterior pituitary via the hypothalamohypophyseal tract.
Source: *Crossman AR, PhD DSc. Hypothalamus, limbic system and olfactory system. Neuroanatomy: an illustrated colour text; 2015. p. 160–70, Chapter 16.*

Table 10.2 Hypothalamic nuclei

Posterior	Middle	Anterior
Posterior	Paraventricular	Preoptic
Mammillary	Dorsomedial	Supraoptic
Tuberomammillary	Lateral	Suprachiasmatic
Dorsal	Ventromedial	
	Arcuate	

Source: *Adapted from Fitzgerald's clinical neuroanatomy and neuroscience, 7th ed.; 2016. p. 253–9.*

arises from this tuber. This stalk is attached to the pituitary gland (hypophysis), which lies within the sella turcica of the sphenoid bone.

- The **supraoptic** and **paraventricular nuclei** of the hypothalamus (located medially) produce **vasopressin** (antidiuretic hormone that helps reabsorb water in the kidneys) and **oxytocin** (that is induced by suckling and stimulates milk production and induces uterine contractions), respectively. Vasopressin and oxytocin are transported to the posterior pituitary in the hypothalamohypophyseal tract.

- The **lateral hypothalamus** (medial and ventral to the subthalamus, also known as **feeding centre**) and the **ventromedial nucleus (satiety centre)** regulate eating and drinking.
- Neurons of the hypothalamic **arcuate nucleus** produce **dopamine** that is released within the neurohypophysis by axons travelling in the hypothalamohypophyseal tract. Dopamine inhibits the release of prolactin by the anterior pituitary gland.
- The **suprachiasmatic nucleus** controls the **diurnal rhythms** and the **sleep–wake cycle**. It receives some afferent fibres directly from the retina.
- **Inputs** to the hypothalamus are both **circulatory** and **neural** (Fig. 10.11).
  - The circulating blood provides **physical** (temperature, osmolality), **chemical** (blood glucose, acid–base state) and **hormonal** signals of the state of the body.

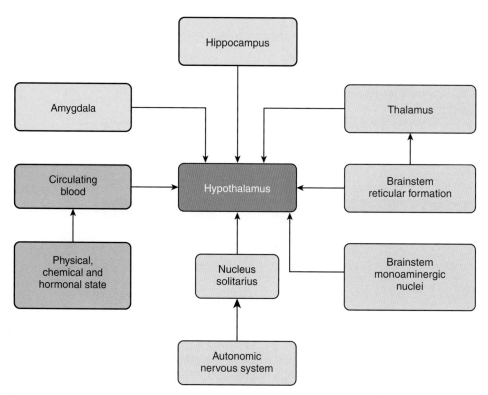

FIGURE 10.11 Neural and nonneural inputs of the hypothalamus.

Source: *Crossman AR, PhD DSc. Hypothalamus, limbic system and olfactory system. Neuroanatomy: an illustrated colour text; 2015. p. 160–70, Chapter 16.*

- Neural signals come from a number of sources with the largest input being from limbic structures, the **hippocampus** and the **amygdala**.
  - Fibres of hippocampal origin constitute the fornix, which terminates in the medial mammillary nucleus within the mammillary body.
  - Fibres from the amygdala to the hypothalamus run in the stria terminalis.
  - The **nucleus solitarius** of the medulla projects to the hypothalamus, transferring information collected by the autonomic nervous system concerning the pressure (using **baroreceptors**) and the chemical constituents of the fluid-filled cavities (using **chemoreceptors**).
  - The **state of arousal** is communicated by connections that originate in the **brainstem**.
- **Outputs** from the hypothalamus are also **circulatory** and **neural** (Fig. 10.12).
  - The hypothalamus has access to the circulation through the **portal system** that allows for the direction of **hormonal synthesis and release**.

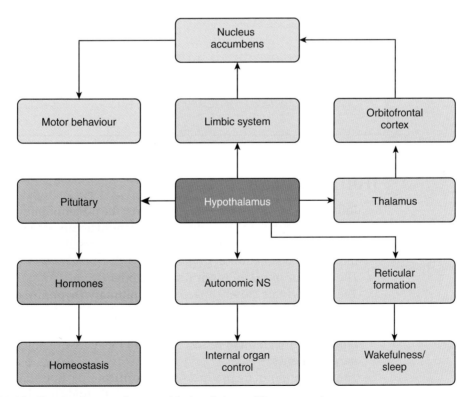

FIGURE 10.12 Neural and nonneural outputs of the hypothalamus. NS, nervous system.
Source: *Crossman AR, PhD DSc. Hypothalamus, limbic system and olfactory system. Neuroanatomy: an illustrated colour text; 2015. p. 160–70, Chapter 16.*

- The neural output of the hypothalamus is directed to various regions of the brain.
    - **Descending** fibres pass to the brainstem and some reach the spinal cord allowing communication with the **reticular formation** and the **preganglionic sympathetic and parasympathetic neurons** of the autonomic nervous system.
    - **Ascending** connections pass to the **limbic system**, both directly and via the thalamus to the orbitofrontal cerebral cortex. These connections help initiate appropriate motor **behavioural responses** of an instinctive kind and at times may allow for more complex adaptive behaviour.

CLINICAL INSIGHT

- **Hypothalamic dysfunction**
    - Tumours and other diseases of the hypothalamus and the associated pituitary gland lead to under- or overproduction of circulating hormones.
    - Disorders of growth (dwarfism, gigantism and acromegaly), sexual function (precocious puberty, hypogonadism) and adrenal cortical control (Cushing disease and adrenal insufficiency) could occur due to abnormalities in the quantity of circulating hormones.
    - **Lateral** hypothalamic lesions cause **aphagia** and **adipsia.**
    - Lesions in the **ventromedial nucleus** cause abnormally **increased food intake.**
    - **Diabetes insipidus** is a disorder of hypothalamic dysfunction due to interruption of the hypothalamohypophyseal pathway caused by tumours in this region or by head injury.

PITUITARY GLAND

The **pituitary gland** consists of two major parts: the posterior pituitary or **neurohypophysis** and the anterior pituitary or **adenohypophysis** (Fig. 10.13).

- The **posterior pituitary** is an expansion of the distal part of the infundibulum and is **neural** in origin.
- The **anterior pituitary** is **not neural** in origin.
- The two parts are closely linked by the **pituitary (hypophyseal) portal system** of vessels.
- Releasing factors synthesized in the hypothalamus pass to the adenohypophysis through these vessels to control the release of anterior pituitary hormones.
- The anterior pituitary produces adrenocorticotropic hormone, luteinizing hormone, follicle-stimulating hormone, thyroid-stimulating hormone, growth hormone and prolactin.

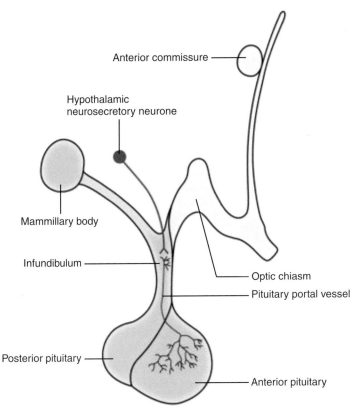

FIGURE 10.13 The anterior and posterior parts of the pituitary gland along with the portal system linking both parts.
Source: *Crossman AR, PhD DSc. Hypothalamus, limbic system and olfactory system. Neuroanatomy: an illustrated colour text; 2015. p. 160–70, Chapter 16.*

CLINICAL INSIGHT

■ **Pituitary adenomas**
  ■ Since the pituitary gland is closely adjacent to the optic chiasm, large tumours of the gland (pituitary macroadenomas) may lead to bitemporal visual field loss.

CASE STUDY DISCUSSION

Unilateral thalamic pain may be seen in lesions or infarcts of the **ventral posterior nuclei of the contralateral thalamus.**

Clinical Features

- Decreased pinprick, temperature, vibration and light touch sensation in the right face and body.
- Decreased two-point discrimination in the right hand.

In the absence of other deficits, sometimes these patients are thought to have psychologically based symptoms in the absence of more objective findings on examination.

However, these symptoms may be seen in lesions in the ventral posterior medial and ventral posterior lateral nuclei of the contralateral thalamus.

Given the sudden onset of symptoms and the multiple risk factors for stroke, the likely diagnosis is an ischaemic infarct of the left thalamus, caused by occlusion of small penetrating arteries resulting in a **lacunar infarct**.

Management

A brain CT showed a small hypodensity in the left thalamus. Subsequent brain MRI showed restricted diffusion in the left lateral thalamus.

The patient was admitted to the neurology service. She had stroke workup that showed no evidence for an embolic stroke. Her hypertension medication was adjusted and she was started on aspirin to prevent further strokes.

Her numbness gradually improved and it completely resolved within few days.

CHAPTER 11

Cerebral Cortex

Rechdi Ahdab

CASE STUDY

Presentation and Physical Examination: A 74-year-old woman known to have colon cancer with liver metastasis presented to the emergency room for two episodes of involuntary movements of the right upper extremity, each lasting for 5 min. She reported jerky movements of the right upper extremity that started in the arm and progressively spread to involve the entire right hemibody. Her neurological examination was normal.

Diagnosis and Management: Brain magnetic resonance imaging (MRI) revealed multiple metastatic lesions (Fig. 11.1). A neurology consult was ordered. After interviewing the patient and reviewing the MRI, the neurologist concluded that she likely experienced partial seizures secondary to her metastatic brain disease; thus, she was started on an anti-epileptic drug. The neurologist identified the lesion that was causing her seizures. His main concern was that with further growth, the culprit lesion would cause right upper extremity paralysis. He recommended treating that specific lesion with stereotactic radiotherapy.

In your opinion, to what lesion was the neurologist referring? Try to answer this question after studying this chapter!

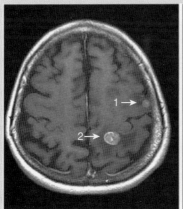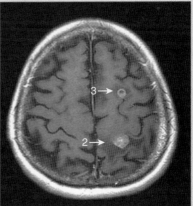

FIGURE 11.1 Axial brain MRI showing three metastatic lesions.
Source: *Courtesy of Rechdi Ahdab, MD. Lebanese American University Medical Center.*

BRIEF INTRODUCTION

The **cerebral cortex** is a thin (2–4 mm) layer of **grey matter** that covers the outer surface of the brain.

- It receives sensory information from the inside and outside world, processes this information, plans and ultimately generates a specific reaction.
- At the macroscopic level, it is organized into complex **sulci** and **gyri**. These folds greatly increase the surface of the cortex without a concomitant increase in volume, which allows the brain to fit in its allocated space within the skull.
- More than two-thirds of the cerebral cortex is buried within the sulci; the latter display a certain degree of variability between subjects. Nevertheless, some are relatively consistent in all individuals and are used as anatomical landmarks to identify specific regions of the cerebral cortex.

Functionally, the cerebral cortex can be divided into multiple separate areas.

- Each area is strategically linked to other cortical areas and fulfils a very precise function.
- These include sensory perception, movement, language, thinking, memory, consciousness and certain aspects of emotions.
- Some cortical regions have a relatively **simple function** and are known as the **primary cortices**. These include areas directly receiving sensory input (such as vision, hearing and somatic sensation) and regions involved in executing a motor command.
- Conversely, the **association cortices** subserve more **complex functions** that require a great deal of data processing.
- Although the sulci delineate some of the functional areas of the cortex, the boundaries of other functional areas do not correspond to any recognizable cortical landmark.

CYTOARCHITECTURE

The neurons of the cerebral cortex are organized into layers. Most cortical areas have **six distinct layers** (Fig. 11.2); each is characterized by the shape, size and density of indwelling neurons as well as the organization of nerve fibres.

The two main cell types that help define the cortical layers are

- **Pyramidal cells** (Fig. 11.3)
  - **Are excitatory** cells.
  - Utilize **glutamate** and **aspartate** as neurotransmitters.
  - Have apical dendrites:
    - Directed towards the surface of the brain.
    - That branch profusely in layer I.
  - Are responsible for the output of the cerebral cortex.
    - Those of **layers II–III** project to other **cortical** areas.
    - Those of **layers V–VI** project to the **thalamus** and other **subcortical** regions.

■ **Stellate cells** (Fig. 11.3)
  ■ Receive inputs from the **thalamus**.
  ■ Have spiny dendrites.
  ■ Output connections are **excitatory**.
  ■ Axons **do not** project out of the cortical layers.
■ Other less common cells can also be found in the cerebral cortex. Examples include Martinotti, fusiform and horizontal cells (Fig. 11.3).

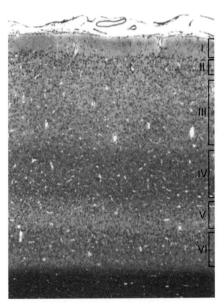

FIGURE 11.2 The six-layered structure of the cerebral cortex.
Source: *Young, Barbara, BSc Med Sci (Hons), PhD, MB BChir, MRCP, FRCPA. Central nervous system. Wheater's functional histology. p. 384–401, Chapter 20.*

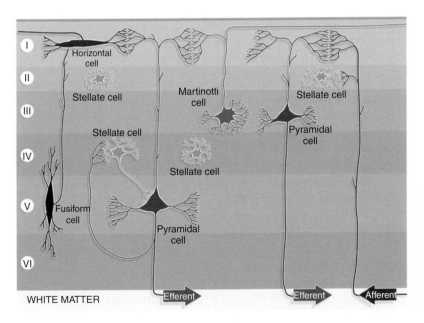

FIGURE 11.3 Schematic showing the five characteristic types of cortical neurons.
Source: *Young, Barbara, BSc Med Sci (Hons), PhD, MB BChir, MRCP, FRCPA. Central nervous system. Wheater's functional histology. p. 384–401, Chapter 20.*

Cortical layers include from outside (pial surface) to inside (white matter) (Figs. 11.2 and 11.3):

- **Molecular layer (layer I)**, which
  - Is rich in synapses and axons that run **parallel** to the surface.
  - Has few cell bodies (mainly neuroglial and nonpyramidal).
- **External granular layer (layer II)**, which is primarily composed of
  - Small pyramidal cells.
  - Numerous stellate cells.
- **External pyramidal layer (layer III)**
  - That is relatively **thick**.
  - Contains pyramidal cells
    - Of medium size.
    - That progressively increase in size towards the deeper part of the layer.
    - That are connected to other regions of the cortex, including the contralateral side of the brain.
- **Internal granular layer (layer IV)**
  - Contains densely packed small cells:
    - Stellate cells (star-shaped).
    - Pyramidal cells.
- **Internal pyramidal (or ganglionic) layer (layer V)**
  - Contains medium-sized and large pyramidal cells.
  - In the region of the motor cortex, some are very large and are known as the **Betz cells**.
  - Gives rise to the bulk of the **corticofugal fibres** (i.e., fibres leaving the cerebral cortex) that project onto the **basal ganglia**, **brainstem** and **spinal cord**
- **Multiform layer (layer VI)**
  - Composed of small neurons (stellate, pyramidal and fusiform).
  - Gives rise to **corticofugal fibres** to the **thalamus** mainly.

Some cortical regions contain **less than six layers** (3–5 layers). Examples include the **olfactory cortex** and the **hippocampus**.

At a more functional level, the cortical layers can be divided into three parts:

- **Supragranular layers (layers I–III)**
  - Are the primary origin and termination of **intracortical** connections.
  - Permits communication between the different cortical areas.
  - Connections are either:
    1. **Intracortical** (connecting areas of the same hemisphere).
    2. **Commissural** (connections to the opposite hemisphere).
- **Internal granular layer (layer IV)**
  - Receives **thalamocortical** connections.
  - **Is most developed** in the **primary sensory** cortices.
  - **Is poorly developed** or **even absent** in **motor** cortices (also called **agranular cortex**).
- **Infragranular layers (layers V and VI)**
  - Primarily connect the cerebral cortex with **subcortical** regions.
  - **Are most developed** in the **motor** cortex.

The six-layered cortical neurons are further organized into columns.

- **Cortical columns** are oriented perpendicularly to the cortical surface.
- These columns are believed to function as separate modules that process incoming information via a complex internal processing chain and appropriately distribute the newly processed information to the proper brain structures.

Variation in Cortical Cytoarchitecture

There are regional variations in the cortex cytoarchitecture. Korbinian Brodmann extensively studied these variations and was able to identify 52 different areas (Fig. 11.4). Although these areas were exclusively defined on the basis of the cellular composition of the cortex, the Brodmann map correlates well with functional maps of the cortex.

More simply, the cortical areas can be subdivided into two major groups:

- **Agranular cortex**
  - Relatively lacks the **granular layers II and IV**.
  - Contains **very well-developed** pyramidal **layers III and V**.
  - Is most frequently associated with motor regions.
- **Granular cortex**
  - **Is a very well-developed granular layer** with numerous small stellate cells.
  - Is associated with regions receiving sensory input from the thalamus.

SULCUS AND GYRUS ANATOMY

The two deepest grooves on the brain are known as fissures.

- The **longitudinal fissure** separates the right and left cerebral hemispheres.
- The **transverse fissure** separates the cerebral hemispheres from the cerebellum.

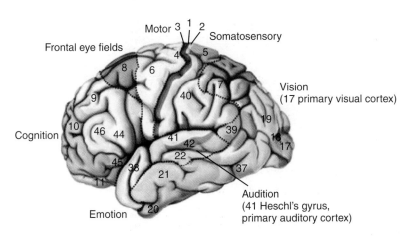

FIGURE 11.4 Brodmann areas and their associated nervous functions. Source: *Shimizu, Yu. Neuronal response to Shepard's tones. An auditory fMRI study using multifractal analysis. Brain Res 1186: 113–123.*

The main sulci of the brain divide the cerebral hemispheres into lobes (Fig. 11.5); the latter are defined by the cranial bones under which they reside and thus are known as the frontal, parietal, temporal and occipital lobes. The main sulci are as follows (Fig. 11.5):

- Central sulcus
- Parieto-occipital sulcus
- Lateral (Sylvian) sulcus
- Calcarine sulcus

The **central sulcus** (Fig. 11.5) divides the **frontal lobe** anteriorly from the **parietal lobe** posteriorly. It is of great functional importance since it

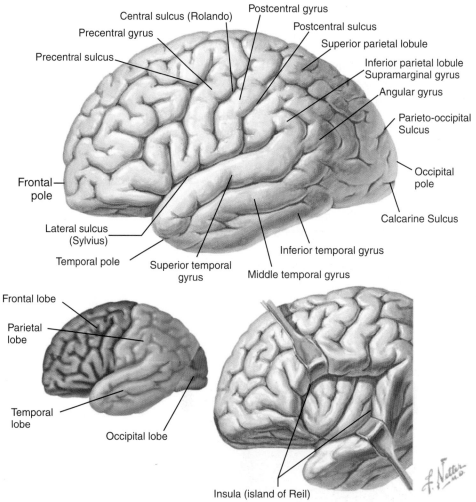

FIGURE 11.5   Surface anatomy of the cerebral cortex showing the four lobes visible on the surface of the brain and one-fifth buried in the depth of the Sylvian fissure.

Source: *Susan E., PhD. Organization and general functions of the nervous system. Mulroney, Netter's essential physiology. p. 48–56, Chapter 4.*

separates the **motor cortex** rostrally from the **somatosensory cortex** caudally. The central sulcus has several characteristic features that render it easy to recognize:

- It runs **uninterrupted** from the lateral fissure to the superior medial border of the hemisphere.
- Its **lower end** is most often separated from the lateral fissure by a **narrow bridge of cortex**.
- Its **upper end** indents the apex at around **1 cm behind the midpoint**.
- It runs forward and downward across the convexity.
- It is bounded rostrally and caudally by two parallel sulci, the pre- and postcentral sulci.

CLINICAL INSIGHT

- **The 'Hand Knob'**
  - The **middle segment** of the central sulcus has a very typical appearance on MRI (Fig. 11.6):
    - It resembles an **inverted omega** or a **doorknob**.
    - This segment is known as the **'hand knob'** since it corresponds to the cortical area that controls the **hand motor function**.
    - At the origin of this aspect, an interdigitation of the walls of the precentral and postcentral gyri is present.
    - The 'hand knob' helps identify the central sulcus, which corresponds to the limit between the frontal and parietal lobes.

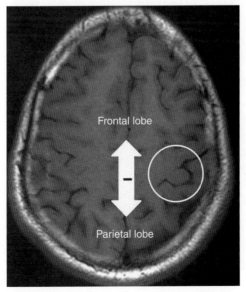

FIGURE 11.6 Central sulcus appearance on MRI with the characteristic motor knob (circle).
Source: *Courtesy of Rechdi Ahdab, MD. Lebanese American University Medical Center.*

The **lateral sulcus (or Sylvian fissure)** is a deep cleft at the **inferolateral aspect** of the hemisphere.

- Its short stem arises at the inferior surface of the hemisphere and divides into three branches (Figs. 11.5 and 11.7):
  - **Anterior horizontal ramus**
  - **Anterior ascending ramus**
  - **Posterior ramus**
- An island of cortex called the **insula** lies deep inside the lateral sulcus.
- The insula cannot be seen from the surface of the brain unless the lips of the lateral sulcus are separated (Fig. 11.5).

The **parieto-occipital sulcus** begins at the superior margin of the hemisphere at about **5 cm rostral** to the occipital lobe (Figs. 11.5 and 11.8).

- It courses inferiorly on the medial surface of the brain.
- It **merges** with the **calcarine sulcus** about **halfway** along its length.

The **calcarine sulcus** is found only on the **medial surface** of the hemisphere (Figs. 11.5 and 11.8).

- It begins under the posterior end of the corpus callosum.
- It courses upwards and backwards until it meets the occipital pole, where it is interrupted abruptly.
- In some subjects, it may continue shortly over the lateral surface of the hemisphere.

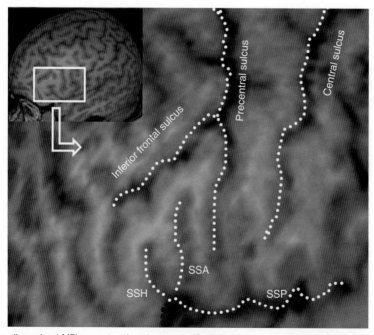

FIGURE 11.7   Three-dimensional MRI reconstruction showing the Sylvian sulcus and its three divisions: anterior horizontal ramus (SSH), anterior ascending ramus (SSA) and posterior ramus (SSP).

Source: *Courtesy of Rechdi Ahdab, MD. Lebanese American University Medical Center.*

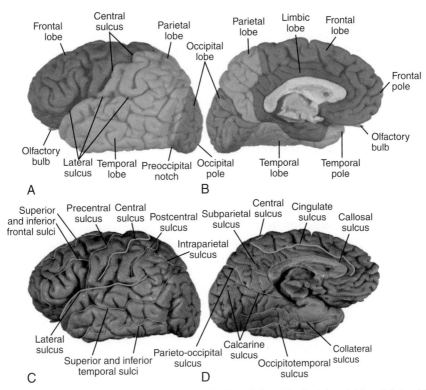

FIGURE 11.8 Lobes and sulci of the cerebral hemisphere. (A) The boundaries of the frontal, parietal, occipital and temporal lobes on the lateral surface of the hemisphere; (B) the boundaries of the frontal, parietal, occipital, temporal and limbic lobes on the medial surface of the hemisphere; (C) major sulci on the lateral surface of the hemisphere; and (D) major sulci on the medial and inferior surfaces of the hemisphere.

Source: *(Dissection courtesy of Grant Dahmer, Department of Cell Biology and Anatomy, University of Arizona College of Medicine.) Vanderah, Todd W, PhD. Gross anatomy and general organization of the central nervous system. Nolte's the human brain. p. 56–83, Chapter 3.*

LOBES OF THE CEREBRAL HEMISPHERES

The **lobes** of the cerebral hemisphere are easy to identify on the **dorsolateral aspect** of the brain but more difficult to define on the medial and inferior surfaces.

Dorsolateral Aspect of the Brain

Frontal Lobes
The **frontal lobes** are bound posteriorly by the central sulcus and inferiorly by the lateral sulcus. The convexity of the frontal lobe is divided into four gyri by three sulci:

- **Precentral sulcus**
- **Superior frontal sulcus**
- **Inferior frontal sulcus**

The **precentral sulcus** runs parallel to the central sulcus and in between both sulci lies the **precentral gyrus**. The precentral sulcus is rarely continuous. It is **typically interrupted** at a dorsoventral level corresponding to the middle frontal gyrus, which is usually continuous posteriorly with the precentral gyrus (Fig. 11.9). Thus, the precentral sulcus is composed of two separate sulci:

- **Superior precentral sulcus:**
  - Corresponds to a posterior bifurcation of the superior frontal sulcus.
  - Rarely reaches the interhemispheric (longitudinal) fissure.
- **Inferior precentral sulcus**, which corresponds to a posterior bifurcation of the inferior frontal sulcus

The **superior** and **inferior frontal sulci** divide the cortical areas that are rostral to the precentral sulcus into three gyri (Fig. 11.10).

- **Superior frontal gyrus**
- **Middle frontal gyrus**
- **Inferior frontal gyrus**

The **superior frontal sulcus** (Fig. 11.10):

- Courses parallel to the interhemispheric fissure.
- Caudally, it merges with the superior precentral sulcus forming a T-shaped branching.

The **inferior frontal sulcus** (Fig. 11.10):

- Courses almost parallel to the Sylvian sulcus.
- Merges caudally with the inferior precentral sulcus.
- Is **frequently interrupted** along its course.

Between the inferior frontal sulcus dorsally and the inferior precentral sulcus lies the posterior part of the **inferior frontal gyrus**, which presents a particular segmentation. The ascending and horizontal branches of the Sylvian

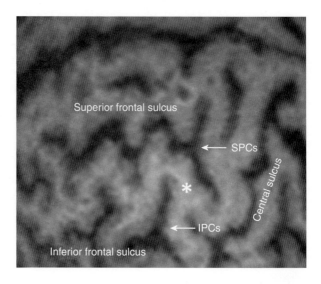

FIGURE 11.9   Three-dimensional MRI reconstruction showing the anatomy of the precentral sulcus. The latter is typically interrupted and composed of a dorsal segment – the superior precentral sulcus (SPCs) – and a ventral segment – the inferior precentral sulcus. Consequently, the middle frontal gyrus is often in communication with the precentral gyrus (asterisk). IPCs, inferior precentral sulcus.

Source: *Courtesy of Rechdi Ahdab, MD. Lebanese American University Medical Center.*

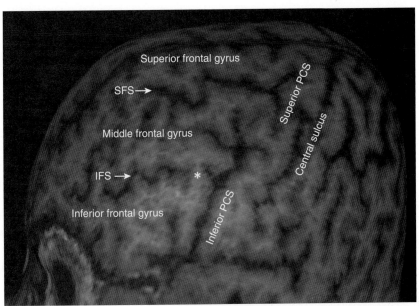

FIGURE 11.10   Three-dimensional MRI reconstruction showing the macro-anatomical landmarks of the frontal lobe. Note that the inferior frontal sulcus is frequently interrupted along its course (asterisk). IFS, inferior frontal sulcus; SFS, superior frontal sulcus; PCS, precentral sulcus. Source: *Courtesy of Rechdi Ahdab, MD. Lebanese American University Medical Center.*

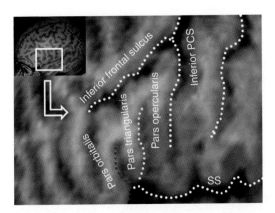

FIGURE 11.11   Three-dimensional MRI reconstruction showing the anatomy of the inferior frontal gyrus. SS, Sylvian sulcus; anterior horizontal ramus (red), anterior ascending ramus (yellow) and posterior ramus (white). PCS, precentral sulcus. Source: *Courtesy of Rechdi Ahdab, MD. Lebanese American University Medical Center.*

fissure subdivide this cortical region into three parts (from anterior to posterior) (Fig. 11.11):

- **Pars orbitalis**
- **Pars triangularis**
- **Pars opercularis**

Parietal Lobe

The **parietal lobe** is defined by the following:

- Central sulcus anteriorly
- Parieto-occipital sulcus posteriorly and inferiorly
- Posterior ramus of the lateral sulcus inferiorly

The dorsolateral surface of the parietal lobe is divided into three gyri by two sulci (Fig. 11.12):

- **Postcentral sulcus:**
    - That runs parallel to the central sulcus.
    - Forms the posterior limit of the postcentral gyrus.
- **Intraparietal sulcus:**
    - Runs parallel to the interhemispheric fissure.
    - Divides the parietal cortex lying caudal to the postcentral sulcus into:
        - **Superior parietal lobule**.
        - **Inferior parietal lobule**, which is mainly composed of two distinct regions:
            - **Supramarginal gyrus**, which arches over the posterior part of the Sylvian fissure, behind the inferior part of the postcentral sulcus.
            - **Angular gyrus**, which is caudal to the supramarginal gyrus.

Temporal Lobe

The **temporal lobe** lies inferior to the posterior ramus of the Sylvian fissure. Its dorsolateral aspect is divided by two sulci, which run parallel to the lateral sulcus, into three gyri (Fig. 11.13):

- **Superior temporal gyrus**
- **Middle temporal gyrus**
- **Inferior temporal gyrus**

Occipital Lobe

The **occipital lobe** occupies a restricted area on the dorsolateral aspect of the hemispheres, caudal to the parieto-occipital sulcus (Fig. 11.14).

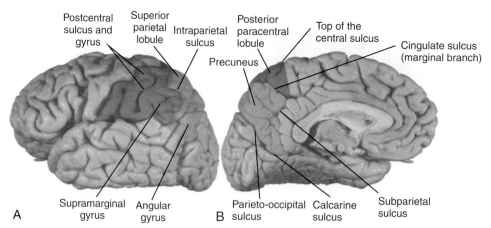

FIGURE 11.12   Lateral (A) and medial (B) surfaces of the parietal lobe.

Source: *(Dissection courtesy of Grant Dahmer, Department of Cell Biology and Anatomy, University of Arizona College of Medicine.) Vanderah, Todd W, PhD. Gross anatomy and general organization of the central nervous system. Nolte's the human brain. p. 56–83, Chapter 3.*

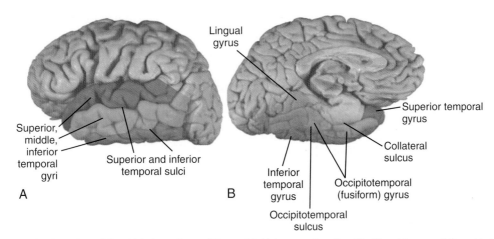

FIGURE 11.13 Lateral, medial and inferior surfaces of the occipital lobe, seen from the side (A) and from medially and below (B).
Source: *(Dissection courtesy of Grant Dahmer, Department of Cell Biology and Anatomy, University of Arizona College of Medicine.) Vanderah, Todd W, PhD. Gross anatomy and general organization of the central nervous system. Nolte's the human brain. p. 56–83, Chapter 3.*

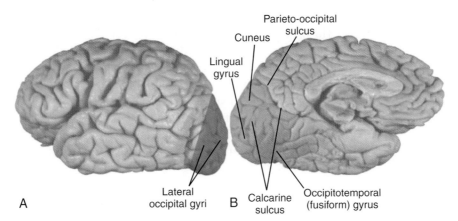

FIGURE 11.14 Lateral, medial and inferior surfaces of the occipital lobe, seen from the side (A) and from medially and below (B).
Source: *(Dissection courtesy of Grant Dahmer, Department of Cell Biology and Anatomy, University of Arizona College of Medicine.) Vanderah, Todd W, PhD. Gross anatomy and general organization of the central nervous system. Nolte's the human brain. p. 56–83, Chapter 3.*

Medial Aspect of the Brain

Several sulci and gyri (Fig. 11.15) mark the medial aspect of the brain.

- **Cingulate sulcus**
  - Its anterior part, **pars subfrontalis**, runs parallel to the corpus callosum.
  - Its posterior part, **pars marginalis**, curves up to the supero-median margin and borders the paracentral lobule posteriorly.
- **Cingulate gyrus**
  - Begins beneath the anterior end of the corpus callosum.
  - Courses parallel to the corpus callosum until it reaches its posterior pole.
  - Is separated from the corpus callosum by the **callosal sulcus**.

- The **paracentral lobule** is the area of cerebral cortex that surrounds the indentation of the central sulcus on the superior border.
  - Its **anterior aspect** is the continuation of the **precentral gyrus**.
  - Its **posterior aspect** is an extension of the **postcentral gyrus**.
- The **precuneus** is an area of the cortex bounded by:
  - The upturn of the posterior end (marginal branch) of the cingulate sulcus superiorly.
  - The parieto-occipital sulcus posteriorly.
  - The calcarine sulcus inferiorly.
- The **cuneus** is a **triangular** area bounded by:
  - Parieto-occipital sulcus superiorly.
  - Calcarine sulcus inferiorly.

Inferior Surface of the Brain

Several sulci and gyri (Figs. 11.15 and 11.16) mark the inferior surface of the brain.
- The **collateral sulcus** runs anteriorly below the calcarine sulcus
  - Between these two sulci lies the **lingual gyrus**.
  - Anteriorly, the collateral sulcus forms the lateral boundary of the parahippocampal gyrus.
  - The parahippocampal gyrus terminates anteriorly as the hook-like uncus.
- The **medial occipitotemporal gyrus** extends from the occipital pole to the temporal pole. It is bounded by the following:
  - **Collateral** and **rhinal sulci** medially
  - **Occipitotemporal sulcus** laterally
- On the inferior aspect of the frontal lobe, the **olfactory bulb** and **tract** overlie a sulcus called the **olfactory sulcus**. The **gyrus rectus** lies medial and a number of **orbital gyri** lie lateral to the olfactory sulcus.

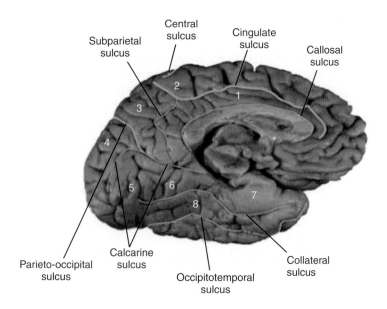

FIGURE 11.15   Major sulci and gyri on the medial and inferior surfaces of the hemisphere. 1, cingulate gyrus; 2, paracentral gyrus; 3, precuneus; 4, cuneus; 5, lingual gyrus; 6, parahippocampal gyrus; 7, uncus; 8, medial occipitotemporal gyrus. Source: *(Dissection courtesy of Grant Dahmer, Department of Cell Biology and Anatomy, University of Arizona College of Medicine.) Vanderah, Todd W, PhD. Gross anatomy and general organization of the central nervous system. Nolte's the human brain. p. 56–83, Chapter 3.*

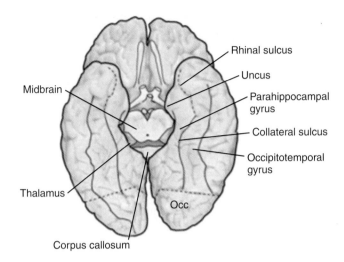

FIGURE 11.16 Sulci and gyri of the inferior surface of the brain (anterior towards the top of the diagram). Occ, Occipital lobe.
Source: *(Dissection by Grant Dahmer, Department of Cell Biology and Anatomy, The University of Arizona College of Medicine.) Nolte, John, PhD. External anatomy of the brain. The human brain in photographs and diagrams. p. 1–21, Chapter 1.*

FUNCTIONAL LOCALIZATION

Functional localization refers to anatomically delineating the functional areas of the cortex. This forms the basis for understanding the clinical correlates of damage to various parts of the brain. Functional maps of the cortex correlate well with the cytoarchitectonic areas defined by Brodmann (BA for Brodmann area).

Sulci and gyri are important cortical landmarks and help to locate functional areas. In some cases, there is a perfect correlation between a sulcus and a specific functional area; this applies to all primary cortices. On the other hand, the exact extent of such cortical areas cannot be determined on the basis of sulcus anatomy, even when dealing with the primary cortices. The following are some examples:

- Although the **primary motor cortex** is always found within the **central sulcus**, its anterior border does not correspond to the precentral sulcus or any other sulcus.
- Similarly, the **primary visual cortex** is always found in the **calcarine sulcus**, but its outer borders do not correspond to a sulcus.
- The **primary auditory cortex** is always found in **Heschl's gyrus**, but its anterior border cannot be defined by a macro-anatomical landmark.

The relationship between functional areas and the surrounding sulci and gyri is even more loosely defined for most secondary cortices and association areas. Here, sulci and gyri are extremely variable, and the exact location of these areas cannot be reliably determined on the basis of macro-anatomical landmarks.

Some cortical functions are not equally distributed between the two hemispheres, one hemisphere being dominant for that specific function. This is the case of **language**, for example, which is a function of the **left hemisphere** in most people.

CLINICAL INSIGHT

■ **Motor Cortex Localization**

A frequent misconception is to consider the precentral gyrus as the primary motor cortex. In fact, the bulk of the primary motor cortex is buried inside the central sulcus, and most of the exposed precentral gyrus corresponds to the secondary motor cortex. Consequently, restricted damage to the more anterior parts of the precentral gyrus may have little impact on motor command.

Sensory Cortex

The **sensory cortex** is organized in an hierarchical manner, and information reaching this area is processed in a very precise order. Sensory information originating in the receptors is conveyed to the thalamus and from there it reaches the different parts of the sensory cortex in the following order:

- **Primary sensory area**
  - Receives input from the **thalamus**.
  - Specialized in detecting and decoding the **basic properties of the stimulus** such as its location and intensity.
- **Secondary sensory cortices** further **analyze the stimulus** in light of previous experiences in an attempt to identify its precise nature.
- **Sensory association areas**
  - **Integrate information** from different sensory modalities.
  - This last stage of processing provides **conscious perception of the stimulus** and helps initiate plans for an appropriate reaction.

Primary Somatosensory Cortex

The **primary somatosensory cortex (SI)** analyzes sensory information such as touch, pressure, joint position, temperature and vibration. This area:

- Is located along the **postcentral gyrus** of the **parietal lobe** (Fig. 11.17).
- Corresponds to **BA 1–3**.
- Receives input from the **ventroposterolateral (VPL)** and **ventroposteromedial (VPM) thalamic nuclei**.
- Is organized in a precise somatotopic fashion (Fig. 11.18).
  - The **face** and **head** are represented **dorsolaterally**.
  - The **lower extremities** are represented **medially**.
  - The **upper extremities** are represented at an **intermediate position**.

Very sensitive areas such as the **hands** and **mouth** have disproportionately **large representations**, which allow for more precise sensory discrimination.

Secondary Somatosensory Cortex

The **secondary somatosensory cortex (SII)** is located in the **upper bank** of the **lateral sulcus**, just inferior to the central sulcus. This area:

- Receives sensory information from:
  - **SI**.
  - Less specific thalamic nuclei.

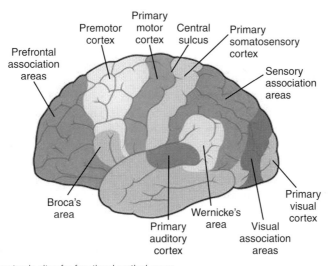

FIGURE 11.17   Classic anatomic sites for functional cortical areas.

Source: *Mangrum, Wells I. Functional magnetic resonance imaging. Duke review of MRI principles: case review series. p. 265–278, Chapter 17.*

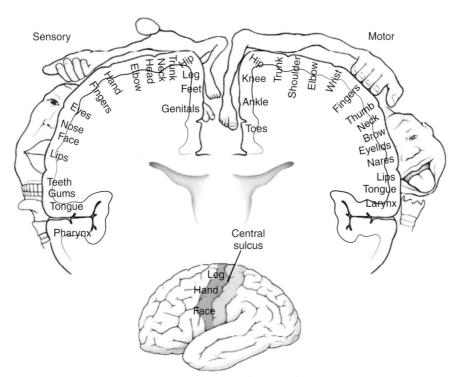

FIGURE 11.18   Somatotopic organization of the primary sensory and motor cortices.

Source: *Waldman, Steven D, MD, JD. The posterior column pathway. Pain review. p. 174–175. Chapter 100.*

- Responds to bilateral stimuli.
- Has a poor somatotopic organization.
- Serves an **integrative function**.

Sensory Association Cortex

The **sensory association cortex** is located in the **posterior parietal cortex (BA 5 and 7)**, directly posterior to **SI**. This area:

- Receives synthesized information from **SI** and **SII**.
- Is involved in:
  - **High-level integration** of sensory information.
  - **Learning process**.
  - **Memory** of the surrounding tactile and spatial environment.

CLINICAL INSIGHT

- **Astereognosis**

When an object is placed in the hand, the somatosensory cortex transforms sensory data into spatial information about the object. One clinical correlate of damage to this part of the cortex is **astereognosis**, which is the inability to discriminate the size and shape of objects. This was the case of a 52-year-old with a cortical bleed in the right postcentral gyrus (Fig. 11.19). The patient was unable to recognize a key or pen by touch when placed in his left hand. He was also found to have **agraphesthesia**, which is the inability to recognize writing on the skin by the touch sensation only.

Visual Cortex

The **primary visual cortex** (or **striate cortex; BA 17**) surrounds the **calcarine sulcus** on the medial aspect of the occipital lobes (Fig. 11.20).

- It discerns the **intensity**, **shape**, **size** and **location of objects** in the visual field.
- It is retinotopically organized.
  - **Upper** visual field is represented **inferior** to the calcarine sulcus.
  - **Lower** visual field is represented **superior** to the calcarine sulcus
  - **Central** vision is represented at the **posterior tip** of the **occipital lobe.**
- Disproportionately large amount of cortex is reserved for the central vision.
- Visual information is then transferred to the **secondary visual areas (prestriate cortex; BA 18 and 19)** and to the **inferior temporal cortex (BA 20 and 21)**.
  - These regions are important for **colour**, **motion** and **depth** perception.
- Visual information ultimately reaches the **visual association cortex**:
  - **Parietal lobe (BA 5 and 7)** for processing of **spatial features** and **movement.**
  - **Temporal lobe** for **object recognition.**

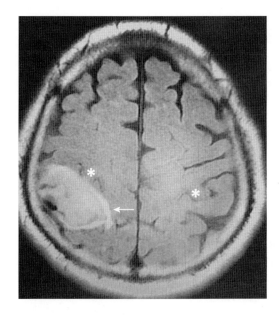

FIGURE 11.19 Axial MRI showing a right parietal cortex bleed (arrow) in the postcentral sulcus. Asterisks mark the central sulcus and its characteristic 'hand knob'.
Source: *Courtesy of Rechdi Ahdab, MD. Lebanese American University Medical Center.*

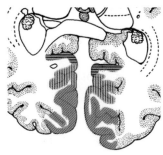

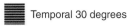 Temporal 30 degrees

10–60 degrees

Central 10 degrees (macular)

FIGURE 11.20 Retinotopic organization of the striate cortex (axial section at the level of the calcarine fissures, viewed inferiorly; the lower bank of the occipital lobe is cut away). Approximately 55%–60% of the surface area of striate cortex, located posteriorly, is responsible for the central 10 degrees of vision. The anterior striate cortex subserves the temporal 30 degrees of the visual field of the contralateral eye.
Source: *Liu, Grant T, MD. Retrochiasmal disorders. Neuro-ophthalmology: diagnosis and management. p. 293–337, Chapter 8.*

Auditory Cortex

The **primary auditory cortex (AI; BA 41)** is located within the **lateral sulcus** on the **upper part** of the **superior temporal gyrus** (Figs. 11.4 and 11.17).

- AI is found in two gyri known as **Heschl's gyri**.
- It is organized tonotopically:
    - **Anterior** auditory cortex receives **high**-frequency sounds.
    - **Posterior** auditory cortex receives **low**-frequency sounds.
- Unilateral sounds are represented in both hemispheres.

The **auditory association cortex (BA 22 and 42)** is located along the **superior bank** of the **middle temporal gyrus**. It is specialized in the classification and memory preservation of sounds.

Motor Cortex

Motor function is mediated by several regions of the **frontal cortex**. Similar to the somatosensory cortex, the motor cortex is subdivided into different regions, each of which is specialized in a specific aspect of movement production.

Primary Motor Cortex (BA 4)

The **primary motor cortex (M1)** occupies the **anterior wall** of the **central sulcus** and only a limited part of the exposed surface of the precentral gyrus, specifically its dorsomedial part (Fig. 11.21).

- Ventrally, M1 is buried in the depth of the central sulcus.
- M1 is the origin of a large proportion of the **corticospinal** fibres.
- Similar to the somatosensory cortex
  - M1 is somatotopically organized with an inverted representation of the body (Fig. 11.18).
  - The hand and mouth have disproportionally large areas.
- It executes **voluntary** movements.

Premotor Cortex

The **premotor cortex (BA 6)** lies rostral to M1 in the frontal lobe (Fig. 11.21). It

- Receives information from the **prefrontal association cortex**.
- Sends output to the brainstem, basal ganglia and cerebellum, in addition to the primary motor cortex.

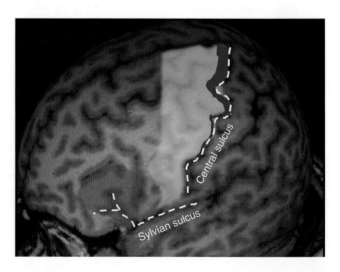

FIGURE 11.21 Cortical location of the primary motor cortex (dark blue), premotor cortex (light blue) and Broca's area (red).
Source: *Courtesy of Rechdi Ahdab, MD. Lebanese American University Medical Center.*

- Is functionally divided into two areas, **ventral** and **dorsal**.
- Is involved in **selecting a specific movement or a sequence of movements** from the repertoire of possible movements.

Supplementary Motor Area

The **supplementary motor area (upper BA 6)** lies on the medial surface of the **superior frontal gyrus**, anterior to the leg representation within M1. It
- Receives input from the **prefrontal association cortex.**
- Is specialized in:
  - **Planning for complex bimanual and sequential movements**.
  - Coordinating motor responses to sensory stimuli.

CLINICAL INSIGHT

- **Apraxia**
  - Damage to the premotor cortex leads to **apraxia**, which is the inability to carry out learned movements despite the presence of normal motor power and sensation. Apraxia is the result of loss of the motor programmes that instruct the motor neurons on how to execute a motor command. These are some apraxic features:
    - How to position one's hand and arm to interact with a tool or object
    - How to orient the limb towards the target
    - How to move the limb in space
    - How to choose the correct speed of the movement
    - How to order a series of acts leading to a goal
    - How to take advantage of the mechanical properties of tools
- Alternatively, apraxia is sometimes the result of lesions that interrupt connections between the parietal association cortex and the premotor cortex

---

Additional Functional Areas

Other important functional areas include:
- **Broca's area (BA 44 and 45)**
  - Corresponds to the **pars opercularis** and **triangularis** of the inferior frontal gyrus in the **dominant** hemisphere (Figs. 11.4, 11.11 and 11.17).
  - Is responsible for the **motor programming of speech**.
  - Injury leads to **expressive (or motor) aphasia**, where patients have difficulty producing written and spoken language.
- **Frontal eye field (BA 8)**
  - Is located rostral to the premotor area in the **prefrontal cortex** (Fig. 11.4).
  - Controls **conjugate horizontal eye movements** on the **contralateral** side.

Cortical Association Areas

Cortical association areas are the parts of the cerebral cortex that do not belong to the primary regions. They function to produce a meaningful perceptual experience of the world, enabling us to interact effectively and **support abstract thinking** and **language**. Cortical association areas integrate and interpret sensory stimuli of all modalities and plan and execute behaviours in response to the stimuli.

Prefrontal Area

The **prefrontal area (BA 9–12)** is extremely well developed in humans (Figs. 11.4 and 11.17).

- It has extensive connections with the various **sensory cortices**, **limbic system** and **thalamus**.
- It is composed of two main portions:
  - **Dorsolateral** prefrontal cortex, which is primarily involved in **executive functions** (planning and execution of a goal).
  - **Orbitomedial** prefrontal cortex, which is involved in **impulse control**, **personality** and **reactivity to mood** and the surrounding.
- The **anterior cingulate gyrus** plays an important role in **mood control**.

CLINICAL INSIGHT

- **Orbitomedial Prefrontal Cortex Injury**

The most striking example of frontal lobe function comes from patients with orbitomedial prefrontal damage. This syndrome comprises a constellation of symptoms that include decreased spontaneous activity, loss of attention, loss of abstract thinking and changes in affect, among others.

Posterior Parietal Area

The **posterior parietal area (BA 5 and 7)** is located posterior to the postcentral gyrus and anterior to the visual cortex.

- This region is connected to:
  - Sensory and visual cortical areas on one side,
  - Premotor and prefrontal association areas on the other.
- Its role is to **process sensory information** from multiple, different modalities and send this integrated view of the environment to the premotor and prefrontal association areas to generate an appropriate response.

CLINICAL INSIGHT

- **Visual Agnosia**

Damage to the visual association cortex in the inferior part of the occipital and temporal lobes causes **visual agnosia**, which is the inability to recognize objects by sight despite normal visual perception. Recognition of objects through modalities other than vision (touch for example) is typically normal. Similar deficits have been observed in patients with auditory (auditory agnosia) or tactile (tactile agnosia) deficits.

CASE STUDY DISCUSSION

Proper knowledge of sulcus and gyrus anatomy provides the key to understanding the clinical correlates of brain damage. The patient experienced a partial motor seizure that initially involved the hand suggesting that the culprit lesion is near the motor 'hand knob' (**lesion 2**). Further growth of this lesion is expected to damage the motor cortex and cause paralysis of the contralateral upper extremity.

CHAPTER 12

Basal Ganglia

Naji Riachi

CASE STUDY

Presentation and Physical Examination: A healthy 63-year-old teacher noted that his handwriting had become smaller. He also complained of a tremor in his right hand when completely relaxed at rest. He was able to accomplish all activities of daily living, but some tasks were slower and a little bit more difficult to accomplish than usual. He had mild difficulty climbing up a ladder or getting up from a low chair. His walking was normal 'but a bit slower than what it used to be'. He had normal cognitive functions. However, his wife mentioned that he had been having 'nightmares' for several years in which he would act out dreams while asleep.

Upon examination, the patient had a normal mental status. He had decreased facial expressions and decreased blink frequency. His voice was soft, low volume and monotonous. The rest of his cranial nerves examination was within normal limits, as was his sensory examination. On motor examination, he had cogwheel rigidity bilaterally, more pronounced on the right side. Motor power and reflexes were normal.

Coordination examination revealed the presence of a right-sided resting tremor of the arm that decreased with activity. Bilateral bradykinesia was found with finger tapping and rapid alternating movements of the hands, more prominent on the right. His posture was stooped upon standing. His gait showed the presence of a reduced right arm swing. Romberg was negative, and he had no retropulsion. He took six steps to turn around with ankles joined.

Diagnosis, Management and Follow Up: Thyroid function tests and brain magnetic resonance imaging (MRI) were normal.

The patient had three of the cardinal features of **Parkinson disease**: resting tremor, bradykinesia and rigidity. He was started on levodopa/carbidopa and was doing much better upon follow-up 3 months later.

After studying this chapter, try to guess the pathophysiology of Parkinson disease, which will be discussed along with the clinical features of the disease at the end of the chapter.

BRIEF INTRODUCTION

The term **basal ganglia** refers to a collection of **five subcortical nuclei** located deep inside the cerebral hemispheres, which are involved in the control of **voluntary movement** and **posture**.

- They act as regulators of the cortical functions via a **loop** that influences the thalamocortical projections and, as a result, the major descending tracts.
- However, unlike the cerebellum, they have **no direct connection** to the spinal cord.
- The loop is formed by connections that go from the cortex to the basal ganglia to the thalamus and back to the cortex (Fig. 12.1).

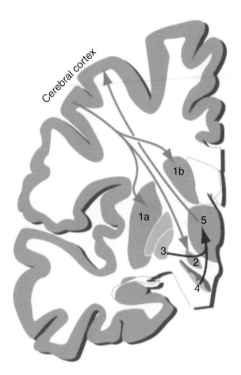

FIGURE 12.1   Basal ganglia. The major inputs come from the cerebral cortex, reaching the putamen (1a), caudate nucleus (1b) and subthalamic nucleus (2). Outputs project from the internal segment of the globus pallidus (3) and the reticular part of the substantia nigra (4) to the thalamus (5), which in turn projects back to the cortex. These connections are mostly uncrossed, but there is some bilaterality (not shown). Excitatory connections are shown in green and inhibitory connections in red.
Source: *Vanderah, Todd W, PhD. Basal nuclei. Nolte's the human brain. p. 475–494, Chapter 19.*

The goal of this chapter is to introduce the anatomy, physiology and connections of the basal ganglia as well as the pathologic processes that govern its associated diseases.

COMPONENTS OF THE BASAL GANGLIA (Figs. 12.2 and 12.3)

The main anatomical components of the basal ganglia are (Fig. 12.4):

- Caudate nucleus
- Putamen
- Globus pallidus
- Two related subcortical nuclei traditionally included in the basal ganglia are
    - Subthalamic nucleus,
    - Substantia nigra.

The caudate nucleus and **putamen** have functional and developmental similarities and are considered as a single structure known as the **striatum**. The **putamen** and **globus pallidus** form a **lens-shape**d structure, sometimes called the **lentiform nucleus**. This term is still used even though the putamen and the globus pallidus have different functions. One may also refer to the **caudate**, **putamen** and **globus pallidus** as the **corpus striatum**.

A traditional classification of the basal ganglia includes the **claustrum**, **amygdala**, **caudate nucleus** and **lentiform nucleus** (Fig. 12.3A).

- The **claustrum** is a thin layer of grey matter separated from the **putamen** by the **external capsule**, and from the **insula** by the **extreme capsule**.

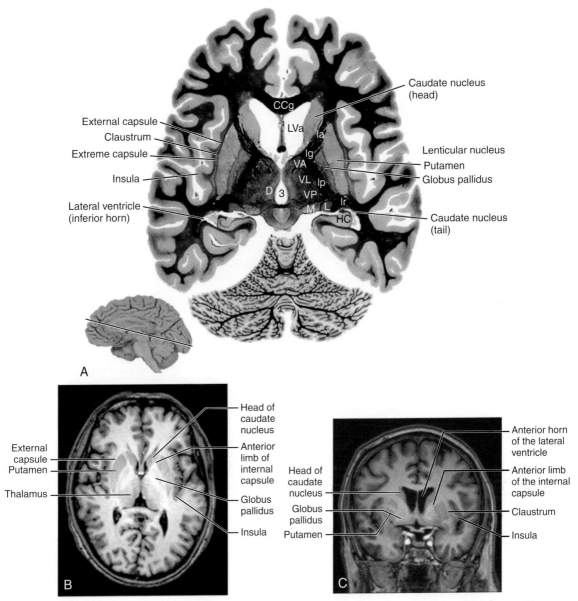

FIGURE 12.2 (A) Basal nuclei and surrounding structures, as seen in an axial section. The claustrum is a plate of grey matter, suspected of playing a role in consciousness, that is layered between the putamen and the insular cortex. The external capsule, between the claustrum and the putamen, is a route through which many projections from the cerebral cortex reach the putamen. The extreme capsule houses association fibres that interconnect different cortical areas. 3, third ventricle; CCg, genu of the corpus callosum; D, dorsomedial nucleus; HC, hippocampus; Ia, Ig, Ip and Ir, internal capsule – anterior limb, genu, posterior limb and retrolenticular part; L, lateral geniculate nucleus; LVa, anterior horn of the lateral ventricle; M, medial geniculate nucleus; VA, VL and VP, ventral anterior, ventral lateral and ventral posterior nuclei. (B) Axial and (C) coronal magnetic resonance images of the brain showing the basal ganglia, thalamus and internal capsule.

Source: *(A) Adapted from Nolte J, Angevine JB Jr. The Human brain in photographs and diagrams, ed 3, St. Louis: Mosby; 2007; Vanderah, Todd W, PhD. Basal nuclei. Nolte's the human brain. p. 475–494, Chapter 19. (B) and (C) Courtesy of Alan Jackson; Standring, Susan, MBE, PhD, DSc, FKC, Hon FAS, Hon FRCS. Basal ganglia. Gray's anatomy. p. 364–372.e1, Chapter 24.*

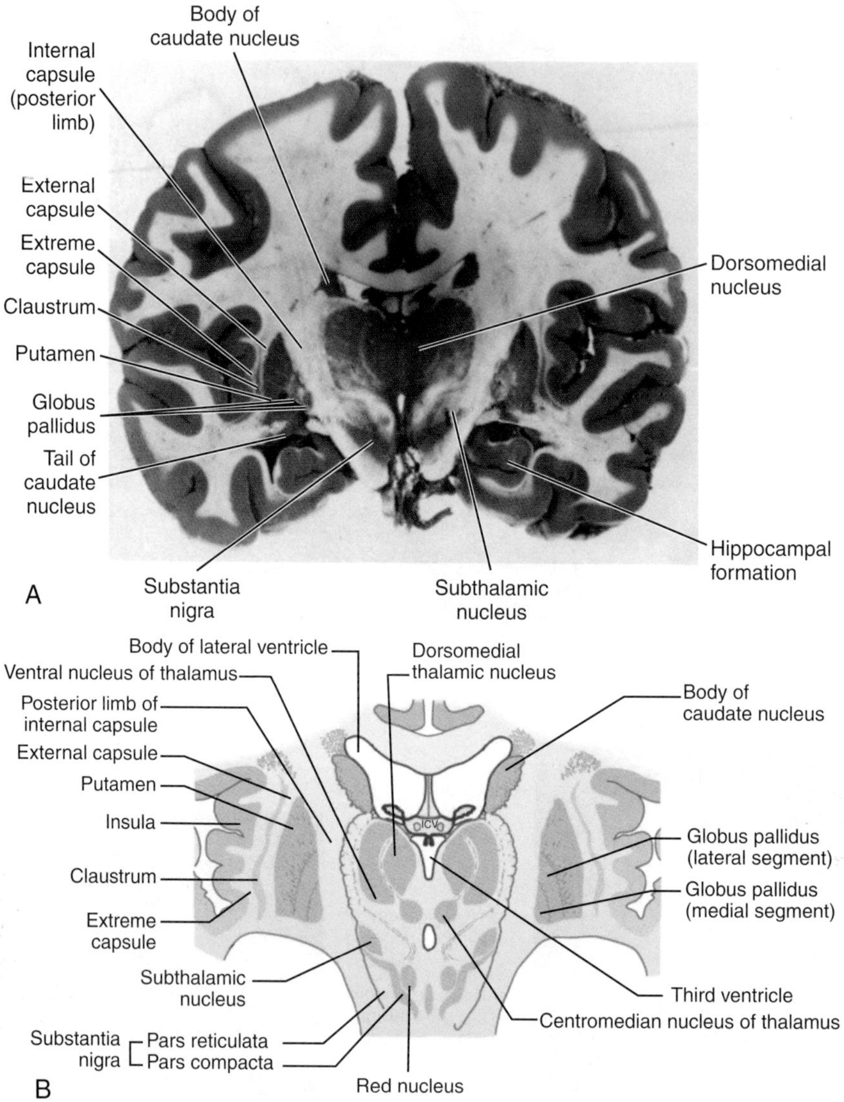

FIGURE 12.3   (A) A coronal section of the anatomical location of various parts of the basal ganglia. (B) Schematic of a coronal section through the diencephalon and basal ganglia. ICV, internal cerebral veins.

Source: *(A) Reprinted from Nolte J. The human brain: an introduction to its anatomy. St Louis: CV Mosby; 1981; Melnick, Marsha E, PT, PhD. Basal ganglia disorders. Umphred's neurological rehabilitation. p. 601–630, Chapter 20. (B) Standring, Susan, MBE, PhD, DSc, FKC, Hon FAS, Hon FRCS. Basal ganglia. Gray's anatomy. p. 364–372.e1, Chapter 24.*

■ The **amygdala** is technically part of the basal ganglia (due to its developmental origin), but functionally, it is part of the limbic system.

When we plan a movement, the prefrontal region is activated. The information is then relayed to the premotor and supplementary motor regions that will project to the basal ganglia. In turn, the basal ganglia relay the information to

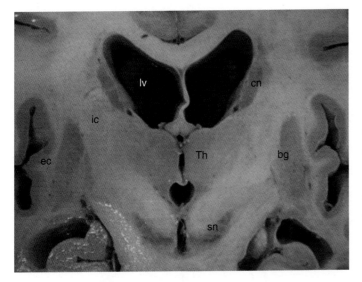

FIGURE 12.4 Coronal cut of a brain specimen tinged with Mulligan's method. Some brainstem structures may be identified: cn, caudate nucleus; lv, lateral ventricle; ic, internal capsule; th, thalamus; bg, basal ganglia; sn, substantia nigra; ec, external capsule.
Source: *Ángeles Fernández-Gil, M. Anatomy of the brainstem: a gaze into the stem of life. Semin Ultrasound CT MR 31(3): 196–219.*

the thalamus, and then the primary motor cortex will become activated. The information will then be carried down through the descending corticospinal and corticobulbar fibres to the lower motor neurons (Fig. 12.5).

Striatum

The **striatum** is composed of the caudate nucleus and the putamen that receive projections from the **telencephalon**. They constitute the **input component** of the basal ganglia.

- The **caudate nucleus** is bordered **laterally** by the **thalamus** and **medially** by the **internal capsule** (Fig. 12.6). It is a **C-shaped** structure that runs antero-posteriorly in the brain in close relation to the lateral ventricle and is composed of three parts related to the main three areas of the **lateral ventricle**:
  - **Head**: forms the lateral wall of the anterior horn of the lateral ventricle.
  - **Body**: forms the floor of the body of the lateral ventricle.
  - **Tail**: continues forward into the temporal lobe in the roof of the inferior horn of the lateral ventricle.
- The **putamen** is the **most lateral** and the **largest structure** of the basal ganglia separated from the caudate nucleus by fibres of the **internal capsule** (Fig. 12.2).

Globus Pallidus (Fig. 12.7)

The **globus pallidus** is derived from the **diencephalon**.

- It is the **smallest nucleus** of the basal ganglia, bordered **laterally** by the **putamen** and **medially** by the **internal capsule**.
- It is divided into an **external (lateral)** and an **internal (medial) parts**, the internal part constituting the **output component** of the basal ganglia.

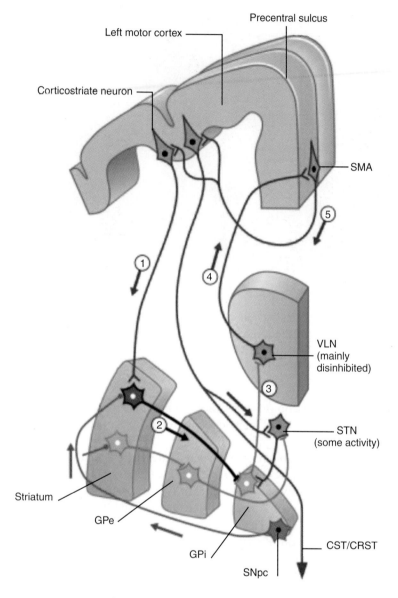

FIGURE 12.5 Activities in the striatal motor loops, prior to movement. The supplementary motor area (SMA) is activated. (1) Corticostriate fibres from the sensorimotor cortex activate the striatum. (2) The activated striatal neurons inhibit internal pallidal (GPi) neurons (3) with consequent disinhibition of the ventral lateral nucleus (VLN) thalamocortical neurons (4) and activation of the SMA (5), which both modifies ongoing corticostriate activity and initiates impulse trains along corticospinal (CST) and corticoreticular (CRST) fibres. GPe, external globus pallidus; SNpc, substantia nigra pars compacta; STN, subthalamic nucleus.
Source: *Mtui, Estomih, MD. Basal ganglia. Fitzgerald's clinical neuroanatomy and neuroscience. p. 314–322, Chapter 33.*

Subthalamic Nucleus (Fig. 12.7)

The **subthalamic nucleus** is a **lens-shaped** nucleus located **at the border** between the **diencephalon** and the **mesencephalon** on the medial side of the internal capsule. It lies just above the **rostral portion** of the **substantia nigra** and continues caudally with the substantia nigra.

Substantia Nigra (Figs. 12.4 and 12.7)

The **substantia nigra** is located in the **mesencephalon**. It is divided into **two regions** with distinct histological and functional characteristics: pars compacta (SNc) and pars reticulata (SNr).

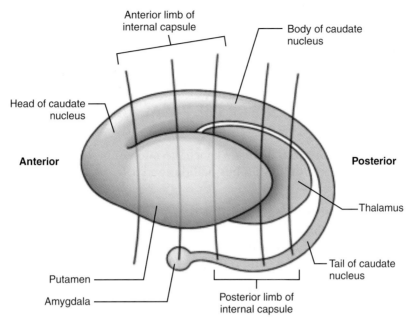

FIGURE 12.6 Lateral aspect of the left caudate nucleus, putamen, amygdala and thalamus. The globus pallidus is obscured by the putamen. The course of the internal capsule is shown in red. The putamen and the head of the caudate nucleus are separated by the anterior limb of the internal capsule, except at their most rostral extent where the two are in continuity. The posterior limb of the internal capsule separates the globus pallidus and the putamen from the thalamus.

Source: *Crossman, Alan R, PhD DSc. Basal ganglia. Neuroanatomy: an ilustrated colour text. p. 146–154, Chapter 14.*

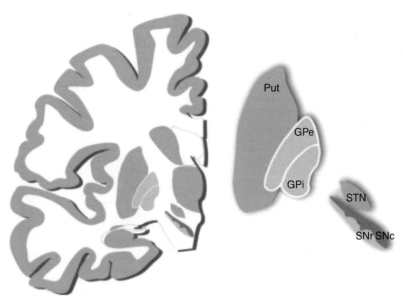

FIGURE 12.7 Gpi, internal segment of the globus pallidus. Gpe, external segment of the globus pallidus; SNc, substantia nigra pars compacta; SNr, substantia nigra pars reticulata; Put, putamen; STN, subthalamic nucleus.

Source: *Vanderah, Todd W, PhD. Basal nuclei. Nolte's the human brain. p. 475–494, Chapter 19.*

- The **SNc** is **dorsal** and composed of **melanin-pigmented** neurons, which give the substantia nigra its dark colour, and hence, its name. The SNc projects rostrally and forms a **side loop to the striatum**.
- The **SNr** shares histological and functional characteristics with the **globus pallidus** and is directly continuous with it.

CONNECTIONS OF THE BASAL GANGLIA
(Figs. 12.8 and 12.9)

All **input** into the basal ganglia terminates in the **striatum**, while all **output** projects from the **globus pallidus** and **SNr**.

Striatum (Fig. 12.10)
Afferents

The striatum has **three** major sources of input:

- **Cerebral cortex**: The **largest source** of input to the basal ganglia; originates from the **motor, sensory** and **association cortices** and is topographically organized.
- **Intralaminar nuclei of the thalamus**: Mostly through the **centromedian nucleus**. Because the cortex projects to the thalamus, the **thalamostriate projections** represent yet another way of how the cortex influences the striatum.
- **SNc: Dopaminergic** neurons project on the striatum. They exert either **inhibitory** or **excitatory** effects on different subpopulations of striatal neurons (*see 'Striatum–Substantia Nigra–Striatum Loop' subsection*).

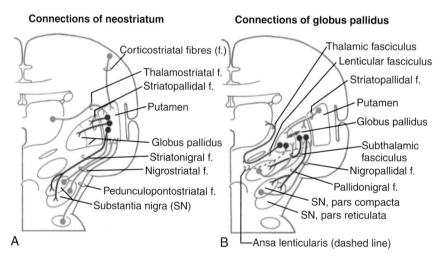

FIGURE 12.8 Schematic representations of the afferent (in green) and efferent (in red) connections of (A) the neostriatum and of the afferent (in green) and efferent (in red and blue) connections of (B) the globus pallidus. The double-headed arrow in (B) represents pallidopallidal fibres.

Source: *Ma, TP. The basal nuclei. Fundamental neuroscience for basic and clinical applications. p. 354–369.e1, Chapter 26.*

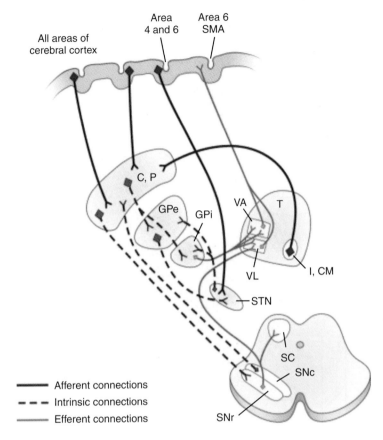

FIGURE 12.9 Schematic drawing of interconnections between the basal ganglia and its afferent and efferent connections. I, CM, Intralaminar, Centromedian nucleus of thalamus; C, P, caudate, putamen (striatum); GPe, lateral (external) globus pallidus; GPi, medial (internal) globus pallidus; SC, superior colliculus; STN, subthalamic nucleus; SNc, substantia nigra pars compacta; SNr, substantia nigra pars reticulata; T, thalamus; VA, ventral anterior; VL, ventral lateral.
Source: *Jankovic, Joseph. Parkinson disease and other movement disorders. Bradley's neurology in clinical practice. p. 1422–1460.e3, Chapter 96.*

Efferents

The striatum projects mainly to the following structures:

- **Globus pallidus**: These fibres contribute to the **cortex–basal ganglia–thalamus–cortex loop** and are topographically organized.
- **Substantia nigra**: **Striatonigral** fibres project to both parts of the substantia nigra.

Globus Pallidus
Afferents

The globus pallidus receives input from the following:

- **Striatum**: Projects topographically to the globus pallidus and to the functionally related SNr.
- **Subthalamic nucleus**

Efferents

The globus pallidus projects to **three** main regions:

- **Ventral lateral (VL) and ventral anterior (VA) thalamic nuclei**: Constitute the major outflow pathway of the basal ganglia through

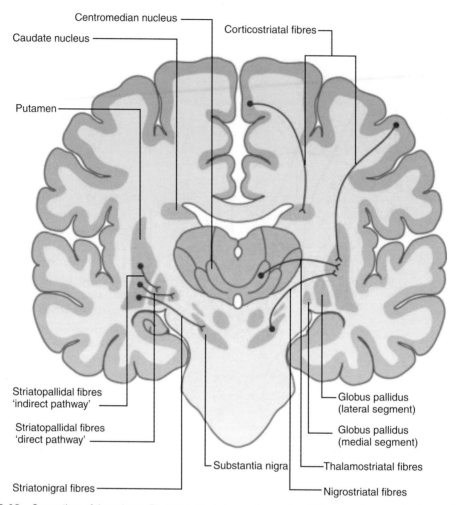

Centromedian nucleus

Caudate nucleus

Corticostriatal fibres

Putamen

Striatopallidal fibres
'indirect pathway'

Striatopallidal fibres
'direct pathway'

Globus pallidus
(lateral segment)

Globus pallidus
(medial segment)

Substantia nigra

Thalamostriatal fibres

Striatonigral fibres

Nigrostriatal fibres

FIGURE 12.10   Connections of the striatum. The major afferent projections to the striatum are shown on the right and major efferent projections from the striatum on the left.

Source: *Standring, Susan, MBE, PhD, DSc, FKC, Hon FAS, Hon FRCS. Basal ganglia. Gray's anatomy. p. 364–372.e1, Chapter 24.*

two fibre bundles, the ansa lenticularis and the lenticular fasciculus (Fig. 12.11).

- The **ansa lenticularis** is a thick fibre bundle that loops **under** (ventral to) the **posterior limb of the internal capsule**. It then heads dorsally to reach the **ipsilateral motor thalamic nuclei (VA/VL)**.
- The **lenticular fasciculus** fibres pass **through** (rather than under) the **posterior limb of the internal capsule**. The fibres then travel **on top of the subthalamic nucleus** before looping dorsally and rostrally towards **VA/VL**.
- On their way to the thalamus, the ansa lenticularis and lenticular fasciculus fibres join other (e.g., cerebellothalamic) fibres and later fuse to reach the thalamus as the **thalamic fasciculus** (Fig. 12.11).

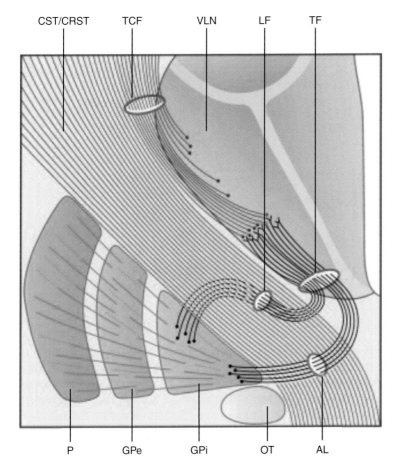

CST/CRST   TCF   VLN   LF   TF

P   GPe   GPi   OT   AL

FIGURE 12.11   Part of the projection from the internal segment of the globus pallidus (GPi) to the ventral lateral nucleus (VLN) and ventral anterior nucleus (VA) of the thalamus sweeps around the base of the internal capsule as the ansa lenticularis (AL); the remainder traverses this region as the lenticular fasciculus (LF). The two parts come together as the thalamic fasciculus (TF) before entering the thalamus. CST/CRST, corticospinal and corticoreticular fibres; GPe, external segment of the globus pallidus; OT, optic tract; P, putamen; TCF, thalamocortical fibres.
Source: *Mtui, Estomih, MD. Basal ganglia. Fitzgerald's clinical neuroanatomy and neuroscience. p. 314–322, Chapter 33.*

- Fibres then project from the thalamus to the **prefrontal** and **premotor cortex** to complete the **cortex–basal ganglia–thalamus–cortex loop**.
- **Subthalamic nucleus**
- **Brainstem reticular formation**: With further projections to the rubrospinal, reticulospinal and vestibulospinal descending tracts.

PHYSIOLOGY AND NEUROCHEMISTRY OF THE BASAL GANGLIA

The basal ganglia are clearly involved in regulation of **voluntary movement** and **posture,** even though their exact motor function is still subject to debate. The cortex is unable to direct motor control properly without the input of information from the basal ganglia. The influence they exert on the cerebral cortex is made via **two important pathways**, the **direct** and the **indirect** pathways (Fig. 12.12).

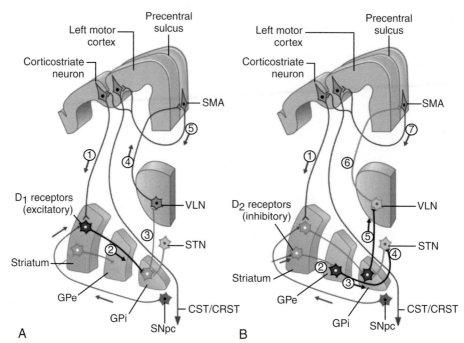

FIGURE 12.12 Coronal section through the motor loop. (A) The sequence of five sets of neurons involved in the 'direct' pathway from the sensorimotor cortex to the thalamus with final return to the sensorimotor cortex via the SMA. (B) The sequence of seven sets of neurons involved in the 'indirect' pathway. The red/pink neurons are excitatory utilizing glutamate. The black/grey neurons are inhibitory utilizing gamma-aminobutyric acid (GABA). The brown, nigrostriatal neuron utilizes dopamine, which is excitatory via D1 receptors on target striatal neurons and inhibitory via D2 receptors on the same and other striatal neurons. CST/CRST, corticospinal, corticoreticular fibres; GPe, GPi, external and internal segments of the globus pallidus; SMA, supplementary motor area; SNpc, compact part of the substantia nigra; STN, subthalamic nucleus; VLN, ventral lateral nucleus of the thalamus.

Source: *Mtui, Estomih, MD. Basal ganglia. Fitzgerald's clinical neuroanatomy and neuroscience. p. 314–322, Chapter 33.*

Direct Pathway: The Cortex–Basal Ganglia–Thalamus–Cortex Loop (Figs. 12.12A and 12.13)

This is the **major loop** utilized by the basal ganglia to affect the cortical neurons. The loop constitutes the **direct pathway**. The following neurotransmitters are released in the direct pathway (Fig. 12.14).

- The **cortical** neurons project on the **striatal** neurons and release **glutamate**, the **excitatory** neurotransmitter. When activated, they **excite** the striatal neurons.
- Within the basal ganglia, the striatal neurons project directly on the **globus pallidus internal (GP (internal))**, which in turn will project on the **thalamus**.
- These two projections contain the **inhibitory** neurotransmitter **gamma-aminobutyric acid (GABA)**. This will create a two-step sequence of a **double inhibition**, which, when disinhibited, will **lead to an excitation**.
- So, the cortical signal excites striatal neurons, which results in **more inhibition from striatum to GP (internal)**. More inhibition of GP (internal) means **less inhibition of motor thalamus (VA/VL)**.

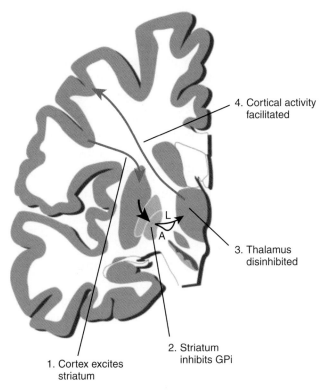

4. Cortical activity
facilitated

L

A

3. Thalamus
disinhibited

2. Striatum
inhibits GPi

1. Cortex excites
striatum

FIGURE 12.13 The 'direct pathway' through the basal ganglia. A, ansa lenticularis; L, lenticular fasciculus. Excitatory connections are shown in blue and inhibitory connections in black.
Source: *Nolte, John, PhD. Basal ganglia. Essentials of the human brain. p. 145–151, Chapter 19.*

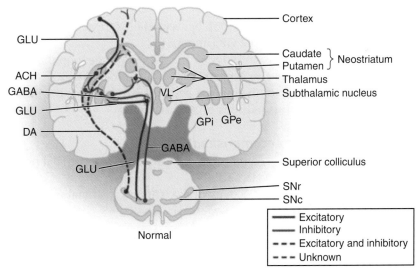

Cortex

GLU

Caudate ⎱
Putamen ⎰ Neostriatum

ACH

Thalamus

GABA

Subthalamic nucleus

GLU

VL

DA

GPi GPe

GABA

Superior colliculus

GLU

SNr
SNc

—— Excitatory
—— Inhibitory
- - - Excitatory and inhibitory
- - - Unknown

Normal

FIGURE 12.14 Anatomy of the basal ganglia and their connections. The feedback loop proceeds from cerebral prefrontal areas to the basal ganglia and eventually back from the basal ganglia to the thalamus to the motor cortex. This ultimately regulates the descending corticospinal motor system. ACH, acetylcholine; DA, dopamine; GABA, γ-aminobutyric acid; GLU, glutamate; GP, globus pallidum (e, external; i, internal); SN, substantia nigra (c, compacta; r, reticulate); VL, ventrolateral.
Source: *Jankovic J. The extrapyramidal disorders: introduction. In Goldman L, Bennett JC, editors. Cecil textbook of medicine, ed 21. Philadelphia: Saunders; 2000, p. 2078.*

- Closing the loop, the **thalamus** will project neurons on the **cortex**. Similar to the corticostriatal neurons, these thalamic neuronal projections contain the **excitatory** neurotransmitter **glutamate**; the increased firing of the VA/VL will, in turn, increase the firing of the **motor cortex**.
- The consequence of the direct pathway is to **increase the excitatory drive from the thalamus to cortex** and to **turn up motor activity**.

Shortly before and during movement, electrical recordings show that the excitatory input from the cortex will activate the double inhibition of the basal ganglia two-step inhibition, which will result in excitation of the thalamocortical projections. This will result in excitation of the cortex.

When no movements are made, electrical recordings show the neurons of the striatum to be quiescent while those of the globus pallidus are active. This will allow the globus pallidus to inhibit the thalamocortical fibres.

Indirect Pathway: Add the Globus Pallidus–Subthalamic Nucleus–Globus Pallidus Loop (Fig. 12.12B)

To form the **indirect pathway**, within the basal ganglia, striatal neurons project on the GP (external), instead of the GP (internal), as is the case in the direct pathway.

- Neurons from the **globus pallidus external (GP (external))** will project **inhibitory GABA** containing neurons onto the **subthalamic nucleus**, and then neurons from the subthalamic nucleus will project **excitatory glutamate** containing neurons back onto the **GP (internal)** (Fig. 12.14).
- This will create a loop between the GP (external), the subthalamic nucleus and the GP (internal).
- This succession of loops, including the side loop through the subthalamic nucleus, is referred to as the indirect pathway. The net result of the side loop of the indirect pathway is to **increase the inhibitory effect of the globus pallidus on the thalamus**.

How is This Accomplished?

- In the indirect pathway, cortical fibres **excite** striatal neurons that project to the GP (external).
- The increased activity of the GABAergic striatal neurons **decreases** activity in the GP (external).
- The GABAergic cells in the GP (external) **inhibit** cells in the subthalamic nucleus. Therefore, the decreased activity of these GP (external) cells (due to increased activity of GABAergic striatal neurons) results in **less inhibition** of cells in the subthalamic nucleus. **Subthalamic** neurons are thus **disinhibited** and **increase their activity**.
- Since the projection from the subthalamic nucleus to the GP (internal) is **excitatory**, the increased activity in the subthalamic nucleus results in **more excitation** to cells in the **GP (internal)**.

- The end result of actions of the indirect loop is an **increase in activity of the GABAergic cells in the GP (internal) that project to VA/VL** or, in other terms, an **increase in inhibition of the thalamic neurons**. The indirect pathway thus **turns down the motor thalamus** and, subsequently, it **turns down the motor cortex** and **motor activity**.

Modulation of Direct and Indirect Pathways

Striatal neurons are modulated by **two** important neuromodulatory systems, the **dopaminergic** and the **cholinergic**. Each of these systems differentially affects the direct and indirect pathways, thereby altering their balance and the amount of motor activity that is produced.

Striatum–Substantia Nigra–Striatum Loop (Fig. 12.15)

In this **side loop**, the **substantia nigra** axon terminals will release **dopamine** into the **striatum**.

- Dopamine is produced by cells in the **SNc**.
- Dopamine has an **excitatory effect** via **D1 receptors** upon cells in the striatum that are part of the **direct** pathway (Fig. 12.12A).
- Dopamine has an **inhibitory effect** via **D2 receptors** upon striatal cells associated with the **indirect** pathway (Fig. 12.12B).

So, the direct pathway (which turns up motor activity) is excited by dopamine while the indirect pathway (which turns down motor activity) is inhibited by dopamine.

- Both of these effects lead to **increased motor activity**.
- To increase motor activity, dopamine will in turn **excite the direct pathway via D1 receptors** and **inhibit the indirect pathway via D2 receptors**.

Cholinergic Interneurons

There is a population of neurons in the striatum called **interneurons** or **local circuit neurons**. These neurons are **cholinergic** and release **acetylcholine (ACh)** (Fig. 12.14).

- The axons of these interneurons **do not leave** the striatum. These cholinergic interneurons synapse on the **GABAergic striatal** neurons that project to the **GP (internal)** and on the **striatal** neurons that project to the **GP (external)**.
- The cholinergic actions **inhibit** striatal cells of the **direct pathway** and **excite** striatal cells of the **indirect pathway**.
- The effects of ACh are **opposite** to the effects of dopamine on the direct and indirect pathways. ACh will thus **inhibit the direct pathway** and **excite the indirect pathway**.
- When activated, the effect of the striatal cholinergic interneurons is then to **decrease motor activity**.

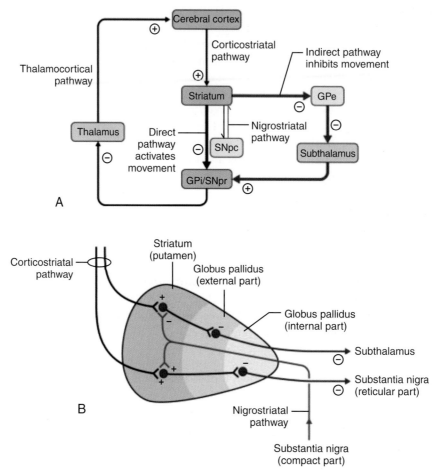

FIGURE 12.15   Basal ganglia. (A) Schematic organization. (B) Differential modulation of direct (thick black arrow) and indirect (red) pathways by dopaminergic neurons from the compact part of the substantia nigra (blue). Excitatory connections, +; inhibitory connections, −; GPi, globus pallidus (internal part); GPe, global pallidus (external part); SNpc, substantia nigra (compact part); SNpr, substantia nigra (reticular part).

Source: *Pentland, Brian. The nervous system. Medical Sciences. p. 337–402, Chapter 8.*

DISORDERS OF THE BASAL GANGLIA

Diseases of the basal ganglia could result in either **hypokinetic (paucity of movement)** or **hyperkinetic (increased movement)** syndromes. While hypokinetic syndromes are usually associated with increased tone or hypertonia, hypotonia or decreased tone is noted with hyperkinetic syndromes. Lesions of the **substantia nigra** result in **hypokinesia**, whereas lesions of the **striatum** or the **subthalamic nucleus** cause **hyperkinesia**. An example of a hypokinesia–hypertonia syndrome is Parkinson disease *(see Case Study Discussion)*, while chorea, ballismus and dystonia are examples of hyperkinetic–hypotonic syndromes.

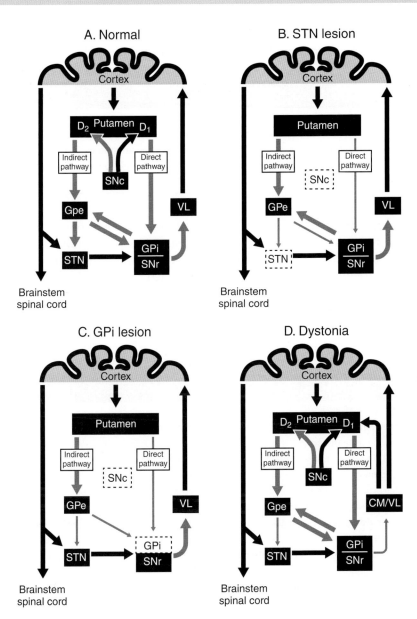

FIGURE 12.16 Functional anatomy of the basal ganglia. (A) Normal physiologic state with balance between the direct and the indirect pathways. (B) Effects of an STN lesion in parkinsonism, decreasing inhibitory input to the VL. (C) Effects of a GPi lesion in parkinsonism, decreasing inhibitory input to the VL. (D) Dystonia. Increased activity along the direct pathway, leading to excessive inhibition of the GPi and decreased inhibitory input to the thalamus. Black arrows indicate excitatory connections, and light grey arrows indicate inhibitory connections. CM, centromedian nucleus of the thalamus; D1, dopamine receptor subtype 1; D2, dopamine receptor subtype 2. Source: *Whitworth, Louis A. Deep brain stimulation in movement disorders: Parkinson's disease, essential tremor, and dystonia. Schmidek and Sweet's operative neurosurgical techniques. p. 1309–1320, Chapter 114.*

What Happens to the Basal Ganglia in a Patient with Hyperkinesia and Hypotonia? (Fig. 12.16)

Hyperkinesia and hypotonia can result from lesions of the striatum or subthalamic nucleus. A variety of abnormal movement syndromes will be seen.

- When the **subthalamic nucleus** is injured (Fig. 12.16B), there is a loss of the projections of the subthalamic nucleus to the globus pallidus, which are excitatory. As a result, the activity of the GABAergic fibres that project from the globus pallidus to the thalamus will be decreased.

The **thalamocortical fibres will then be disinhibited** and will increase the output to the cortex, thus **movement will be increased**.

CLINICAL INSIGHT

- **Ballismus**
  - **Flinging, violent choreic movements** that involve mostly the proximal extremities. They can result in injury since they are of **high velocity** and **amplitude**. They are usually **unilateral (hemiballism)** and result from lesions of the **contralateral subthalamic nucleus**.

- When the **striatum** is injured (Fig. 12.16C), the GABAergic output to the globus pallidus will be decreased or lost. This will disinhibit the GABAergic fibres that project from the globus pallidus to the subthalamic nucleus, which will result in a diminished activity of the subthalamic nucleus projections, which will then lead, as in the previous situation, to a **disinhibition of the thalamocortical projections**, thus leading to an **increase in movement**.

CLINICAL INSIGHTS

- **Chorea**
  - **Abnormal, involuntary, jerky, rapid** and **arrhythmic movements** (Fig. 12.17) involving distal muscles at first, and then spreading to involve the proximal and facial muscles and even the tongue. These abnormal movements will be superimposed on the normal movements and will thus distort them, as patients tend to try to incorporate them together to make the abnormal movements less apparent. Motor power is usually **not affected**.
  - **Huntington chorea** is a degenerative, progressive genetic condition that will cause **chorea** associated with psychiatric and cognitive manifestations. It is associated with a striking loss of the **caudate nucleus** that can be observed on brain imaging.
- **Athetosis**
  - **Slow, involuntary movements** that are more continuous than the ones seen in chorea. They appear **sinuous** and may result in **extreme, sustained postures**. They involve the face, neck, tongue and extremities and may be unilateral or bilateral.
- **Dystonia**
  - **Sustained, slow involuntary movements** or **postures** that usually involve the large truncal and limb girdle muscles. It can be generalized, focal, multifocal or segmental. Some clinical examples include **torticollis (cervical dystonia)** (Fig. 12.18), **blepharospasm (continuous blinking or closure of the eyes),** or writer's cramp. Some of these conditions can be treated with **botulinum toxin** injections.

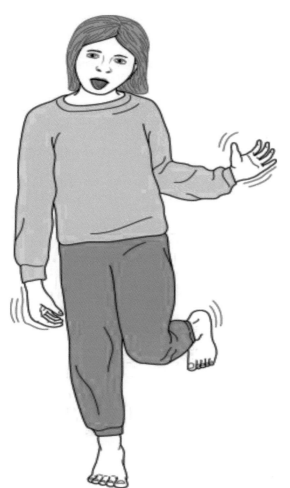

FIGURE 12.17 Patients with chorea may appear to have coy smiles and brief grimaces, and walk with a playful sashay. However, the pathologic nature of their movements – chorea – can be made obvious if they attempt to maintain a fixed position, such as standing at attention, standing on the ball of one foot or protruding their tongue.
Source: *Kaufman, David Myland, MD. Involuntary movement disorders. Kaufman's clinical neurology for psychiatrists. p. 397–453, Chapter 18.*

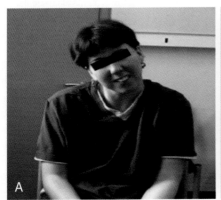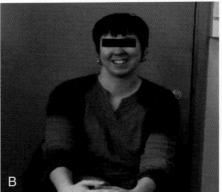

FIGURE 12.18 Photograph of patient with focal cervical dystonia (torticollis) (A) before and (B) 3 months following botulinum toxin injections to neck muscles.
Source: *Hu, Michele TM. Other movement disorders. Medicine 36(12): 636–639.*

CASE STUDY DISCUSSION

What Happens to the Basal Ganglia in a Parkinson Disease Patient? (Figs. 12.19 and 12.20)

In **Parkinsonism**, a **paucity of dopamine** in the brain is observed, which results from **degeneration of the SNc**. Since dopamine increases the inhibitory effect of the striatum on the globus pallidus, this inhibitory effect will be lost in a patient with Parkinsonism. This will result in an **increase in the activity of the globus pallidus**, which in turn, will **increase the inhibition of the thalamocortical neurons**, thus resulting in **hypokinesia** and **hypertonia**.

Clinical Features

Parkinsonism is characterized by hypokinesia, rigidity and a resting tremor.

- The slowness of movements progressively interferes with activities of daily living, which manifests as difficulty in walking, getting up from a chair or turning in bed, eating and dressing, as well as decreased head turns.

- The voice becomes hypophonic (decreased volume) and monotonous, and the facial expressions are lost (masked facies).

- With time, the gait will become increasingly more difficult, with difficulty found at initiating gait. It will become characterized by a narrow base and short accelerating steps, with the trunk flexed forward, a phenomenon referred to as **'festination'**.

- The patient will assume a stooped posture (Fig. 12.21) and with time will become more prone to falls due to postural instability.

- The **tremor** has a frequency of 4–6 Hz, is very obvious at rest, and **disappears** or **is greatly reduced with activity**.

- The rigidity has a **cogwheel pattern**, present from the beginning to the end of the passive movement, with the muscle giving way in little jerks when stretched.

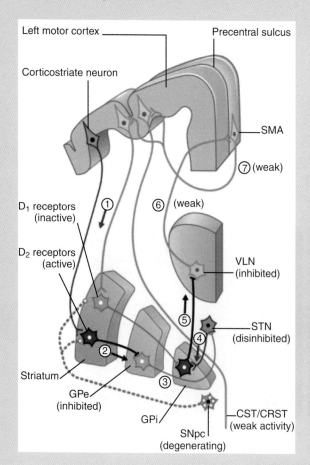

FIGURE 12.19   Consequences of degeneration of the pathway from the compact part of the substantia nigra (SNpc) to the striatum (S) in Parkinson disease. The effects arise from loss of tonic facilitation of spiny striatal neurons bearing D1 receptors, together with loss of tonic inhibition of those bearing D2 receptors. The direct pathway is disengaged, and the indirect pathway is activated by default. (1) Corticostriate neurons from the sensorimotor cortex now strongly activate those GABAergic neurons (2) in the striatum that synapse upon others (3) in the external pallidal segment (GPe). The double effect is disinhibition of the subthalamic nucleus (STN). The STN discharges strongly (4) onto the GABAergic neurons of the internal pallidal segment (GPi); these, in turn, discharge strongly (5) into the ventral lateral nucleus (VLN) of the thalamus, resulting in reduced output along thalamocortical fibres (6) travelling to the supplementary motor area (SMA). Inputs (7) from SMA to corticospinal and corticoretic-ular fibres (CST/CRST) become progressively weaker, with consequences for initiation and execution of movements.

Source: *Mtui, Estomih, MD. Basal ganglia. Fitzgerald's cinical neuroanatomy and neuroscience. p. 314–322, Chapter 33.*

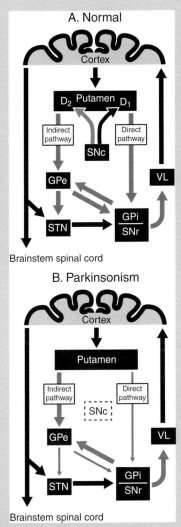

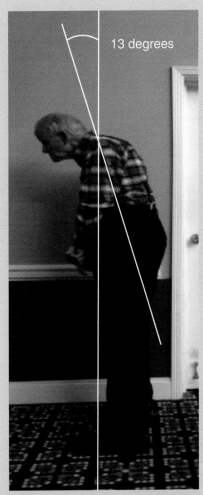

13 degrees

FIGURE 12.21 Abnormal posture of a patient with Parkinson disease. Measurement of the flexion angle.
Source: *Nair, Prajakta, MS. Reliability and validity of nonradiologic measures of forward flexed posture in Parkinson disease. Arch Phys Med Rehabil 98(3): 508–516.*

FIGURE 12.20 Functional anatomy of the basal ganglia. (A) Normal physiologic state with balance between the direct and the indirect pathways. (B) Parkinson disease. Loss of dopaminergic input from the SNc leads to increased activity along the indirect pathway and decreased activity along the direct pathway, resulting in increased inhibitory input to the ventral lateral thalamic nucleus (VL). D1, dopamine receptor subtype 1; D2, dopamine receptor subtype 2.
Source: *Whitworth, Louis A. Deep brain stimulation in movement disorders: Parkinson's disease, essential tremor, and dystonia. Schmidek and Sweet's operative neurosurgical techniques. p. 1309–1320, Chapter 114.*

CHAPTER 13

Visual System

Ali A. Haydar

CASE STUDY

Presentation and Physical Examination: A 48-year-old male, smoker and known to have hypothyroidism (on thyroid hormone replacement therapy), presented to the neuro-ophthalmology unit complaining of severe (9/10) left-sided headaches. Headaches were throbbing in nature, radiating to the left eye, jaw and teeth, lasting for 2 hours, associated with rhinorrhoea, and occurred on multiple episodes in the 4 weeks prior to presentation. Initially, the patient was treated for sinusitis by his family physician. Ten days later, the patient revisited his physician with persistent complaints. Again, he described the headaches as excruciating, left-sided, throbbing in nature, episodic, not relieved by rest and unrelated to noise and light. He was diagnosed with cluster headaches and was started on non-steroidal anti-inflammatory drugs (NSAIDs) with only slight improvement. One week later, the patient's daughter reported a 'sunken and droopy eye' on the left hemi-face and face flushing during the attacks. The patient was referred to the ophthalmology ward for further evaluation.

During examination, the patient was found to have ptosis, reverse ptosis (lower eyelid higher than normal) and anisocoria (miosis in the left eye).

Diagnosis, Management and Follow-Up: A cocaine test was performed to investigate the presence of Horner syndrome. The left pupil dilated less to cocaine drops than the normal right pupil; persistent anisocoria confirmed the diagnosis of Horner syndrome. No response was elicited on the hydroxy-amphetamine test, thus indicating a third-order neuron lesion.

Additional workup included magnetic resonance imaging (MRI) and chest computed tomography (CT) scans to rule out masses compressing the sympathetic pathway and complete blood count (CBC), all of which were negative. The preliminary diagnosis was **Horner syndrome secondary to a cluster headache**.

The patient was treated by oxygen therapy, triptans and calcium channel blockers for cluster headaches. Few days later, he reported substantial relief of symptoms and better quality of life.

BRIEF INTRODUCTION

Vision is a vital sense in humans. As part of the central nervous system (CNS), the **visual system** performs various complicated functions, including reception of light and creation of monocular images, execution of a binocular perception, appreciation and classification of visual objects, estimating distances towards and between objects, and balancing body movements.

The process of transmitting visual information to the brain involves multiple steps:
- The **cornea** and the **lens** focus an image of the environment onto the **retina**, a light-sensitive layer coating the back of the eye.
- The **photoreceptors** of the retina, **cones** and **rods**, detect light photons focused by the lens and convert them to neuronal signals.
- These signals are then communicated and integrated by numerous structures of the brain in a hierarchical manner.

The aim of this chapter is to introduce the structures and pathways of the visual system and highlight important neuro-ophthalmologic conditions causing visual dysfunction.

EYE ANATOMY

The **eye**, composed of **three layers**, is the organ of vision (Fig. 13.1).

- The **outer** layer is composed of the **sclera**, the whitish part of the eye, and the **cornea**, a transparent cover over the pupil and the iris.
- The **pigmented middle** layer is formed by the **uvea** and divided into **anterior (iris and ciliary body)** and **posterior (choroid)** parts.
- The **inner** layer is formed by the retina, a light-sensitive tissue, functioning as a camera film.

Retina

An **ectodermal** derivative, the retina originates as an outgrowth of the **diencephalon**, specifically the **optic vesicle**. The retina

- Is connected to the brain via the **optic nerve** (cranial nerve [CN] II).
- Is composed of **10 layers**.
- Can detect light with wavelengths roughly ranging from **400 nm (violet)** to **700 nm (red)**.

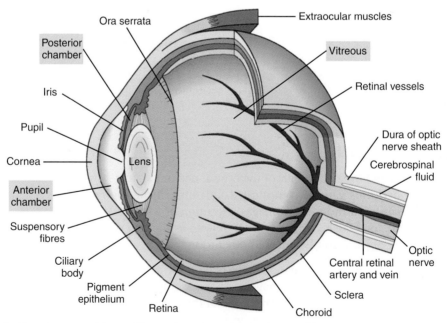

FIGURE 13.1 Normal anatomy of the eye. The anterior and posterior chambers are filled with aqueous humour and are anterior to the lens. The vitreous is a specialized support tissue, not merely a gelatinous fluid.

Source: *Stevens, Alan, MB BS, FRCPath. Ophthalmic pathology. Core pathology. p. 495–504, Chapter 22.*

Fundus of Eye (Fig. 13.2)
Optic Disc

- Is positioned 3–4 mm **medial** to the **fovea**.
- Possesses a central depression called the physiologic **cup**, with normal **cup/disc ratio ≤ 0.3** (Fig. 13.3).
- Is formed by **ganglion cell axons** converging from the retina to form the **optic nerve**.
- Lacks rods or cones (**blind spot**).
- Is a canal for central retinal vessels.

CLINICAL INSIGHT

- **Papilloedema**
  - Since the optic nerve is surrounded by an extension of the brain meninges, any **rise in intracranial pressure** will increase cerebrospinal fluid (CSF) pressure around the nerve and compress the thin walls of the retinal vein. This leads to congestion of the retinal vein and **oedema of the optic disc**, a condition known as **papilloedema**.
  - Bilateral presentation and vision is generally preserved.
  - Aetiologies: pseudotumour cerebri, neoplastic, haematoma and hydrocephalus.
  - Associated symptoms: visual problems, headache and vomiting.

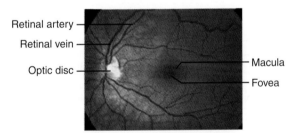

Retinal artery
Retinal vein
Optic disc
Macula
Fovea

FIGURE 13.2   Fundus of the left eye.
Source: *Kumar, Parveen, CBE BSc MD DM(HC) FRCP(L&E) FRCPath. The special senses. Kumar and Clark's clinical medicine. p. 1047–1065, Chapter 21.*

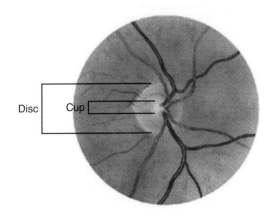

Disc   Cup

FIGURE 13.3   Optic disc and optic cup in fundus image.
Source: *Haleem, Muhammad Salman. Automatic extraction of retinal features from colour retinal images for glaucoma diagnosis: A review. Comput Med Imaging Graph 37(7–8): 581–596.*

Macula Lutea
■ Is an oval yellowish **pigmented area** (yellow spot) near the retinal centre.
■ Contains xanthophyll carotenoid pigments that protect the eye against ultraviolet light.

Fovea Centralis
■ Is a small pit in the centre of the macula.
■ Possesses **cone photoreceptors** at a maximum concentration with **no rods**.
■ Provides **sharp central vision**, which is required for reading, driving, etc.
■ Has **no vessels** and depends on the choriocapillaris, the capillary layer of the choroid, for nutrients.

Cell Types of the Retina (Fig. 13.4)
The major circuit of information transmission to the brain is based on a **three-neuron chain**: photoreceptors, bipolar cells and ganglion cells.

Photoreceptors: Rods and Cones (Table 13.1)
■ Are **first-order** neurons synapsing with bipolar cells.
■ Possess **visual pigments** that act by absorbing light and initiating neuroelectrical impulses (graded potentials).
■ Utilize **glutamate** as a neurotransmitter.

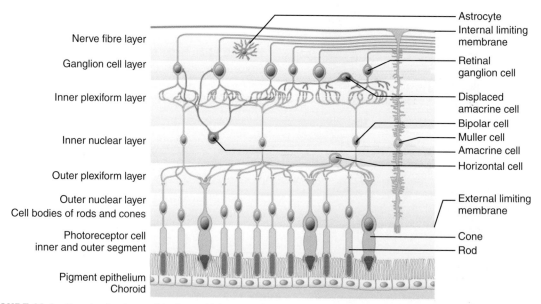

FIGURE 13.4   Neural cells whose cell bodies and interconnections account for the layered appearance of the retina in histological section. Also shown are the two principal types of neuroglial cells in the retina (although microglia are also present, they are not shown). Source: *Standring, Susan, MBE, PhD, DSc, FKC, Hon FAS, Hon FRCS. Eye. Gray's anatomy. p. 686–708.e1, Chapter 42.*

Table 13.1 Rods versus cones	
Rods	**Cones**
Achromatic vision (one photosensitive pigment)	Colour vision (three photosensitive pigments)
High sensitivity; works best in the dark (scotopic vision)	Low sensitivity; works best in daylight (photopic vision)
Poor visual acuity (many rods linked to one bipolar cell)	Good visual acuity (every cone linked to one bipolar cell)
Concentrated in peripheral retina	Concentrated in central retina
Around 120 million cells	Around 7 million cells

Bipolar Cells

■ Are **second-order** neurons that transmit signals from photoreceptors to ganglion cells.
■ Are positioned between the **inner** and **outer plexiform layers**.
■ Utilize **glutamate** as a neurotransmitter.

Ganglion Cells

■ Are **third-order** neurons that leave the retina and **form the optic nerve**.
■ Are the only cells in the retina capable of generating **action potentials**.
■ Terminate in the lateral geniculate nucleus, hypothalamus, superior colliculus and pretectum.
■ Utilize **glutamate** as a neurotransmitter.

Association Neurons

■ **Horizontal cells**
  ▪ Are **inhibitory interneurons** that regulate the input from photoreceptor cells by lateral inhibition.
  ▪ Alter the responses of bipolar cells.
  ▪ Have a role in **colour discrimination**.
  ▪ Are positioned in the **nuclear** and **plexiform layers**.
  ▪ Utilize **gamma amino butyric acid (GABA)** as a neurotransmitter.
■ **Amacrine cells**
  ▪ Execute lateral inhibition of ganglion cells by acting at the bipolar–ganglion cell synapses.
  ▪ Are positioned between the inner nuclear and outer plexiform layers.
  ▪ Utilize GABA, dopamine, glycine and acetylcholine as neurotransmitters.
  ▪ Are believed to lack axons; however, new studies proved that some of these cells do have axons.

VISUAL PATHWAYS (Figs. 13.5 and 13.6)

The visual image is transmitted from the retina to the primary visual cortex through different structures and checkpoints. These are the optic nerve, optic chiasm, optic tract and lateral geniculate nucleus (LGN).

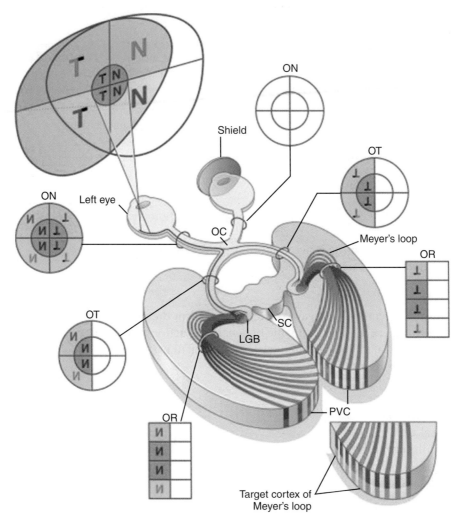

FIGURE 13.5   Pathway from the visual field of the left eye to the primary visual cortex. T denotes the temporal (outer) half of the left visual field; N denotes the nasal (inner) half of the left visual field. In the left retina and optic nerve (ON), the neural representation of the image is reversed side to side. It is also inverted top to bottom. The right retina and optic nerve are inactive because this eye is shielded. At the optic chiasm (OC), the axons forming the nasal half of the left optic nerve cross the midline and form the medial half of the right optic tract (OT). Those forming the lateral half of the nerve form the lateral half of the left optic tract. Each set synapses in the corresponding lateral geniculate body (LGB). The optic radiations (OR) are fan-like, with the axons carrying the foveal input initially in the middle of the fan. As they approach the occipital pole, the foveal axons (red) in both hemispheres move to the back and enter the posterior part of the primary visual cortex (PVC). Note the striped pattern of delivery to the cortex on both sides. The blank intervals between are the same width and contain the axons and cortex responsible for the visual field of the right eye. SC, superior colliculus.
Source: *Mtui, Estomih, MD. Visual pathways. Fitzgerald's clinical neuroanatomy and neuroscience. p. 265–273, Chapter 28.*

Optic Nerve (CN II)

- Part of the CNS, the myelinated optic nerve is derived from the diencephalon (optic stalks).
- All meningeal layers (dura, arachnoid and pia mater) cover the optic nerve.
- Blood supply is mainly from the central retinal, choroidal, scleral (circle of Zinn–Haller) and pial vessels.

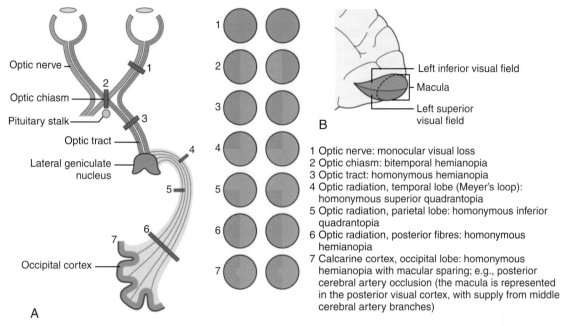

1 Optic nerve: monocular visual loss
2 Optic chiasm: bitemporal hemianopia
3 Optic tract: homonymous hemianopia
4 Optic radiation, temporal lobe (Meyer's loop): homonymous superior quadrantopia
5 Optic radiation, parietal lobe: homonymous inferior quadrantopia
6 Optic radiation, posterior fibres: homonymous hemianopia
7 Calcarine cortex, occipital lobe: homonymous hemianopia with macular sparing; e.g., posterior cerebral artery occlusion (the macula is represented in the posterior visual cortex, with supply from middle cerebral artery branches)

FIGURE 13.6 Schematic diagram of the visual pathway and the associated field defects with its disruption at different points on the pathway.
Source: *Reproduced from Butler P, Mitchell A, Healy J. Applied radiological anatomy 2nd ed. Cambridge, UK: Cambridge University Press; 2012.*

CLINICAL INSIGHT

- **Optic neuritis**
  - An **inflammation** of the optic nerve.
  - Strongly associated with **multiple sclerosis**.
  - Patients suffer from **episodic blindness** and **eye pain** upon movement.
- **Glaucoma**
  - Causes increased intraocular pressure that damage the optic nerve.
  - Leads to retinal ganglion cells injury, causing loss of peripheral vision.

Optic Chiasm

- Also derived from the diencephalon, the optic chiasm is located superior to the hypophysis (pituitary gland).
- Fibres from the nasal retina cross over to the contralateral optic tract.
- Fibres from the temporal retina travel ipsilaterally.
- Blood supply is mainly from the anterior cerebral artery, branches of the internal carotid artery (ICA), and anterior and posterior communicating arteries.

CLINICAL INSIGHTS

- **Pituitary tumour**
  - **Midsagittal** transection of the optic chiasm leads to **bitemporal hemianopia**.
  - Trans-sphenoidal hypophysectomy is the optimal treatment of large pituitary tumours.
- **Internal carotid artery (ICA) calcification**
  - **Bilateral lateral** compression of the optic chiasm by calcified ICAs results in **binasal hemianopia**.
  - **Unilateral** ICA calcification may lead to **contralateral nasal hemianopia**.

Optic Tract

- The **left optic tract** correlates with the **right visual field** and vice versa.
- Each contains fibres from the **ipsilateral temporal retina** and the **contralateral nasal retina**.
- The tract transmits visual information to the **ipsilateral** LGN, pretectal nuclei and superior colliculus.
- Main blood supply is from the **anterior choroidal artery** (branch of ICA).
- Any lesion in the optic tract due to stroke, tumour, surgery or infection will lead to **contralateral homonymous hemianopia**.

Lateral Geniculate Nucleus

- **The primary relay nucleus** for visual pathway, it is located in the **posterior** part of the **thalamus**.
- LGN is composed of **six layers**:
  - Layers **1, 4 and 6** obtain fibres from the **contralateral nasal retina**.
  - Layers **2, 3 and 5** obtain fibres from the **ipsilateral temporal retina**.
- In addition, layers can be classified by cell size:
  - Layers **1 and 2** contain the **magnocellular** ganglion cells: responsible for detection of **movement**.
  - Layers **3–6** contain the **parvocellular** ganglion cells: responsible for detection of **colour texture** and **depth**.
- All layers project to the **primary visual cortex** (Brodmann area [BA] 17) via **optic radiations**.
- LGN receives **dual blood supply** from the **lateral choroidal artery** (branch of the posterior cerebral artery) and **anterior choroidal artery**.
- Lesion in LGN leads to **contralateral homonymous hemianopia**.

Optic Radiations (Geniculocalcarine Tract)

- They have axons extending from the **LGN**, reaching the **retrolenticular part of the internal capsule**, and ending at **the primary visual cortex (BA 17)**.
- They receive blood supply via the middle cerebral artery, posterior cerebral artery (calcarine branch) and anterior choroidal artery.
- Mainly two divisions of the optic radiation, upper and lower, transmit the visual information (Table 13.2).

Table 13.2 Upper versus lower divisions of the optic radiation

	Upper Division	**Lower Division**
Projection	Upper bank (cuneus) of the calcarine fissure	Lower bank (lingual gyrus) of the calcarine fissure
Pathway	Parietal	Temporal (Meyer's loop)
Input	Superior retinal quadrants	Inferior retinal quadrants
Visual field	Inferior visual field	Superior visual field
Lesion (unilateral)	Contralateral lower homonymous quadran-tanopia (pie on the floor)	Contralateral upper homonymous quadran-tanopia (pie in the sky)
Lesion (bilateral)	Lower altitudinal[a] hemianopia	Upper altitudinal hemianopia

[a]*Altitudinal defect: complete loss of upper or lower half of the visual field.*

Primary Visual Cortex (BA 17)
The **primary visual cortex** is positioned around the **calcarine sulcus** in the occipital lobe.
- Retinal information is received through the **ipsilateral** LGN.
- Lesion leads to contralateral homonymous hemianopia **with macular sparing**.
- Visual cortex retinotopic organization:
  - **Posterior part** interprets the **central** vision (**macular input**).
  - **Intermediate part** interprets the **peripheral** vision (**paramacular input**).
  - **Anterior part** interprets the **monocular input.**
- Note that the **macular area is spared** in vascular lesions of the occipital cortex due to **dual blood supply** (middle and posterior cerebral arteries).

Secondary Association Areas (BA 18 and 19)
Secondary association areas are located in the occipital lobes and surround the primary visual cortex.
- They process visual information received from BA 17 such as colour, form and motion detection.
- They are responsible for **pursuit eye movements** (tracking of a mobile object) (Table 13.3).
- **Stimulation** leads to **contralateral conjugate** eye deviation.
- Lesion leads to **visual agnosia**, i.e., the patient will see the visual stimuli, but will not be able to understand their meaning.

Frontal Eye Fields (BA 8)
Frontal eye fields are located rostral to the premotor cortex.
- They are responsible for **saccadic eye movements** (rapid, abrupt movement) (Table 13.3)
- **Stimulation** leads to **contralateral conjugate** eye deviation
- Lesion leads to **ipsilateral conjugate** eye deviation

Table 13.3 Types of eye movements			
Type of Eye Movement	**Function**	**Stimulus**	**Clinical Tests**
Vestibular	Maintain steady fixation during head rotation	Head rotation	Fixate on object while moving head; calorics test *(see Clinical Insight of Caloric Reflex Test)*
Saccades	Rapid refixation to eccentric stimuli	Eccentric retinal image	Voluntary movement between two objects; fast phases of OKN or of vestibular nystagmus *(see chapter 14)*
Smooth pursuit	Keep the moving object image on fovea	Retinal image slip	Voluntarily follow a moving target; OKN slow phases
Vergence	Disconjugate, slow movement to maintain binocular vision	Binasal or bitemporal disparity; retinal blur motion	Fusional amplitudes; near point of convergence

Notes: *OKN, optokinetic nystagmus: a physiologic reflex involving smooth pursuit followed by saccade, provoked by episodic visual stimuli wandering across the individual's visual field.*
Source: *Hoyt, CS, & Taylor, D. Pediatric ophthalmology and strabismus, expert consult-online and print. 4 ed. UK: Elsevier Health Sciences; 2012.*

VISUAL PATHWAYS BLOOD SUPPLY

Blood supply to the visual pathways is depicted in Fig. 13.7.

PUPILLARY LIGHT REFLEXES (Fig. 13.8)

- Pupillary light reflexes control the **pupil diameter** in response to **light intensity**.
  - A **high** intensity light will cause pupillary **constriction (miosis)**, permitting less light to enter.
  - A **low** intensity light will cause pupillary **dilation (mydriasis)**, permitting more light to enter.
- If you shine a light into one eye, both eyes will constrict by **direct** (stimulated eye) and **consensual** (unstimulated eye) pupillary light reflex.
- **CN II** is the **afferent** limb pathway, and **CN III** (oculomotor nerve) is the **efferent** limb.
- **Mechanism:** Optic fibres carry light impulses from the retina towards the LGN passing through the optic nerve, chiasm and tract. Prior to reaching the LGN, some of these fibres relay to the **ipsilateral pretectal nucleus**, which in turn projects onto the **Edinger–Westphal nuclei bilaterally**. **Preganglionic fibres** from each Edinger–Westphal nucleus project onto the **ipsilateral ciliary ganglion**. The **short ciliary nerve** carries **postganglionic fibres** that innervate the **constrictor pupillae muscle**, which will finally constrict the pupil. Both pupils constrict simultaneously upon shining light on one eye; however, the direct reflex is usually more pronounced than the consensual reflex.

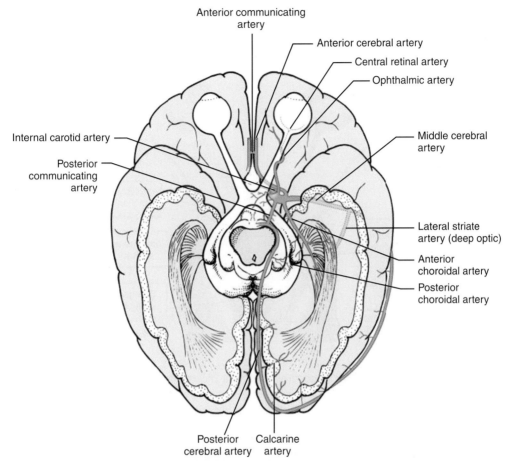

FIGURE 13.7 Diagram of a brain dissected to display the visual pathways as seen from the ventral aspect. The blood supply to the various parts of the visual pathways is shown in red on the right-hand side of the diagram (corresponding to the left side of the brain). Note the blood supply to the following areas: intracranial optic nerve, ophthalmic artery (an important inferior relation) and pial branches of the hypophyseal artery; optic chiasm, adjacent related vessels including the superior hypophyseal, internal carotid, posterior communicating, anterior cerebral and anterior communicating artery; lateral root of the optic tract, anterior choroidal artery; lateral geniculate body, anterior choroidal artery and branches of the posterior cerebral artery; commencement of the optic radiation (geniculocalcarine tract), anterior choroidal artery; posteriorly directed fibres, lateral striate (deep optic) branch of the middle cerebral artery; termination of the geniculocalcarine tract and visual cortex, perforating branches of the cortical arteries, principally the calcarine branch of the posterior cerebral, although the middle cerebral artery may anastomose and aid in the supply of the cortex at the anterior end of the calcarine sulcus and at the posterior pole.

Source: *Forrester, John V, MB ChB MD FRCS(Ed) FRCP(Glasg) (Hon) FRCOphth(Hon) FMedSci FRSE FARVO. Anatomy of the eye and orbit. The eye: basic sciences in practice. p. 1–102.e2, Chapter 1.*

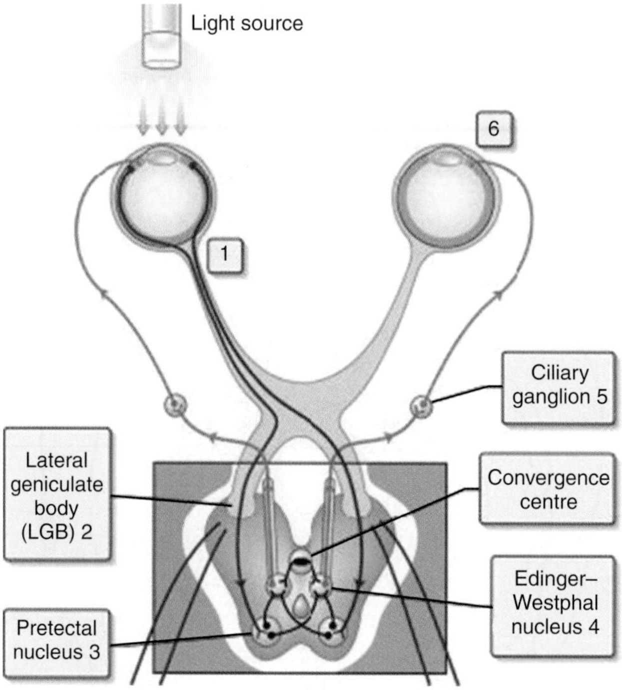

FIGURE 13.8 Pupillary light reflex. Afferent pathway: (1) light activates optic nerve axons; (2) axons (some decussating at the chiasm) pass through each lateral geniculate body; and (3) synapse at pretectal nuclei. Efferent pathway: (4) action potentials pass to Edinger–Westphal nuclei of the oculomotor nerve, then, (5) via parasympathetic neurons in the oculomotor nerves to cause (6) pupil constriction. Source: *Kumar, Parveen, CBE BSc MD DM(HC) FRCP(L&E) FRCPath. Neurological disease. Kumar and Clark's clinical medicine. p. 1067–1153, Chapter 22.*

CLINICAL INSIGHT

- **Marcus Gunn pupil (relative afferent pupillary defect)**
    - Is caused by a lesion to the **afferent** optic nerve.
    - Is commonly found in **multiple sclerosis** due to retrobulbar neuritis.
    - **Swinging flashlight test** is the diagnostic tool (Fig. 13.9).
- **Argyll Robertson pupil (pupillary light–near dissociation)** (Fig. 13.10)
    - **Bilateral** small, irregular pupils that **lack miotic response** to light, whether **direct** or **consensual**.
    - **Miotic response** to **near objects**, i.e., **accommodation** is **preserved.** This is because the pathways controlling accommodation do not involve the pretectal nuclei.
    - It is caused by a lesion in the **rostral midbrain (pretectum)** in close proximity to the aqueduct of Sylvius.
    - Most common aetiology is **neurosyphilis** but may occur in diabetes and lupus as well.
- **Adie's tonic pupil** (Fig. 13.10)
    - **Unilateral** dilated, irregular pupil, more frequently seen in women.
    - **There is absence of reaction to bright light and incomplete constriction to convergence.**
    - It is due to denervation of the **sphincter pupillae.**
    - It is occasionally associated with absent tendon reflexes.

Normal   Defect

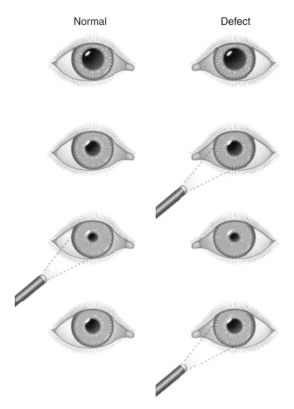

FIGURE 13.9   Relative afferent pupillary defect (Marcus Gunn pupil). This patient has an abnormal left optic nerve. In ambient light (top row), the pupils are equal. As the abnormal eye is illuminated (second row), only modest constriction is noted. As the light is swung to the normal eye (third row), the pupils constrict briskly. When the light is swung back to the abnormal eye (bottom row), paradoxical dilation is noted.

Source: *From Friedman NJ, Kaiser PK, Pineda A. Massachusetts ear & eye infirmary illustrated manual of ophthalmology. 3rd ed. Philadelphia: Saunders; 2009.*

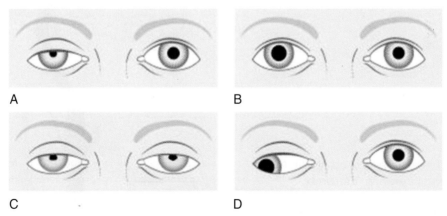

A

B

C

D

FIGURE 13.10   Pupillary defects. (A) Right Horner syndrome (ptosis and miosis). (B) Right Adie's tonic pupil. (C) Argyll Robertson pupils with bilateral ptosis and small irregular pupils. (D) Right oculomotor nerve palsy (looking down and out, ptosis and a dilated pupil).

Source: *Olson, John. The visual system. Macleod's clinical examination. p. 275–295, Chapter 12.*

PUPILLARY REFLEX DILATATION (Fig. 13.11)

This pathway is composed of three neurons carrying sympathetic innervations to **ipsilateral** sweat glands, eye dilator muscles, and upper and lower eyelids muscles. Fig. 13.12 summarizes the oculosympathetic pathway that is responsible for the pupillary reflex dilatation.

CLINICAL INSIGHT

■ **Horner syndrome** (Figs. 13.10 and 13.11) *(see Case Study Discussion)*
  ■ Horner syndrome is caused by transection of the **sympathetic pathway** at any level.
  ■ Symptoms develop ipsilaterally: **miosis, partial ptosis, anhidrosis** and possible **enophthalmos**.
  ■ Diagnosis is achieved by using **4% cocaine eye drops**; cocaine will **dilate a normal eye**, but will not do so in Horner syndrome.

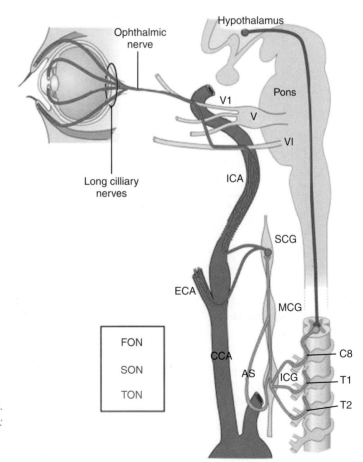

FIGURE 13.11 Anatomy of the oculosympathetic pathway. AS, ansa subclavia; CCA, common carotid artery; ECA, external carotid artery; ICA, internal carotid artery; ICG, inferior cervical ganglion; MCG, middle cervical ganglion; SCG, superior cervical ganglion; FON, first-order neuron; SON, second-order neuron; TON: third-order neuron. Source: *Reede, Deborah L., MD. Horner's syndrome: Clinical and radiographic evaluation. Neuroimaging Clin N Am 18(2):369–385.*

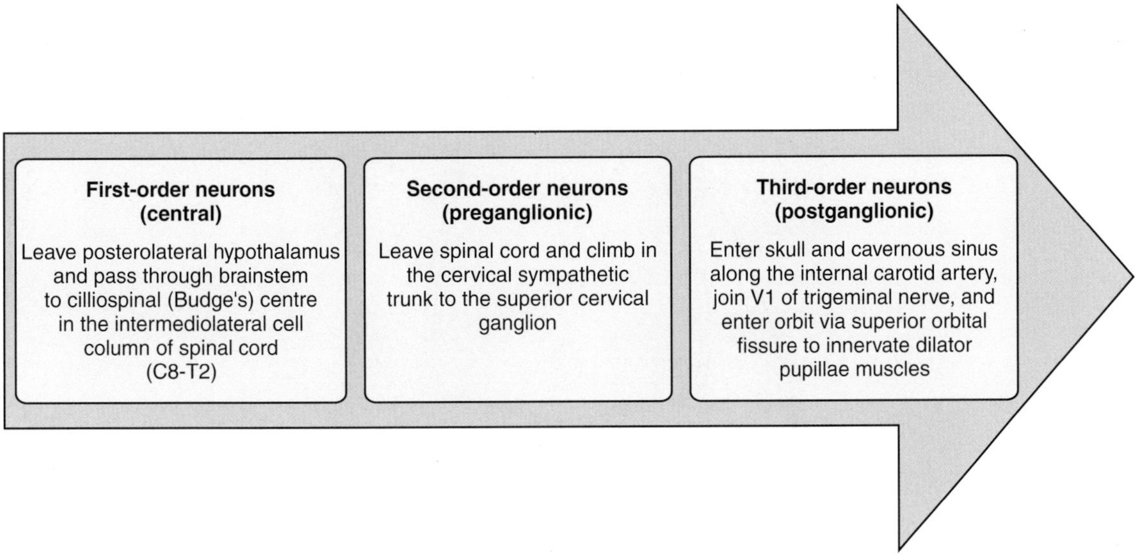

FIGURE 13.12 Summary of the oculosympathetic pathway.
Source: *Courtesy of Ali A. Haydar, MD. Lebanese American University Medical Center.*

PUPILLARY NEAR REFLEX/ACCOMMODATION (Fig. 13.13)

The **pupillary near reflex/accommodation** involves three simultaneous adaptive mechanisms:

- **Convergence:** contraction of both **medial recti**
- **Lens thickening:** contraction of both **ciliary muscles**, causing the **lens to thicken** and thus increasing its refractive power
- **Pupillary constriction:** contraction of both **pupillary sphincters**, thus increasing the optical performance

Accommodation is a **parasympathetic reflex** that occurs upon visual **transition from far to near sight**. The visual impulse travels through the normal visual pathway to the **visual cortex**, which will in turn project to visual association cortices. The visual association cortices then project through **corticobulbar tracts** to:

- **Both motor nuclei** of oculomotor nerves, which will conduct the command to **both medial recti** to contract and converge the eyes.
- **Both Edinger–Westphal nuclei**, whose preganglionic fibres project to the **ciliary ganglion**. Postganglionic fibres of the short ciliary nerves innervate the **constrictor pupillae muscles** causing constriction of the pupils, and the ciliary muscles causing contraction, thus thickening of the lenses.

Note that all the near reflex efferent actions are mediated via **CN III**.

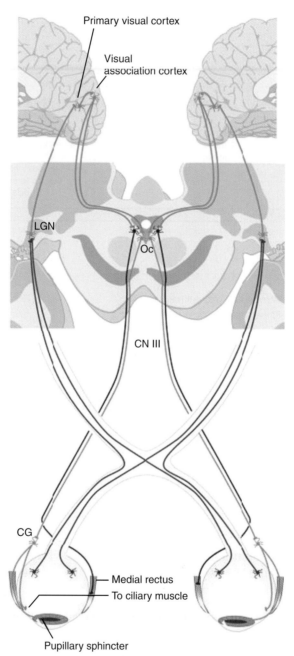

FIGURE 13.13   Pathway of the near reflex. The afferent limb is the same as in the standard visual pathway (through the LGN to the primary visual cortex). The efferent limb involves the visual association cortex, with projections to the oculomotor nuclei. The oculomotor nerve finally carries the near reflex command to the medial rectus, ciliary muscle and pupillary sphincter. CG, ciliary ganglion; CN III, oculomotor nerve; LGN, lateral geniculate nucleus; Oc, oculomotor nucleus.

Source: *Modified from Nolte J. Elsevier's integrated neuroscience. Philadelphia: Mosby Elsevier; 2007.*

TYPES OF EYE MOVEMENTS (Fig. 13.14 and Table 13.3)

CLINICAL INSIGHT

- **Caloric reflex test**
  - **Warm water (≥44°C)** causes the endolymph within the ipsilateral horizontal canal to rise, resulting in increased vestibular afferent nerve firing. Both eyes will turn in the direction of the contralateral ear, associated with **horizontal nystagmus towards the ipsilateral ear.**
  - **Cold water (≤30°C)** causes the endolymph within the semicircular canal to fall, resulting in reduced vestibular afferent nerve firing. Both eyes will turn in the direction of the ipsilateral ear, associated with **horizontal nystagmus towards the contralateral ear**.
  - Mnemonic is **COWS**: **C**old is **O**pposite, **W**arm is **S**ame.

Conjugate Horizontal Gaze Centre (Fig. 13.15)

- It is known as **paramedian pontine reticular formation (PPRF).**
- After receiving stimulation from the **contralateral frontal conjugate gaze centre**, the PPRF relays to:
  - **Ipsilateral abducens nerve nucleus**, innervating the relevant lateral rectus muscle.
  - **Contralateral oculomotor nerve nucleus** via the **medial longitudinal fasciculus (MLF)**, innervating the relevant medial rectus muscle.
- The outcome is a perfectly coordinated conjugate gaze to one side, with adduction of one eye and abduction of the other.

CLINICAL INSIGHTS

- **Internuclear ophthalmoplegia (MLF syndrome)** (Fig. 13.16)
  - It is caused by injury to the **MLF between** the **abducens** and **oculomotor nuclei**.
  - It results in **ipsilateral weak adduction** (medial rectus palsy) and **contralateral abducting nystagmus**.
  - **Convergence** is **preserved**
  - It is frequently encountered in **multiple sclerosis**.
- **One-and-a-half syndrome** (Fig. 13.16)
  - It is caused by lesions in the **ipsilateral MLF** and **PPRF**.
  - It consists of **ipsilateral horizontal gaze palsy** and **internuclear ophthalmoplegia**: ipsilateral adduction and abduction failure and contralateral adduction failure.
  - The unaffected lateral rectus can abduct with **nystagmus**.

Conjugate Vertical Gaze Centre

- It is controlled by the **rostral interstitial nucleus of the MLF (riMLF)**, which receives diffuse projections from cortical areas.
- riMLF then projects to the **oculomotor** and **trochlear nuclei (bilaterally)**, with fibres travelling through the **posterior commissure**.

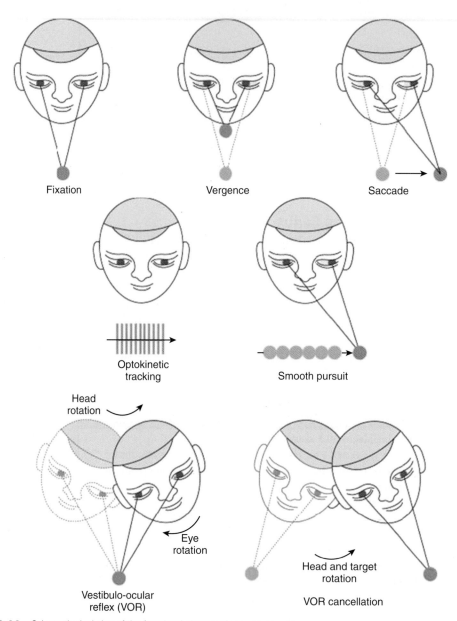

FIGURE 13.14 Schematic depiction of the functional classes of eye movements.
Source: *Hullar, Timothy E. Evaluation of the patient with dizziness. Cummings otolaryngology. p. 2525–2547.e3, Chapter 164.*

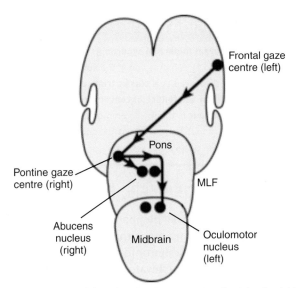

FIGURE 13.15   When looking to the right, the left frontal conjugate gaze centre stimulates the right (contralateral) pontine gaze centre, the pontine paramedian reticular formation (PPRF). The pontine gaze centre, in turn, stimulates the right (adjacent) abducens nerve nucleus and, upwards through the left medial longitudinal fasciculus (MLF), the left (contralateral) oculomotor nerve nucleus, which sits in the midbrain.

Source: *Kaufman, David Myland, MD. Visual disturbances. Kaufman's clinical neurology for psychiatrists. p. 261–285, Chapter 12.*

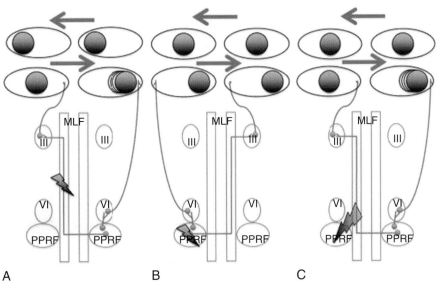

A   B   C

FIGURE 13.16   Lateral eye movement disorders: (A) the clinical features of internuclear ophthalmoplegia due to a lesion of the MLF, the lesion is on the side of adduction failure; (B) lateral gaze palsy due to a lesion in the PPRF, the side of the lesion corresponds to the side of lateral gaze failure; and (C) 'one-and-a-half' syndrome due to a lesion affecting both the MLF and PPRF; the side that can still abduct (albeit with nystagmus) is contralateral to the side of the lesion. MLF, medial longitudinal fasciculus; PPRF, paramedian pontine reticular formation; VI, abducens nucleus; III, oculomotor nucleus.

Source: *Sakai, Koji, PhD. Brainstem white matter tracts and the control of eye movements. Semin Ultrasound CT MR 35(5): 517–526.*

CLINICAL INSIGHT

- **Parinaud (dorsal midbrain) syndrome**
  - It is caused by compression of the **superior colliculus** and **pretectal area**.
  - It is characterized by a **classic triad: upward gaze palsy, pupillary light–near dissociation** and **failure of convergence**.
  - **Pineal tumour** is the most common aetiology.
  - A large tumour may compress the aqueduct and lead to symptomatic increased intracranial pressure.

BLEPHAROPTOSIS (Fig. 13.17)

Simply known as **ptosis**, blepharoptosis is an abnormal drooping of the upper eyelid margin, covering **more than 1.5 mm** of the superior corneal limbus.

- **Aponeurotic** blepharoptosis: most common type, due to stretching or disinsertion of the **levator aponeurosis** from the tarsus; frequently encountered in the **elderly**
- **Myogenic** blepharoptosis: seen in **myasthenia gravis** and **myotonic dystrophy**

CLINICAL INSIGHT

- **Myasthenic ptosis**
  - Ptosis is **proportionally** related to **fatigue**
  - Presents **bilaterally**, but asymmetrical
  - Diagnosis is confirmed when ptosis improves after **cholinesterase inhibitor injection**
- **Neurogenic** blepharoptosis: seen in **Horner syndrome** and **CN III palsy**
- **Traumatic** blepharoptosis: results from **eyelid laceration** seen in blunt injury and postocular surgery
- **Mechanical** ptosis: seen after surgery or **inflammation** of the eyelid, or in the presence of an **ocular mass** such as a haemangioma or neurofibroma

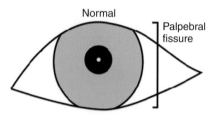

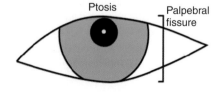

FIGURE 13.17   Normal eye versus eye with ptosis. Source: *Tuli, Sanjeev Y., MD. Blepharoptosis: assessment and management. J Pediatr Health Care 26(2): 149–154.*

CASE STUDY DISCUSSION

Horner syndrome occurs due to a lesion in the sympathetic pathway to the eye. Aetiologies differ depending on the age of the patient and site of the lesion. Thorough investigation is crucial to detect life-threatening conditions.

Clinical Features and Pathophysiology

- **Mild ptosis**: Results from **paralysis of Muller muscle**, which contributes to upper eyelid elevation, but levator palpebrae superioris muscle function is preserved.
- **Miosis**: Due to **paralysis of iris dilator muscle**.
- **Anhidrosis** or absence of sweating: Results from **loss of innervation** of the **sweat glands**.
- **Enophthalmos**: Due to paralysis of **orbitalis muscle**.

Differential Diagnosis

The differential diagnosis list is very long. It can be narrowed, however, by knowing which sympathetic pathway neurons are affected. **Cocaine** and **hydroxyamphetamine tests** are **the initial tests of choice**.

- **Cocaine test:** Cocaine (concentration of 4%) eye drops are used. Cocaine will **block norepinephrine reuptake** from the synaptic cleft and cause a pupil with intact sympathetic tone to dilate. **Failure to dilate confirms the diagnosis of Horner syndrome**.
- **hydroxyamphetamine test:** Hydroxyamphetamine causes **active release of norepinephrine** from the presynaptic nerve ending, which will dilate the pupil. A **positive response (pupillary dilation)** indicates that the lesion is in the **first-** or **second-order neurons**. In our patient, the left **pupil did not respond** to hydroxyamphetamine, thus indicating a **third-order neuron lesion**.

A number of differentials, depending on the neuron order, are listed herein:

- **First-order neuron:** Stroke, meningitis, multiple sclerosis, syringomyelia and hypothalamic lesions
- **Second-order neuron:** Aortic aneurysm, central venous catheterization, chest tubes, neuroblastoma, and Pancoast tumour, a tumour of the pulmonary apex
- **Third-order neuron:** Cluster or migraine headache, carotid artery dissection, herpes zoster and otitis media

Management and Prognosis

There is no specific treatment for Horner syndrome. Management and prognosis depend on the different aetiologies.

CHAPTER 14

Auditory and Vestibular Systems

Jade Nehmé, Michel Kmeid, Nabil Moukarzel

CASE STUDY

Presentation and Physical Examination: A 47-year-old male athlete presented with chronic disequilibrium and unsteadiness of 7 years duration; the condition was very disabling with inability to work normally. He also complained of a pulsatile oscillopsia since 5 years described as 'my eyes are jumping' when exercising. One year earlier, he started to have episodes of true vertigo precipitated by loud sounds and after coughing and sneezing; each episode lasted around 1 min and resolved spontaneously. He also mentioned the presence of hearing loss in the right ear as well as the sensation of hearing his own voice, breathing and chewing sounds while eating. He had no previous medical history.

On physical examination, otoscopy was normal for both ears. He had an upbeating rotatory nystagmus precipitated by Valsalva manoeuvres, pressure over the right external auditory canal and loud sounds (Fig. 14.1). The rest of the neurological and ear–nose–throat (ENT) examination was unremarkable.

Diagnosis, Management and Follow-Up: A pure tone audiometry was done and showed the presence of a conductive hearing loss in the right ear, specifically on the low frequencies (Fig. 14.2). Tympanometry and acoustic reflexes were intact bilaterally, whereas cervical vestibular-evoked myogenic potentials (cVEMPs) showed a low threshold level of 60 decibels (dB) in the right ear and a normal threshold level of 95 dB in the left one (Fig. 14.3).

Due to the presence of chronic disequilibrium, a brain magnetic resonance imaging (MRI) was done and ischaemic brain lesions were ruled out. However, a right superior canal

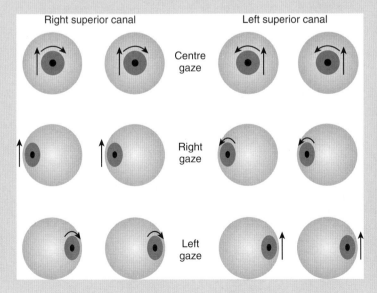

FIGURE 14.1 Direction of the slow phase of eye movements with superior canal excitation. Eye movement occurs in the plane of the superior canal regardless of the direction of gaze. There are both vertical and torsional components when the patient is looking directly ahead (centre gaze). The torsional and vertical components can be separated by having the patient look to the right or left during stimulation.
Source: *Weinreich, Heather M. Superior semicircular canal dehiscence syndrome. Otologic surgery. p. 445–457, Chapter 42.*

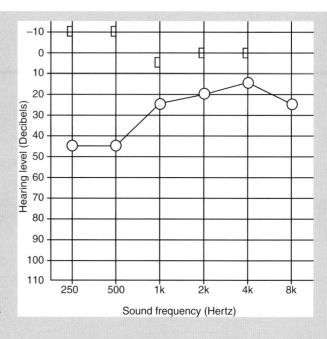

FIGURE 14.2   Typical audiogram in a patient with right-sided superior canal dehiscence syndrome. Circles represent air conduction and brackets represent bone conduction. Note that there is a negative bone conduction threshold at 250 and 500 Hz, and the air–bone gap is largest at low frequencies. Source: *Weinreich, Heather M. Superior semicircular canal dehiscence syndrome. Otologic surgery. p. 445–457, Chapter 42.*

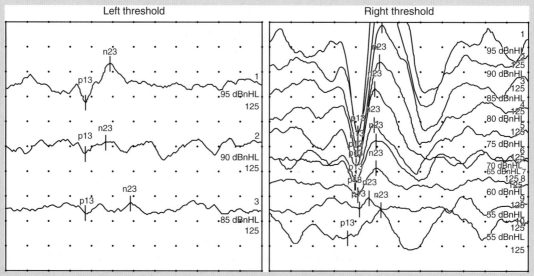

FIGURE 14.3   Typical cervical vestibular evoked myogenic potential (cVEMP) results in a patient with right-sided superior canal dehiscence syndrome and an intact left side. The cVEMP is initially measured with clicks at 95 dB above normal adult hearing level (dB nHL), and the stimulus amplitude is decreased until the response is no longer measurable. In the left ear, the patient has a cVEMP response at 95 dB but not with lower amplitude stimuli. In the right ear, the amplitude of the cVEMP is much larger at 95 dB, and the response continues to be detectable at amplitudes as small as 60 dB. Thus, in this example, the cVEMP threshold is 95 dB nHL on the left and 60 dB nHL on the right. Source: *Weinreich, Heather M. Superior semicircular canal dehiscence syndrome. Otologic surgery. p. 445–457, Chapter 42.*

dehiscence was suspected; a temporal bone computed tomography (CT) scan with reconstruction in the plane of the superior canal confirmed the presence of a 4 mm defect in the roof of the right superior canal (Fig. 14.4). Thus, the patient was diagnosed with **superior semicircular canal (SCC) dehiscence**, also known as 'Minor syndrome'.

The patient underwent a **right superior canal plugging procedure** via a middle cranial fossa approach (Fig. 14.5). After surgery,

the patient perceived a significant improvement of his disequilibrium and auditory symptoms. Reduction in the air–bone gap on the audiogram and normalization of the cVEMPs thresholds in the right ear were also noted 2 months postsurgery.

Try to guess what is the pathophysiology, clinical features and management of Minor syndrome after studying this chapter.

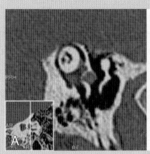
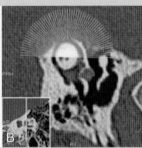
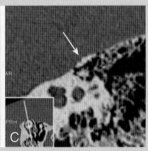

FIGURE 14.4 Computed tomographic (CT) scan demonstrating superior canal dehiscence (SCD). (A) CT image is reformatted in the plane of the superior canal. An area of dehiscence between the superior canal and middle fossa is present. (B) Orthogonal reconstructions are performed at 3° intervals for 180° around the superior canal. These planes of reconstruction are shown as white lines. (C) An orthogonal reconstruction demonstrating SCD. The region of the reconstruction is shown in small view in the lower left.

Source: *Weinreich, Heather M. Superior semicircular canal dehiscence syndrome. Otologic surgery. p. 445–457, Chapter 42.*

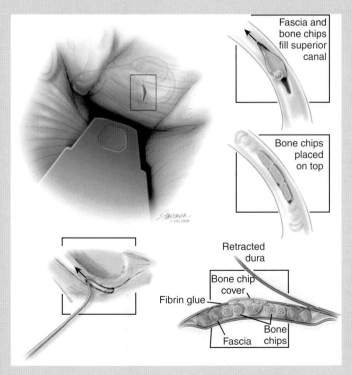

FIGURE 14.5 Plugging of the superior canal dehiscence. The area of the superior canal is identified while the dura is retracted. Fascia and bone chips are used to plug both ends of the superior canal.

Source: *Weinreich, Heather M. Superior semicircular canal dehiscence syndrome. Otologic surgery. p. 445–457, Chapter 42.*

BRIEF INTRODUCTION

The **ear** is located within the temporal bone. The **inner ear** lies in the **petrous bone**, in close contact with the middle and posterior cranial fossae. It is encased in a bony labyrinth that is divided into two parts:

- Anterior labyrinth, which is formed by the cochlea, the auditory organ.
- Posterior labyrinth, which is formed by the vestibule and SCCs that function in maintaining balance and equilibrium.

The auditory and vestibular systems are extensively interconnected. As a result, several pathologies related to the ear will end up affecting both systems at variable degrees. These pathologies can result from injury to the bony labyrinth, the membranous labyrinth or the corresponding peripheral and central neuronal pathways.

The goal of this chapter is to describe the anatomy of the auditory and vestibular systems as well as the interconnections between the central and peripheral auditory and vestibular pathways and to highlight some pathologies related to the inner ear.

INNER EAR ANATOMY

Gross inner ear anatomy is depicted in Fig. 14.6.

Bony Labyrinth

The **bony labyrinth** is the **outer** part of the inner ear. It protects the whole labyrinth and consists of two subdivisions:

- **Anterior** bony labyrinth, which gives the architecture of the **cochlea** assuming the function of **hearing**.
- **Posterior** bony labyrinth, which gives the architecture of the **vestibule** and **SCCs** assuming the function of **balance** and **equilibrium**.

Anterior Bony Labyrinth

- The bony labyrinth of the cochlea forms a **coiled (2½ turns)**, 35 mm long duct with a wide base, and a narrow apex.
- The core of the cochlea is called the **modiolus**; its pores allow the passage of **auditory nerve fibres**.
- The osseous spiral lamina is a bony ridge extending from the modiolus towards the periphery. It curls around the centre of the cochlea causing partial division of the bony anterior labyrinth into an **upper** chamber, the **scala vestibule**, and a **lower** chamber, the **scala tympani**. These two scalae communicate at the apex of the cochlea at what is known as the **helicotrema**.
- The anterior labyrinth communicates with the middle ear through the **round window**. At this level, a thin membrane separates the aqueous environment of the scala tympani of the cochlea from the air-filled middle ear cavity.

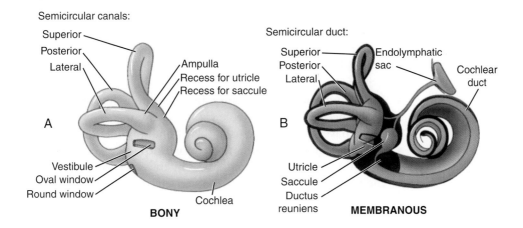

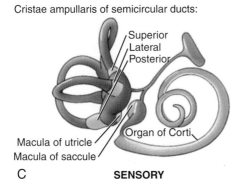

FIGURE 14.6   Cochlea of the inner ear. (A) Anatomy of the bony labyrinth. (B) Anatomy of the membranous labyrinth. (C) Anatomy of the sensory labyrinth. The labyrinth is divided into two parts: anterior and posterior. The anterior labyrinth is the cochlea. It assumes the function of hearing. The anterior labyrinth has one window connecting it to the middle ear (the round window) and one aqueduct connecting it the subarachnoid space of the posterior fossa (the cochlear aqueduct, not shown in the figure). The sensory neuroepithelium of the cochlea is the organ of Corti. The posterior labyrinth consists of the vestibule (saccule and utricle) and the three semicircular canals. It assumes the function of balance and equilibrium. The posterior labyrinth also has a window connecting it to the middle ear (the oval window) and one aqueduct connecting it to the endolymphatic sac (the vestibular aqueduct that contains the endolymphatic duct). The sensory neuroepithelium of the vestibule is called the maculae whereas that of the semicircular canals is found in the ampulla of the canal and is called the crista ampullaris.

Source: *From Gartner LP, Hiatt JL. Color textbook of histology, 3rd ed. Philadelphia: Saunders; 2007, p. 528.*

■ The anterior labyrinth is also connected to the **subarachnoid space** of the posterior cranial fossa through the **cochlear aqueduct**.

Vestibule and SCCs (Posterior Labyrinth)

■ The vestibule has two parts: **sacculus** and **utriculus**. These are organized into two perpendicular planes: **horizontal** for the utriculus and **vertical** for the sacculus.

■ The **three SCCs** are classified as the following:

  ■ Two **vertical** canals, **anterior (superior)** and **posterior (inferior)**: These are at 45° relative to the **sagittal plane**; the anterior canal is at 45° anterior to the interaural line (the straight line connecting the external auditory meatus of each ear), whereas the posterior canal is at 45° posterior to it.

- One **horizontal** (lateral) canal: It is tilted upwards at **30°** from the horizontal plane.
- At one end, each SCC becomes dilated forming the **ampulla**. The SCCs are connected to the vestibule via **five crura**; the superior and posterior canals have a **common crus** at their **nonampullated** end.
- In the **posterior labyrinth**, the **oval window** connects the scala vestibuli of the cochlea to the middle ear by the stapes footplate.
- The posterior labyrinth is also connected to the endolymphatic sac through the **vestibular aqueduct**.

Membranous Labyrinth

The **membranous labyrinth** is a complex arrangement of communicating membranous canaliculi and sacs filled with **endolymph** and surrounded by **perilymph**, located within the bony labyrinth; its main constituents are the **cochlear duct** in the **anterior** labyrinth and the **vestibule** and SCCs in the **posterior** labyrinth.

Cochlea

- The membranous labyrinth within the spiral bony cochlear duct forms a **third chamber**: the **scala media**. It is encased between the scala vestibuli (superiorly) and the scala tympani (inferiorly).
- The scala media contains the **organ of Corti**, the **sensory organ** of the cochlea. It is bordered by the following structures.
  - **Superiorly: Reissner membrane**, separating it from the scala vestibuli.
  - **Inferiorly: basilar membrane**, separating it from the scala tympani. The basilar membrane supports the organ of Corti. It is narrow at the base and wide at the apex and is attached to the spiral lamina.
  - **Laterally:** spiral ligament.
- Within the **lateral wall** of the membranous labyrinth lies the **striae vascularis**, responsible for regulating the metabolic milieu of the scala media and supporting cochlear function.

Vestibule and SCCs

- The sacculus and utriculus are known as the **otolith organs**; their **sensory epithelium** is called the **maculae**. They detect and monitor **linear accelerations** in three axes: **interaural, nasal–occipital** and **rostral–caudal**.
- Within the ampulla of each SCC lies the **crista ampullaris**, the SCC **sensory organ**. The SCCs are sensitive to **angular accelerations**, and thus are grouped into functional pairs:
  - Two lateral canals
  - Right anterior with the left posterior canal
  - Left anterior with the right posterior canal

- Angular head movement activates the pair of SCCs present in the same plane as the movement occurs. As a result, the endolymph of the paired SCCs flows in opposite directions relative to their ampullae.
  - **Ampullopetal (towards** the ampulla) flow is **excitatory**.
  - **Ampullofugal (away** from the ampulla) flow is **inhibitory**.
- Relative to their resting firing rates, neuronal impulses are therefore increased in one vestibular nerve and decreased in the other.

Membranous Ducts

- **Endolymphatic duct:** Connects the endolymphatic compartments to the endolymphatic sac.
- **Periotic duct:** Connects the scala tympani to the subarachnoid space of the posterior cranial fossa within the cochlear aqueduct.
- **Ductus reuniens:** Narrowest segment between the cochlea and the sacculus.

CLINICAL INSIGHTS

- Defects of the bony and membranous labyrinths
  - **Superior canal dehiscence (Minor) syndrome** is related to a bony defect in the **roof** of the superior SCC, resulting in an abnormal communication between the middle cranial fossa and the labyrinth. This creates a **third mobile window** in the inner ear with altered flow of endolymph within the membranous labyrinth, leading to various vestibular and auditory symptoms. Minor syndrome will be discussed in more detail at the end of this chapter.
  - Dehiscence of the **posterior** SCC is a rare entity and is usually related to **fibrous dysplasia** or a **high-riding jugular bulb**.
  - Dehiscence of the **lateral** SCC is seen in association with **chronic otitis media** with or without a cholesteatoma (abnormal noncancerous skin growth within the middle ear).
- Infectious and tumoural processes affecting the bony and membranous labyrinths
  - Infections of the middle ear can spread to the labyrinth resulting in suppurative labyrinthitis. From there, involvement of the meninges and bacterial meningitis may ensue from haematogenous seeding, direct contiguous spread, or via the cerebrospinal fluid (CSF) (through the cochlear aqueduct).
  - Tumoural processes affecting the temporal bone can also involve the bony and membranous labyrinths. Examples include paragangliomas, endolymphatic sac tumours and metastasis (adenocarcinoma, squamous cell carcinoma, melanoma).

FLUID SYSTEMS OF THE LABYRINTH

Two different types of fluids are present within the labyrinth: **perilymph** and **endolymph** (Fig. 14.7).

- **Perilymphatic compartment:**
  - **The perilymphatic space** lies **between the osseous and membranous labyrinth** (scala tympani and scala vestibuli of the cochlea).
  - It contains **perilymph**, which is a liquid similar in composition to CSF and **extracellular fluid** (high in sodium and low in potassium).

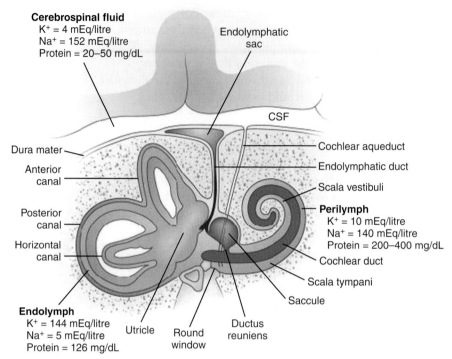

Cerebrospinal fluid
K+ = 4 mEq/litre
Na+ = 152 mEq/litre
Protein = 20–50 mg/dL

Endolymphatic sac

CSF

Dura mater
Anterior canal
Posterior canal
Horizontal canal

Cochlear aqueduct
Endolymphatic duct
Scala vestibuli
Perilymph
K+ = 10 mEq/litre
Na+ = 140 mEq/litre
Protein = 200–400 mg/dL
Cochlear duct
Scala tympani
Saccule

Endolymph
K+ = 144 mEq/litre
Na+ = 5 mEq/litre
Protein = 126 mg/dL

Utricle
Round window
Ductus reuniens

FIGURE 14.7   Anatomy of the inner ear. This figure illustrates the fluid compartments of the inner ear. The perilymphatic compartment is found between the bony and membranous labyrinth (light brown area in the figure). It has a composition similar to that of plasma and CSF (high in sodium and low in potassium). The endolymphatic compartment is found within the membranous labyrinth (dark blue area for the anterior labyrinth and light blue area for the posterior labyrinth). It has a composition similar to intracellular fluid (high in potassium and low in sodium). CSF, cerebrospinal fluid.
Source: *From Baloh, R.W. Dizziness, hearing loss, and tinnitus. Philadelphia: F.A. Davis Company; 1998, Figure 6, p. 16.*

- Perilymph of the scala tympani communicates with the CSF of the subarachnoid space of the posterior fossa via the **periotic duct** that runs through the cochlear aqueduct located at the basal turn of the cochlea.
- **Endolymphatic compartment:**
  - The **endolymphatic space** lies within the **membranous labyrinth** (scala media of the cochlea and the posterior labyrinth).
  - It contains **endolymph** with a composition similar to **intracellular fluid** (high in potassium and low in sodium).
  - The ionic composition is maintained by the **striae vascularis**. This difference in ionic composition creates a **positive direct current** of 80 mV in the scala media that slightly decreases from base to apex.
  - Located partly within the petrous bone and partly within the layers of the dura of the posterior fossa, the **endolymphatic sac** acts as a regulator of endolymph volume and pressure. It is connected to the vestibule via the **endolymphatic duct** that runs through the **vestibular aqueduct**.

CLINICAL INSIGHT

- **Perilymphatic fistula**
  - A **perilymphatic fistula (PLF)** is an abnormal connection between inner ear **perilymph** and the **middle ear** or **mastoid cavity**. Loss of perilymph and decreased impedance of the vestibular fluid lead to **endolymphatic hydrops** *(discussed below)* and **abnormal endolymphatic flow**. Variable **vestibular** and **auditory symptoms** can be seen in PLF. These include disequilibrium, positional vertigo, vertigo and nystagmus induced by positive pressure transmitted through the external ear canal, fluctuating hearing loss and tinnitus.
- **Endolymphatic hydrops**
  - **Meniere syndrome** is characterized by a constellation of clinical findings that starts with **aural fullness, tinnitus, episodic vertigo** and **hearing loss**. Hearing loss is initially fluctuating with partial or complete recovery in between episodes but then becomes progressive and irreversible with further damage to the labyrinth. It is thought to be related to **endolymphatic hydrops,** i.e., excessive build-up of endolymph fluid with dilation of the membranous labyrinth secondary to increased endolymphatic pressure.
  - Endolymphatic hydrops could be the result of **excessive endolymph production, decreased resorption** or **altered flow**. The exact pathogenesis of the disease is not well defined; however, many authors believe that it is the result of **inflammation** and **fibrosis of the endolymphatic sac**.
  - The **idiopathic** form of endolymphatic hydrops is termed **Meniere disease**. Secondary causes include viral infections (mumps, influenza), meningitis, otosyphilis, congenital abnormalities, autoimmune inner ear disease and trauma.

SENSORY NEUROEPITHELIUM OF THE INNER EAR

The inner ear functions as the sensorineural receptor organ of the auditory and vestibular systems. It converts an **acoustic waveform** into an **electrochemical stimulus** that can be transmitted to the central nervous system (CNS). While performing this sensory transduction process, the inner ear (**organ of Corti**) analyzes a sound stimulus in terms of its **frequency, intensity** and **temporal properties**, and transmits the information to the CNS for further processing and interpretation. Transduction also occurs at the level of the vestibular sensory neuroepithelium and functions in maintaining balance and equilibrium.

Organ of Corti (Fig. 14.8)

- Major cellular structures of the organ of Corti:
  - **One row of inner hair cells (IHCs)**
  - **Three rows of outer hair cells (OHCs)**
  - Supporting cells: Hensen, Claudius and Deiters cells
  - Tectorial membrane
- Hair cells of the organ of Corti:
  There exist two types of cells in the organ of Corti: IHCs and OHCs.
  - IHCs: Act as the **principal transducer of energy** from the basilar membrane to generate a nerve impulse.

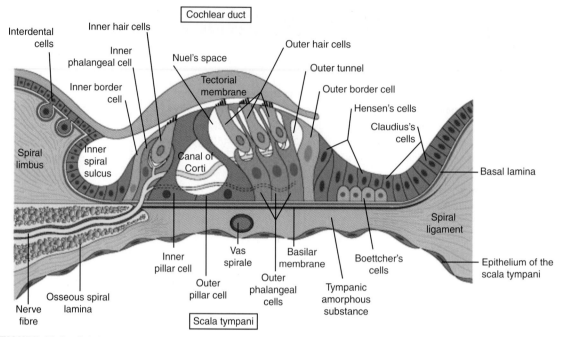

FIGURE 14.8   Spiral organ (organ of Corti); schematic drawing. This is a simplified presentation of the complex afferent and efferent innervation of the hair cells. The organ of Corti represents the actual cochlear organ. Cochlear sensory cells (hair cells) together with different supporting cell types rest on the basilar membrane and a gelatinous membrane (tectorial membrane) covers their apical cell surface. The organ of Corti stretches along the whole length of the cochlear duct.
Source: *Paulsen, F. Ear. Sobotta atlas of human anatomy, vol. 3. p. 133–160, Chapter 10.*

- **OHCs:** Act as a **motor unit to amplify motion** of the basilar membrane (**cochlear amplifier**).

  The differences between IHCs and OHCs are summarized in Table 14.1.

- Hair cells have **stereocilia,** i.e., bundles of actin filaments. Stereocilia are graduated in length with the **longest** on the **strial side** and the **shortest** on the **modiolar side**. They move as a unit as they are connected to each other by filamentous links, cross-links and tip links.

- On the apex of hair cells, a rudimentary **kinocilium** (9+2 arrangement of microtubules) is found.

- The **longest stereocilia** of OHCs are firmly embedded in the **tectorial membrane**, which lies above them, whereas those of IHCs are not attached or loosely connected to the membrane.

- **Transduction** is triggered by **displacement of the basilar membrane** by a traveling wave through the perilymph from the base to the apex. The maximal amplitude of basilar membrane displacement is frequency dependent; this is due to the 'tonotopic organization' of the cochlea:

  - **High frequency** sounds cause **maximal displacement** at the **base** where the basilar membrane is stiff; they **do not reach the apex** of the cochlea.

Table 14.1 Functional and ultrastructural differences between IHCs and OHCs

Characteristics	IHCs	OHCs
Morphology	Flask-shaped	Cylindrical
Number	3500 organized in one row on the medial (modiolar) side of the tunnel of Corti	12,000 organized in three rows on the lateral (strial) side of the tunnel of Corti
Ultrastructure	Rich in organelles (Golgi apparatus and mitochondria) with high metabolic activity	Rich in microfilaments and microtubules
Role	Passive transducers of the auditory system	Frequency specific contractile activity
Afferent innervation	Type I fibres – 27,000 (95%)	Type II fibres – 2100 (5%)
Efferent innervation	From lateral superior olivary complex	From medial superior olivary complex

Note: *IHCs, inner hair cells; OHCs, outer hair cells.*

- - **Low frequency** sounds **travel the total length** of the basilar membrane with **maximal displacement** near the **apex**.
- The deflection of stereocilia with basilar membrane movements results in closure of nonspecific ion channels and current inflow of potassium inside the cell leading to cellular depolarization.
- The sharp-tuned, frequency-selective response of the cochlea is related to the contractile activity of OHCs. It facilitates the movement of the basilar membrane at frequencies near the best frequency of the specific cochlear location. **OHCs** are therefore referred to as **cochlear modifiers**.
- Supporting cells provide nutrients and support to the organ of Corti.
- Tectorial membrane is a fibrogelatinous structure arising from the bony spiral lamina. The tips of the stereocilia of the OHCs are partially embedded in the tectorial membrane; as a result, vibration of the basilar membrane by sound waves causes shearing forces within the tectorial membrane that result in stimulation of hair cells.

CLINICAL INSIGHTS

- **Acoustic otoemissions** (AOE)
  - **Acoustic signals** are generated by **OHCs**; they can be either spontaneous or in response to an acoustic stimulus (evoked). These signals are transmitted to the middle ear and external ear canal where they can be recorded by a microphone.
  - The presence of AOE indicates OHCs integrity, and this can be used as a **screening test for neonatal hearing loss**. They can also be used to differentiate between cochlear and retrocochlear pathologies in sensorineural hearing loss as well as for monitoring purposes (ototoxicity, exposure to loud noise, intraoperative).
- **Presbycusis**
  - **Presbycusis** is a bilateral **progressive sensorineural hearing loss** associated with **ageing**. OHC degeneration begins at the basal end of the cochlea; as a result, perception of **high frequency** sounds is usually affected (**3000 Hz and above**).

- **Noise-induced hearing loss**
  - Hearing loss can occur as a result of a single intense exposure to noise (gunfire or explosion) or a chronic repetitive exposure to loud sounds. This predominantly affects the **anterior basal turn** of the cochlea, i.e., the region that processes **3000–4000 Hz** sound waves.
- **Sudden sensorineural hearing loss**
  - It is the sudden loss of hearing **exceeding 35 dB in at least three adjacent frequencies** that **occurs over less than 3 days**; it is typically unilateral when the aetiologies are viral or vascular, and bilateral when the cause is autoimmune; this hearing loss has a bad prognosis when associated with vestibular symptoms.
- **Ototoxicity**
  - Ototoxicity refers to a drug-related injury to the cochlea, the vestibular system or both.
  - Some drugs are predominantly cochleotoxic targeting the organ of Corti, whereas other drugs are vestibulotoxic *(see Clinical Insight box, p. 351)*.
  - Cochlear structures at risk of injury are mainly the **inner row of OHCs** at the cochlear basal turn (aminoglycosides, cisplatin) and the **striae vascularis** (loop diuretics).
  - The most important cochleotoxic drugs are aminoglycoside antibiotics (neomycin, tobramycin, kanamycin and amikacin), loop diuretics, quinines, salicylates and platinum-based chemotherapy.
  - Patient usually develops **bilateral symmetrical high frequency hearing loss** and **tinnitus**.

Posterior Labyrinth
Cristae Ampullaris *(Fig. 14.9)*
- They are specialized **neuroepithelium of the SCCs.**
- They consist of hair cells and supporting cells organized into central, intermediate and peripheral zones.
- On the **apical surface** of hair cells, **stereocilia** and a **single long kinocilium** are found.
- Kinocilia are arranged in a regular direction giving a specific polarization to hair cells:
  - In **horizontal cristae**, kinocilia are located on the **side closest to the utriculus.**
  - In **vertical cristae**, kinocilia are located on the **side furthest from the utriculus.**
- Overlying the cristae is a gelatinous membrane consisting of mucopolysaccharides: the **cupula**. The cupula has a density equal to 1 (similar to the endolymph), which prevents it from floating upwards; this makes the cristae relatively insensitive to gravity changes.

Maculae *(Fig. 14.10)*
- Are specialized **neuroepithelium of the otolith organs.**
- Located on the **medial wall of the sacculus** and the **floor of the utriculus.**

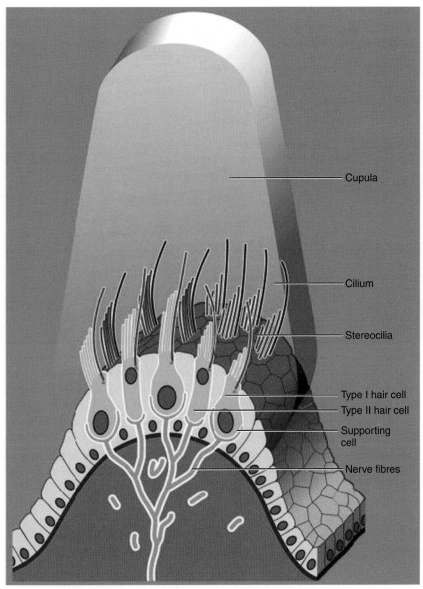

Cupula

Cilium

Stereocilia

Type I hair cell
Type II hair cell
Supporting
cell
Nerve fibres

FIGURE 14.9   At one end of each semicircular canal is a dilated portion, the ampulla, which contains a receptor organ called the crista ampullaris. Each crista ampullaris is an elongated epithelial structure situated on a ridge of supporting tissue, arising from the membranous wall of the ampulla and oriented at right angles to the direction of flow of the endolymph in the semicircular canal. The hair cells are of the same two morphological forms, type I and type II cells, the former being invested with a basket of sensory dendrites and the latter having small dendritic endings at the base only. The hair cells are supported by a single layer of columnar cells that is continuous with the simple cuboidal epithelium lining the rest of the membranous labyrinth. Like those of the maculae, the hair cells of the cristae have numerous stereocilia and a single kinocilium, the kinocilium being situated at the margin of the cell nearest to the utricle. The stereocilia and the kinocilia of the hair cells are embedded in a ridge of gelatinous glycoprotein, which is tall and cone-shaped in cross-section, giving rise to the term cupula. In contrast to the macula, the cupula does not contain otolithic crystals.
Source: *Young, Barbara, BSc Med Sci (Hons), PhD, MB BChir, MRCP, FRCPA. Special sense organs. Wheater's functional histology.*
p. 402–427, Chapter 21.

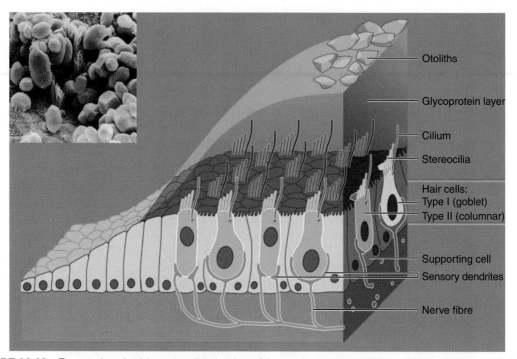

FIGURE 14.10 The saccule and utricle are two dilated regions of the membranous labyrinth, lying within the vestibule of the inner ear and filled with endolymph. The walls of each are composed of a fibrous membrane, which is bound down in places to the periosteum of the vestibule and, in other areas, is attached to the periosteum by fibrous strands, the intervening space being filled with perilymph. Internally, the saccule and utricle are lined by simple cuboidal epithelium but, in each, there is a small region of highly specialized epithelium called the macula, containing receptor cells that contribute part of the sensory input to that part of the brain responsible for maintaining balance and equilibrium. The macula of the utricle is oriented at right angles to that of the saccule. The maculae are made up of two basic cell types: sensory hair cells and support cells. The support cells are tall and columnar with basally located nuclei and microvilli at their free surface. The hair cells lie between the support cells, with their larger nuclei placed more centrally. Each hair cell has a single eccentrically located cilium of typical conformation, often called the kinocilium, and many stereocilia. The 'hairs' are embedded in a thick, gelatinous plaque of glycoprotein, probably secreted by the supporting cells. At the surface of the glycoprotein layer is a mass of crystals mainly composed of calcium carbonate and known as otoliths.
Source: *Young, Barbara, BSc Med Sci (Hons), PhD, MB BChir, MRCP, FRCPA. Special sense organs. Wheater's functional histology. p. 402–427, Chapter 21.*

- Consist of hair cells and supporting cells. The cilia of hair cells are attached to the **otolithic membrane** overlying the maculae; this membrane contains calcium carbonate crystals (**otoliths** or **otoconia**) increasing its density above 1 (2.71–2.94).
- At the centre of the maculae, the **striola** is found. It is a region in the otolithic membrane where the otoliths are very small and the thickness of the membrane is reduced in the utriculus and increased in the sacculus.
- **Kinocilia** are polarized:
  - In **utricular** macula, they are oriented **towards the striola**.
  - In **saccular** macula, they are oriented **away from the striola**.

CLINICAL INSIGHT

- **Benign paroxysmal positional vertigo (BPPV)**
  - BPPV is the most common form of **peripheral vertigo**.
  - Vertigo occurs due to **inappropriate stimulation of the SCC** by the **movement of particles** (detached otoconia from the otolithic membrane) in response to **gravity**. These otoconia can be seen attached to the cupula of the SCC, termed 'cupulolithiasis', but are more often free floating within the endolymph, termed 'canalolithiasis'.
  - Vertigo lasts **10–30 s** and is triggered by a **specific head position**. No hearing loss or neurological symptoms are noted.
  - The **posterior SCC** is most commonly involved (90%), followed by the lateral SCC.
  - Diagnosis is established by eliciting characteristic **vertigo** and **nystagmus** (latent, upbeating, geotropic, fatigable) with the **Dix–Hallpike manoeuvre** (Fig. 14.11).
  - **Canalith repositioning manoeuvres** are the mainstay of treatment. Different types of manoeuvres can be used: **Epley** (Fig. 14.12) or **Semont manoeuvres** for the **posterior canal**, and **barbecue manoeuvre** for the **lateral canal**.
  - Surgical occlusion of the posterior SCC is used in extreme cases with intractable BPPV.

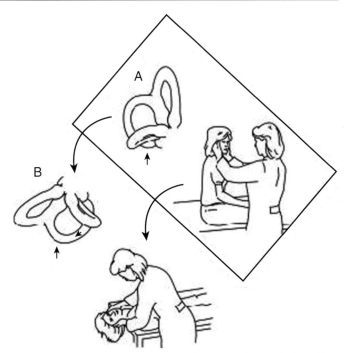

FIGURE 14.11   Dix–Hallpike test for BPPV. (A) In this test, the patient sits on the examination table and the head is turned 45° horizontally. (B) The head and trunk are quickly brought straight back en bloc so that the head is hanging over the edge of the examination table by 20°. Nystagmus is looked for and the patient is asked if they have vertigo. Although not shown in the figure, the patient is then brought up slowly to a sitting position with the head still turned 45° and nystagmus is looked for again. This test is repeated with the head turned 45° in the other direction. The figure also shows movement of debris in the right posterior semicircular canal (black arrows) during the test. In this example, the patient would have nystagmus and vertigo when the test is performed on the right side, but not when the test is performed on the left side.
Source: *From Tusa RJ. Vertigo. Neurol Clin 2001;19:39; with permission.*

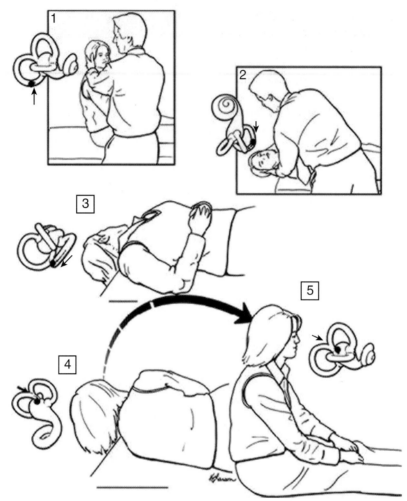

FIGURE 14.12 The Epley manoeuvre for the treatment of posterior canal BPPV. Steps (1) and (2) of the Epley manoeuvre are the steps of a positive Dix–Hallpike test. After holding for 20 s in position 2, the head is turned 90° towards the unaffected side (3). After holding for 20 s in position 3, the head is turned again 90° in the same direction to a nearly face-down position with the body also turned to accommodate the head movement (4). After holding for 20 s in position 4, the patient is brought to a sitting up position (5). The movement of the otolith material within the labyrinth is depicted with each step, showing how otoliths are moved from the semicircular canal to the vestibule. Source: *Adapted from Fife TD, Iverson DJ, Lempert T, et al. Practice parameter: therapies for benign paroxysmal positional vertigo (an evidence-based review): report of the Quality Standards Subcommittee of the American Academy of Neurology. Neurology 2008;70:2069; with permission.*

Hair Cells of the Maculae and Cristae Ampullaris

- Hair cells are **mechanosensitive** through filamentous tip links that connect mechanoelectrical (MET) channels in a short stereocilium with the membrane of an adjacent, longer stereocilium.
  - When stereocilia move **towards** the kinocilium, the tension on the tip links increases leading to opening of the MET channels with resulting potassium influx inside the cell and **cellular depolarization**.

- When stereocilia **move away** from the kinocilium, the tension on the tip links loosens leading to closure of the MET channels and **cellular hyperpolarization**.
- When stereocilia are displaced in a direction **perpendicular to the polarization axis**, **little** or **no electrical response** is noted in the hair cells.

CLINICAL INSIGHT

- **Vestibular ototoxicity**
  - Some drugs are predominantly vestibulotoxic, targeting the vestibular end organs. These include streptomycin and gentamicin (aminoglycoside antibiotics). The patient may experience **disequilibrium** and **positional vertigo** and may later develop **gait ataxia** and **oscillopsia** (secondary to bilateral vestibular hypofunction).
  - These drugs, because of their vestibulotoxicity, can be used in the treatment of Meniere disease when medical treatment fails to cure the episodes.

ANATOMY OF THE VESTIBULOCOCHLEAR NERVE (CN VIII)

The anatomy of the **vestibulocochlear nerve** and **internal auditory canal (IAC)** is depicted in Fig. 14.13.

Cochlear Nerve and Auditory Afferents

- **Auditory afferents:** Two types of auditory afferent nerve fibres are found within the cochlear nerve:
  - **Type I (90%–95% of fibres): Large, myelinated** fibres with a **direct** independent synapse on the body of a single IHC (**one IHC receives around 20 type I fibres**).
  - **Type II (5%–10% of fibres): Thin, myelinated** and **unmyelinated** fibres. Each fibre forms branches synapsing with **multiple (around 10) OHCs.**

  Around **30,000 afferent auditory neurons** innervate the cochlear hair cells. These neurons are **bipolar** and their **cell bodies** are present in the **spiral ganglion**, located in the Rosenthal canal within the **modiolus**.

  The neurotransmitter of the afferent system is predominantly **glutamate**.
- **Cochlear nerve:** The cochlear nerve travels through the **anteroinferior quadrant of the IAC** and then enters the brainstem at the **pontomedullary junction** within the foramen of Luschka. From there, primary auditory axons enter the **ventral cochlear nucleus** on the ventrolateral side of the inferior cerebellar peduncle.

Vestibular Nerves and Vestibular Afferents

- **Vestibular afferents:** These consist of fibres from **bipolar neurons** whose **cell bodies** reside in the **Scarpa ganglion** (superior and inferior vestibular ganglia), located at the bottom of the IAC.

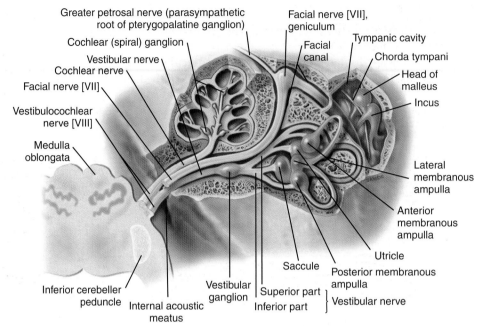

FIGURE 14.13   Vestibulocochlear nerve [VIII], course in the petrous part of the temporal bone; superior view; the petrous part has been opened. The cochlear nerve is composed of nerve fibres generated in the organ of Corti of the cochlea. The perikarya (cell bodies) of these fibres are located in the cochlear (spiral) ganglion within the modiolus (bipolar neurons) and the central axons form the cochlear nerve. The vestibular organ also possesses bipolar neurons. Like the cochlear neurons, they receive sensory input from hair cells. Their perikarya reside in the vestibular ganglion which is located at the floor of the internal acoustic meatus. The central neuronal projections form the vestibular nerve. The nerve merges with the cochlear nerve to form the vestibulocochlear nerve [VIII] (clinically frequently referred to as the statoacoustic nerve) at the internal acoustic meatus and enters the brainstem at the cerebellopontine angle. Also demonstrated is the course of the facial nerve [VII] in the internal acoustic meatus and the facial canal.

Source: *Paulsen, F. Brain and spinal cord. Sobotta atlas of human anatomy, vol. 3. p. 211–342, Chapter 12.*

- From the **superior vestibular ganglion,** arises the **superior vestibular nerve**; it supplies the **anterior (superior)** and **horizontal (lateral) cristae** and the **utricular macula**.
- From the **inferior vestibular ganglion,** arises the **inferior vestibular nerve**; it supplies the **posterior crista** and the **saccular macula**.
The neurotransmitter of the afferent system is **glutamate**.
- **Vestibular nerves:**
  - The two vestibular nerves (inferior and superior) course through the **postero-superior** and **postero-inferior quadrants of the IAC**. They enter the brainstem at the **ventrolateral pontomedullary junction**.
  - In the brainstem, fibres pass between the inferior cerebellar peduncle and the descending tract of the trigeminal nerve and then diverge into rostral and caudal branches before reaching the **vestibular nuclear complex**.
    - The **rostral branch** supplies the **superior** and **medial vestibular nuclei** and gives off a collateral branch to the cerebellum.
    - The **caudal branch** supplies the **inferior, medial** and **ventrolateral vestibular nuclei**.

CLINICAL INSIGHTS

- **Vestibular neuritis**
  - It is a self-limiting disorder consisting of sudden onset of **rotatory vertigo** associated with **vegetative symptoms (diaphoresis, nausea, vomiting)** that are exacerbated by movement. The patient typically denies any auditory or neurological symptoms. The pathogenesis is not well defined, but it is thought to be related to a **viral origin** (reactivation of **herpes simplex virus type 1**). Episodes vary in their severity and usually last for a few days. Treatment is mainly **symptomatic**.
- **Vestibular schwannoma (VS)**
  - VS is a **benign nerve sheath tumour** of the superior and inferior **vestibular nerves**.
  - It arises from the **transitional zone** (Obersteiner–Redlich zone) between the **peripheral** Schwann myelin and the **central** myelin at the medial IAC or the lateral cerebellopontine angle (CPA).
  - There is equal prevalence regarding the origin from the superior and inferior vestibular nerves.
  - Eighty per cent of CPA tumours and 8% of all intracranial tumours are VS.
  - Ninety-five per cent are sporadic and 5% are familial or occur in the setting of **neurofibromatosis type 2 (bilateral VS).**
  - **Hearing loss** is the most common symptom (95% of cases), followed by **tinnitus** (65%) and **disequilibrium** (60%); disequilibrium is usually well-tolerated as the brain compensates for the slowly progressing vestibular injury.
  - With large tumours, involvement of the sensory branches of the trigeminal nerve (midface numbness) and the facial nerve (numbness of the posterior external auditory canal, i.e., Hitselberger sign) are noted. Motor fibres of the facial nerve are fairly resistant to external compression; haemifacial paralysis or spasm is seen in only 10%–20% of patients and occurs late in the course of the disease.
  - With very large tumours, visual changes, signs of increased intracranial pressure, hydrocephalus, and involvement of lower cranial nerves (IX, X, XI and XII) may be seen.
  - **MRI** is the **gold standard for diagnosis** (Fig. 14.14). Thus, the role of auditory brainstem responses (ABRs) in diagnosing VS (fully or partially absent waves, delayed absolute latency of wave V or increased interaural wave V latency more than 0.2 ms) has significantly diminished.
  - Management of patients with VS includes observation, surgical excision and stereotactic radiation. Observation is reserved for small, nongrowing or slowly growing tumours, especially in older patients.
- **Vestibulocochlear nerve compression syndromes**
  - Compression syndromes can be secondary to different disease processes depending on the site of nerve compression:
    - At the level of the CPA: The three most common lesions are VS, meningiomas and epidermoid cysts.
    - At the level of the IAC: VS are the most common, followed by facial nerve schwannomas, meningiomas, intracanalicular vascular lesions (haemangiomas, arteriovenous fistulas, arterial loops) and intracanalicular metastasis (melanoma, lymphoma, breast cancer, etc.).
  - Symptoms are variable and include **vertigo**, **disequilibrium**, **hearing loss** and **pulsatile tinnitus**.

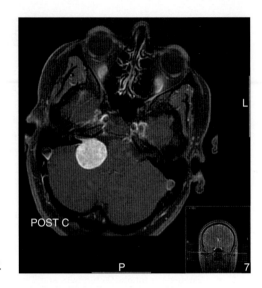

FIGURE 14.14   Benign vestibular schwannoma.
Source: *Marsh, Henry. Brain tumours. Surgery 27(3): 135–138.*

CENTRAL AUDITORY AND VESTIBULAR PATHWAYS

Central Auditory Pathways (Fig. 14.15)

Several nuclei and fibre bundles are involved in the auditory pathway.

- **Cochlear nucleus:**
  - Is located within the **floor of the lateral recess of the 4th ventricle**.
  - Is composed of two parts – ventral and dorsal:
    - **Ventral cochlear nucleus (large):** Is also divided into anterior, posterior and ventral nuclei.
      - The **anterior nucleus** plays a role in **sound localization**.
      - The **posterior** and **ventral nuclei** function in **encoding sound frequency**, **intensity** and **spectral shape**.
    - **Dorsal cochlear nucleus (small):** **Laminar** and **tonotopically organized**, it does not function in sound localization; it appears to have a role in **orientation towards a sound source** and can be a potential site for generation of tinnitus.
- **Superior olivary complex (SOC):**
  - Is located in the **caudal pons**, lateral to the medial lemniscus and dorsal to the spinothalamic tract.
  - Is composed of three subdivisions:
    - Medial superior olive (MSO)
    - Lateral superior olive (LSO)
    - Medial nucleus of the trapezoid body (vestigial in humans)
  - Is the first site of **binaural innervation**. As a result, its main function is **sound localization** and **recreation of the auditory space**.
- **Lateral lemniscus (LL):**
  - Is located in the **rostral pons** and **midbrain**.
  - Receives input from **ipsilateral** and **contralateral cochlear nuclei** and **SOC**.

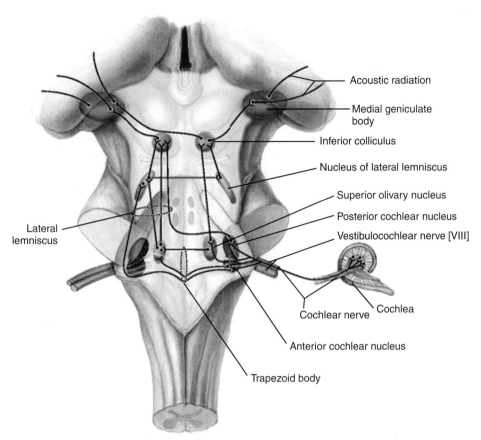

FIGURE 14.15   Auditory pathway; overview. The function of the ascending auditory pathway is to transmit acoustic signals to the brain, to process this information centrally and to create an acoustic awareness. First neuron: bipolar cells in the spiral ganglion of the cochlea; after exiting the small apertures of the tractus spiralis foraminosus deep within the internal acoustic meatus, the fibres from the cochlear nerve unite with the vestibular nerve at the floor of the internal acoustic meatus to form the vestibulocochlear nerve [VIII]; fibres from the basal cochlear part traverse to the posterior cochlear nucleus and those from the apical parts terminate in the anterior cochlear nucleus. Second neuron: multipolar cells of the cochlear nuclei; fibres from the anterior cochlear nerve pass mainly to the olivary complex on the same or opposite side; a part of the fibres crosses to the opposite side and, without synapsing, runs in the lateral lemniscus to the inferior colliculus; fibres that reach the olivary complex on the same side, either ascend to the nucleus of the lateral lemniscus, synapse, cross to the opposite side, synapse again and then reach the inferior colliculus or they ascend directly in the lateral lemniscus to reach the inferior colliculus. Third or fourth neuron: from the inferior colliculus, connections are made to the medial geniculate body. Fourth or fifth neuron: the acoustic radiation connects the medial geniculate body with the transverse temporal Heschl's gyri or convolutions and Wernicke's centre in the temporal lobe.
Source: *Paulsen, F. Ear. Sobotta atlas of human anatomy. vol. 3. p. 133–160, Chapter 10.*

- Projects onto the **central nucleus of the inferior colliculus**.
- Has a role in **sound localization** and **processing**.
- **Inferior colliculus:**
  - Is located in the **midbrain**.
  - Plays a role in **head** and **body orientation** in response to auditory stimuli and processes the **physical characteristics** and **localization of sounds** for auditory perception.

- Medial geniculate body (MGB):
  - Is located on the **inferior surface of the thalamus.**
  - Is **bilaterally innervated** – each hemisphere receives bilateral auditory input.
- **Acoustic radiation:**
  - A pathway through which fibres project from the MGB to the **auditory cortex.**
  - Its location can be variable from one hemisphere to another and from subject to another.
  - Usually passes through the **sublenticular part of the internal capsule,** and then bends around the inferior sulcus of the insula before reaching **Heschl's gyrus.**
- **Auditory cortex (Heschl's gyrus)** (Fig. 14.16):
  - It is located **deep within the Sylvian fissure on the superior surface of the temporal lobe.**
  - The **tonotopic organization** seen throughout the auditory system is preserved at this level. The **primary (AI)** and **secondary (AII)** auditory cortices (**Brodmann areas 41 and 42,** respectively) are found within the **transverse gyrus of Heschl,** at the posterior part of the superior temporal gyrus.
  - The secondary auditory cortex (AII) is called **planum temporale;** it is **larger in the dominant hemisphere** (usually the **left** one).
  - AII is surrounded by an extensive area of auditory cortex as well as **Wernicke's area (Brodmann area 22),** which functions

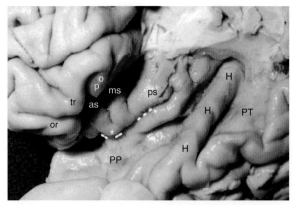

FIGURE 14.16 Superior temporal plane and the primary auditory cortex (H). Resection of the frontal lobe posterior to the inferior frontal gyrus opens a view of the upper surface of the temporal lobe, designated the superior temporal plane, the transverse temporal gyrus of Heschl (H), Heschl's sulcus immediately behind the gyrus and two broad flat planes of tissue anterior and posterior to Heschl's gyrus and sulcus. From the temporal pole anteriorly to the front of Heschl's gyrus, the flat surface is designated the planum polare (PP). From Heschl's sulcus to the posterior end of the temporal surface, the flat surface is designated the planum temporale (PT). The PT is usually triangular, with its point medial and its base directed laterally. It is usually larger in the language-dominant temporal lobe. Note that Heschl's gyrus commonly bifurcates at its lateral end. The partes orbitalis (or), triangularis (tr) and opercularis (op) of the inferior frontal gyrus overhang the anterior lobule of the insula. The anterior lobule displays the anterior short (as), middle short (ms) and posterior short (ps) gyri. These converge to the apex (asterisk) of the insula inferiorly. The central sulcus of the insula (dashed white lines) separates the anterior lobe from the posterior lobe of the insula and then swings medially under the apex towards the suprasellar cistern.
Source: *Naidich, Thomas P. Surface anatomy of the cerebrum. Imaging of the brain. p. 127–153, Chapter 9.*

in **receptive language** and is usually **dominant** in the **left** hemisphere.

- Posterior to Wernicke's area and specifically in the **inferior parietal lobe**, the **angular** and **supramarginal gyri** are found (**Brodmann areas 39 and 40**, respectively). They **integrate auditory**, **visual** and **somatosensory inputs** and play a major role in **reading** and **writing**.

- The primary auditory cortex is connected via transcortical pathways to other cortical areas in the temporal lobe, mediocaudal across the insula to the parietal lobe and to frontal eye fields. The targets in the parietal lobe are thought to play a role in **spatial processing** (information about the **sound source position** and **motion**). This function of **sound localization** appears to be **dominant** in the **right** hemisphere.

- Although activity in the auditory cortices is bilaterally equal, processing of **language** is **dominant** in the **left** hemisphere, whereas processing of **musical stimuli** (perception of pitch intervals and variation of meter and rhythm) is lateralized to the **right** hemisphere.

- Other areas connected to the auditory cortex are: the **prefrontal cortex**, the **limbic system** and the **cerebellum**. These can be implicated in the generation of **tinnitus**. They usually contribute to the processing of complex auditory information such as **music**.

CLINICAL INSIGHTS

- **Auditory brainstem response (ABR)** (Fig. 14.17)
  - An objective test that elicits and registers **brainstem potentials** in response to **click** or **tone burst acoustic stimuli**.
  - A **waveform** is recorded with peaks (**waves I through VII**) representing generator sites: waves **I** and II (**distal** and proximal ends of the **cochlear nerve** (CN VIII), respectively), **III** (**lower brainstem** near the cochlear nucleus and the trapezoid body), IV (SOC), **V (LL)** and VI/VII (inferior colliculus). The **most reliable** are **waves I, III and V**.
  - **Threshold ABR** is used to estimate hearing threshold in the paediatric population (**screening and diagnosis of neonatal hearing loss**). ABR is also used to evaluate the integrity of the auditory neural pathways: detection of CPA tumours (i.e., VS) and brainstem lesions, assessment of patients suspected to have demyelinating diseases such as multiple sclerosis, and for prognostic purposes in comatose patients.
  - ABR can also be used for **intraoperative monitoring** of the VIII nerve and auditory brainstem status during posterior fossa surgery (acoustic neuroma resection, brainstem implants, vascular decompression of CN VIII, etc.)
- **Brainstem lesions affecting the auditory pathways**
  - Hearing disorders secondary to brainstem lesions are rare because of the bilateral projections of the auditory pathways. Nevertheless, an **extensive midline pontine lesion** either from a stroke or from a tumoural process eliminates the crossed input to the SOC on both sides. As a result, the patient exhibits a **deficit in localizing sound waves** and in determining the **direction of moving objects**. Processing auditory temporal information as well as analyzing sound frequency and amplitude remain intact.
- **Central auditory hearing disorders (CAHD)**
  - **Prethalamic lesions** along the auditory pathways (**peripheral to the MGB**) will result in **hearing loss**, whereas **post-thalamic lesions (central to the MGB)** will result in **auditory agnosia**.

- Auditory agnosia refers to the **inability to recognize or understand environmental sounds, words** and **music** that the patient is said to hear. It is the result of **bilateral lesions of the primary auditory cortices (cortical deafness)** or **bilateral lesions of the acoustic radiations (subcortical deafness)**.
- When the deficit is **only linguistic**, it is called **pure word deafness**. Lesions affecting the **left superior temporal lobe** cause this type of deficit.
- When the deficit is **specific to environmental sounds**, it is called **nonverbal auditory agnosia**. **Unilateral** or **bilateral**, **cortical** or **subcortical temporoparietal lesions** cause this type of deficit.
- When the deficit is **specific to music**, it is called **amusia** and is usually caused by **lesions in the right insula**.
- **Central auditory processing disorders (CAPD)**
  - According to the American Speech–Language–Hearing Association, **CAPD** is defined as:
    - A neurobiological disorder affecting the **process of central auditory perception**: localization, lateralization, speech discrimination, music interpretation and identification of auditory patterns, etc.
    - Not attributable to a cognitive or higher-order disorder
  - Can affect **children** and **adults of all ages**: up to half of children with learning disabilities have been diagnosed with some form of CPAD. It can be related to a **neurological insult**, **neurotoxins**, **genetic disorder** or **brain trauma**. In many cases, no specific organic neuropathology can be identified.
  - Diagnosed using **behavioural** and **electrophysiologic central auditory tests.**
  - Management should be individualized according to each case and each deficit and consists of central auditory training activities and environmental modifications.

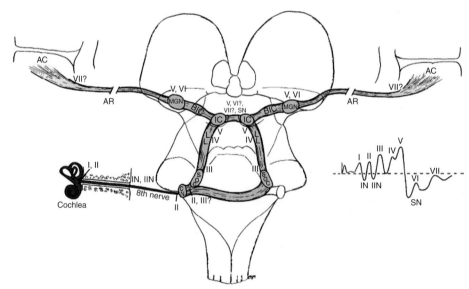

FIGURE 14.17 Diagram showing the probable generators of the human brainstem auditory evoked potentials. SN, slow negativity after wave V; AC, auditory cortex; AR, auditory radiations; BIC, brachium of the inferior colliculus; CN, cochlear nucleus; IC, inferior colliculus; LL, lateral lemniscus; MGN, medial geniculate nucleus; SOC, superior olivary complex.
Source: *From Legatt AD, Arezzo JC, Vaughan HG, Jr. The anatomic and physiologic bases of brainstem auditory evoked potentials. Neurol Clin 1988; 6:681, with permission.*

Central Pathways of the Vestibular System

- **Vestibular nuclear complex** (Fig. 14.18)
  - Is composed of **four main subdivisions**: **superior, lateral, medial** and **inferior**, with minor cell groups (f, l, x, y, z and e) summarized in Table 14.2.
- **Inputs to the vestibular nuclear complex** (Figs. 14.18 and 14.19)
  - **Vestibular nerve**
  - **Visual system**: Optokinetic input via the **nucleus of the optic tract** and the **accessory optic nuclei (midbrain pretectal nuclei)**. The SCCs are not sensitive to low frequency movements of the head (<0.05 Hz) but the visual system is. Such information is supplemented to the vestibular nuclear complex via projections from the visual system.
  - **Oculomotor-related inputs** through:
    - Prepositus nucleus
    - Interstitial nucleus of Cajal
    - Pontine and medullary reticular formation
  - Input related to **central autonomic function, alertness** and **behavioural state**

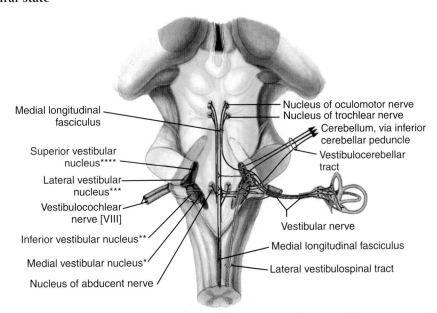

FIGURE 14.18 Equilibrium (balance) pathway; overview. The equilibrium (balance) pathway coordinates eye movements and movements of the torso, neck and extremities. First neuron: the afferent fibres of the vestibular ganglion mainly project into the medial vestibular nucleus (Schwalbe's nucleus), the superior vestibular nucleus (nucleus of Bekhterev) and the inferior vestibular nucleus (Roller's nucleus); afferent fibres of the ampullary crests of the semicircular canals mainly course to the nucleus of Bekhterev and Schwalbe's nucleus as well as into the vestibulocerebellum via the direct sensory cerebellar pathway; afferent fibres of the utricle project into the medial vestibular nucleus, and afferent fibres of the saccule project into the lateral vestibular nucleus; the lateral vestibular nucleus (Deiters' nucleus) also receives collateral fibres from the vestibular pathways and, in particular, connections from the cerebellum. Second neuron: from the vestibular nuclei efferent fibres project to the cerebellum (vestibulocerebellar tract); to the spinal cord (vestibulospinal tract); to the nuclei controlling the extraocular muscles (medial longitudinal fasciculus); to the thalamus (via the vestibulothalamic tract to the inferior posterior ventral nucleus and from there via the thalamic radiation to the postcentral gyrus). *Schwalbe's nucleus, **Roller's nucleus, ***Deiters nucleus, ****nucleus of Bekhterev. Source: *Paulsen, F. Ear. Sobotta atlas of human anatomy. vol. 3. p. 133–160, Chapter 10.*

Table 14.2 Characteristics of the divisions of the vestibular nuclear complex

Vestibular Nucleus	Anatomy	Projections	Function
Superior (Bechterew or Bekhterev)	Dorsal and rostral	To oculomotor nuclei via MLF	VOR pathway
Lateral (Deiters)	Two parts: ■ Dorsolateral: contains the giant cells of Deiters ■ Ventrolateral	■ Dorsolateral: lateral vestibulospinal tract ■ Ventrolateral: vestibulooocular pathways, medial vestibulospinal tract and vestibulothalamic pathways	Principal nucleus for the VSR pathways
Medial (Schwalbe)	Extends rostrocaudally from abducens nucleus to hypoglossal nucleus	■ Rostral part: to oculomotor nuclei ■ Caudal part: to cerebellum ■ Also gives rise to the medial vestibulospinal tract	■ Involved in the VSR pathways ■ Coordinates simultaneous head and eye movements
Inferior (Roller, descending or spinal)	Merges rostrally with the ventral lateral vestibular nucleus	To spinal cord, cerebellum and reticular formation	Role in the vestibulospinal pathways

Notes: *MLF, medial longitudinal fasciculus; VOR, vestibulooocular reflex; VSR, vestibulospinal reflex.*

- ▨ Inhibitory commissural input from the **contralateral vestibular nucleus**
- ▨ Input from the **cervical spinal cord:**
  - To the lateral and medial vestibular nuclei
  - Role in the **cervicoocular reflex (COR).** The COR is mediated through neck proprioceptors; it helps the **vestibulooocular reflex (VOR)** in stabilizing gaze during head movements, and its role becomes apparent when the vestibule is damaged.
  - Role in the **development of vertigo** and **nystagmus** after neck injury in some patients
- ▨ Input from the **cerebellum:**
  - The cerebellum monitors and adjusts the performance of the vestibular system.
- ■ **Output of the vestibular nuclear complex** (Figs. 14.18 and 14.19)
  Two major outputs from the vestibular nuclear complex exist: one for the VOR and another for the vestibulospinal reflex (VSR).
  - ▨ **Output for the VOR pathway** (Fig. 14.20):
    - **Bilateral** projections from the **medial, superior** and **ventrolateral vestibular nuclei** to the **ocular motor nuclei, interstitial nucleus of Cajal** and **prepositus nucleus** through two white matter tracts:
      - **Ascending tract of Deiters:** Projects to the ipsilateral abducens nucleus during horizontal head movements.
      - **Medial longitudinal fasciculus (MLF):** MLF involvement can be seen in patients with multiple sclerosis resulting in central vestibular symptoms.
    - **Two types** of VOR are described:
      - **Compensatory:** Stabilizes gaze during **angular head motion,** mediated by the **SCCs.**

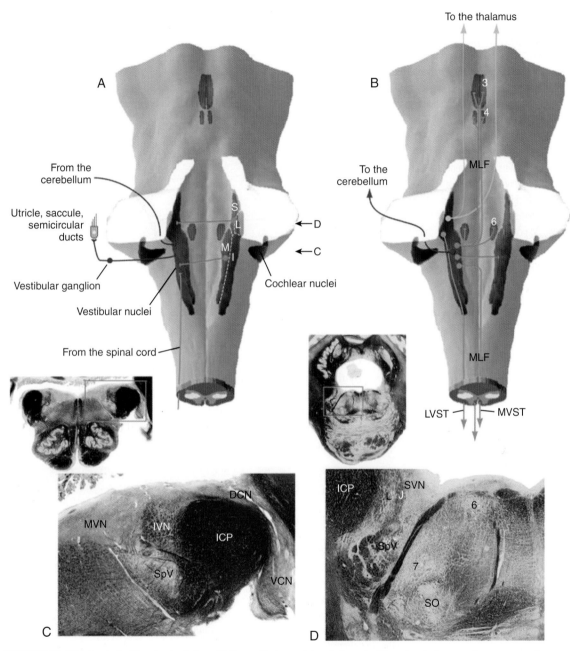

FIGURE 14.19 Inputs to (A) and outputs from (B) the vestibular nuclei; not shown in (A) are inputs from small accessory optic nuclei in the midbrain. C and D in (A) refer to the planes of the brainstem cross-sections in (C) and (D), showing the vestibular nuclei. 3, oculomotor nucleus; 4, trochlear nucleus; 6, abducens nucleus; 7, facial motor nucleus; DCN, dorsal cochlear nucleus; I and IVN, inferior vestibular nucleus; ICP, inferior cerebellar peduncle; J, juxtarestiform body; L, lateral vestibular nucleus; LVST, lateral vestibulo-spinal tract; M and MVN, medial vestibular nucleus; MLF, medial longitudinal fasciculus; MVST, medial vestibulospinal tract; S and SVN, superior vestibular nucleus; SO, superior olivary nucleus; SpV, spinal trigeminal nucleus; VCN, ventral cochlear nucleus.
Source: *Vanderah, Todd W., PhD. Hearing and balance: the eighth cranial nerve. Nolte's the human brain. p. 348–382, Chapter 14.*

FIGURE 14.20 Vestibuloocular reflex. When the head is turned to the right, inertia causes the fluid in the horizontal semicircular canals to lag behind the head movement. This bends the cupula in the right semicircular canal in a direction that increases firing in the right vestibular nerve. The cupula in the left semicircular canal bends in a direction that decreases the tonic activity in the left vestibular nerve. Neurons whose activity level increases with this movement are indicated in solid lines. Neurons whose activity level decreases are indicated in dotted lines. For simplicity, the connections of the left vestibular nuclei are not shown. Via connections between the vestibular nuclei and the nuclei of cranial nerves III and VI, both eyes move in the direction opposite to the head turn.

Source: *From Lundy-Ekman L; Neuroscience: fundamentals for rehabilitation, ed 3. Philadelphia: Saunders; 2007.*

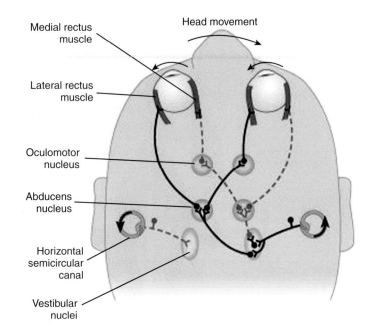

- Orienting: Aligns the eye with the **gravitational axis**, mediated by the **otolith organs**.
- The neural integrator of the VOR system is the **nucleus prepositus**, located just below the **medial vestibular nucleus**. It transforms and integrates velocity information into positional data. Injury to the vestibuloocular neural integrator results in **gaze-evoked nystagmus**.

CLINICAL INSIGHT

- **Nystagmus** (Fig. 14.21)
  - Head rotations that exceed 30° in their amplitude are too large be compensated by the VOR. As a result, **back and forth eye movements** take place with a **slow** component in one direction and a **fast** component in the opposite direction. This movement is called **nystagmus** and can be **vertical**, **horizontal** or **torsional**. Stimulation of the vestibular and visual systems can lead to a normal **physiological nystagmus**, but spontaneous or excessive nystagmus is a sign of a central or peripheral vestibular disorder.
  - **Output for the VSR pathway:**
    Three major pathways connect the **vestibular nuclei** to the **anterior horn cells** of the spinal cord:
    - **Medial vestibulospinal tract:** Have a role in stabilization of **head position** by generating neck muscle contractions in response to inputs from the SCCs.
    - **Lateral vestibulospinal tract:** Responsible for protective, antigravity **activation of ipsilateral extensor muscles** in the trunk and lower extremities. With unilateral peripheral vestibular injury, patients tend to fall towards the side of the lesion.
    - **Reticulospinal tract:** Have a role in **postural changes** in response to **nonvestibular sensory stimuli** (auditory, visual, tactile, etc.).

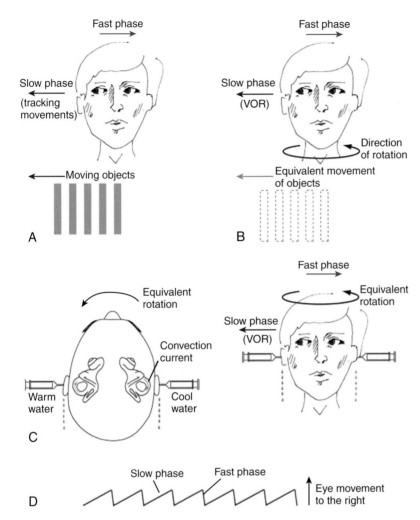

FIGURE 14.21 Three different ways to cause nystagmus with its fast phase to the left. (A) Movement of a series of objects to an individual's right causes slow tracking eye movements to the right, followed by rapid 'reset' movements to the left. (B) Rotation to the left is equivalent, as far as retinal image movement is concerned, to movement of objects to the right. The result is nystagmus to the left, as in (A). If the individual's eyes are open, visual movement continues throughout the rotation, and the nystagmus may persist. If the eyes are closed, the nystagmus is mediated only by the vestibular system and is transient. The direction of nystagmus reverses at the end of rotation in either condition. (C) Warm water instilled into the left ear (or cool water in the right) causes the same movement of endolymph in the left (or right) horizontal semicircular duct as does the rotation in (B). Again, the result is nystagmus to the left. (D) Idealized electrical recording of horizontal nystagmus with its fast phase to the left. VOR, vestibulo-ocular reflex.
Source: *Vanderah, Todd W., PhD. Hearing and balance: the eighth cranial nerve. Nolte's the human brain. p. 348–382, Chapter 14.*

BLOOD SUPPLY TO THE AUDITORY AND VESTIBULAR SYSTEMS

The **vertebrobasilar vascular system** supplies the posterior region of the brain, which includes the **brainstem**, **cerebellum** and **inner ear**. The vascularization of the inner ear is summarized in Fig. 14.22.

- The cochlear nucleus receives rich vascular supply from both the **anterior–inferior cerebellar artery (AICA)** and the **posterior–inferior cerebellar artery (PICA)**.
- The **vestibular nuclear complex** receives its blood supply mainly from:
  - **PICA**: supplies the inferior surfaces of the cerebellar hemispheres and the dorsolateral medulla.
  - **Basilar artery**: main artery of the pons; supplies central vestibular structures via perforator, short and long circumferential branches.

Blood supply to the inner ear

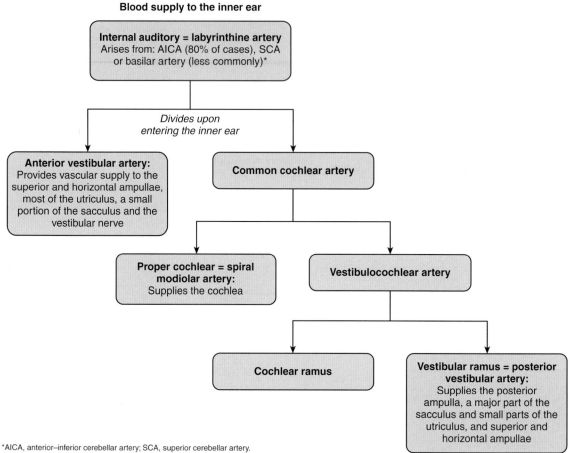

*AICA, anterior–inferior cerebellar artery; SCA, superior cerebellar artery.

FIGURE 14.22   Vascularization of the inner ear.
Source: *Courtesy of Jade Nehmé, MD. Bellevue Medical Center.*

CLINICAL INSIGHT

- **Labyrinthine infarction**
  - Manifests with acute onset of **unilateral loss of auditory** and **vestibular functions**: deafness, acute vertigo, nausea, vomiting and tinnitus.
  - Most commonly related to thromboembolic disease of the **AICA** or **basilar artery**. However, it may also occur with migraine, fat embolism, thromboangiitis obliterans and other causes of a hypercoagulable state such as polycythaemia vera, macroglobulinaemia, leukaemia and sickle cell disease.
  - The **cochlea** is much more susceptible to **anoxic injury** than vestibular end organs. OHCs and spiral ganglion neurons exhibit an alteration in their electrical activities after only 60 s of vascular occlusion with irreversible loss of function within 30 min.
  - **Rotatory vertigo** can be the presenting manifestation of a stroke or transient ischaemic attack involving the territory of the **vertebrobasilar vascular system**. However, **anterior circulation (internal carotid) infarcts** can be associated with **lightheadedness** but do not present with true rotational vertigo.

CASE STUDY DISCUSSION

Superior canal dehiscence syndrome is a rare **vestibular disorder** that was first described by Minor and colleagues in 1998. It is caused by a defect in the temporal bone that overlies the superior SCC, creating a **communication between the membranous labyrinth and the temporal lobe**.

Clinical Features

Clinical features can be either vestibular, auditory or a mixture of both.

- **Vestibular symptoms:** Vertigo, chronic disequilibrium, oscillopsia. Vertigo and characteristic nystagmus (vertical and torsional in the plane of the superior SCC) are induced by sound (Tullio phenomenon), pressure changes in the external auditory canal (Hennebert sign) and Valsalva manoeuvres.
- **Auditory symptoms:** Hearing loss (conductive, affecting the mid and low frequencies), autophony and tinnitus. Patients may experience hyperacusis.

Pathophysiology

The defect in the **roof of the SCC** creates a **third mobile window** (normally the inner ear has two windows: oval and round). It can be congenital, acquired (intracranial hypertension) or a combination of both.

The third mobile window leads to:

- Increased sensitivity to acoustic and mechanical stimulation resulting in **sound-** and **pressure-induced vestibular symptoms**.
- Increased sensitivity to bone-conducted sounds (**pulse sounds, neck and eye movements' sounds**, and **breathing sounds are abnormally heard by the patient**).
- Decreased sensitivity to air-conducted sounds – as part of the acoustic energy – which will be dissipated through the abnormal window; this results in **conductive hearing loss**.

Investigations

- Tympanometry and acoustic reflexes are normal.
- **Audiogram**: **conductive hearing loss** in the mid and low frequencies.
- Vestibular-evoked myogenic potentials (VEMPs):
  - Consists of recording changes in myogenic activities in response to an acoustic stimulus (loud sound):
    - **Cervical VEMPs: relaxation potentials in ipsilateral sternocleidomastoid muscle**.
    - **Ocular VEMPs: excitatory activity in contralateral inferior rectus and inferior oblique muscles.**
  - Thresholds for eliciting a response are reduced, whereas the amplitude of the response is increased.

Management

Plugging or **resurfacing of the superior canal** via the middle cranial fossa surgical approach is the standard treatment for Minor syndrome. It is indicated in patients with disabling auditory or vestibular symptoms.

CHAPTER 15

Limbic and Olfactory Systems

Ahmad Sweid

CASE STUDY

Presentation and Physical Examination: A 54-year-old heavy smoker (60 pack-years), hypertensive and diabetic man presented to the emergency department (ED) with acute confusion, complex partial seizures and change in personality over 2 weeks prior to the presentation. The family reported that he had frequent falls, unsteady gait, slurred speech and difficulty finding words. They also described a number of episodes of staring blankly for >20 s without response, after which he returns to his normal state. The patient complained of tremors and difficulty performing learned tasks. Upon examination, there was an upper limb intention tremor, horizontal gaze nystagmus and ataxia; the remainder of the neurological examination was normal.

Diagnosis, Management and Follow-Up: Brain computed tomography (CT) scan was normal. The patient was admitted to the intensive care unit (ICU) for monitoring and was planned for a lumbar puncture to test the cerebrospinal fluid (CSF), as well as brain magnetic resonance imaging (MRI) to rule out abnormalities that could not be detected on the CT scan.

Axial cuts of the fluid attenuation inversion recovery (FLAIR) sequence on MRI showed hyperintense signals from the medial temporal lobe on the left and right sides (Fig. 15.1), consistent with the radiological diagnosis of **limbic encephalitis**. CSF testing revealed elevated protein level.

After ruling out viral and bacterial infections on CSF tests, the patient was started on empirical steroids and intravenous immunoglobulins (IVIG) for paraneoplastic limbic encephalitis as a working diagnosis. A full body CT scan with contrast was performed and confirmed the presence of lung malignancy that was not appreciated on initial chest radiographs. The lung tumour was biopsied and revealed squamous cell carcinoma.

While studying this chapter, try to understand the anatomy and function of the limbic system in order to correlate it to the clinical presentation of limbic encephalitis, the pathophysiology of which will be discussed at the end of this chapter.

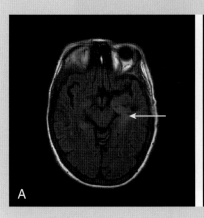
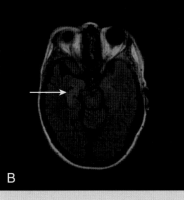

FIGURE 15.1 Axial fluid attenuation inversion recovery (FLAIR) MRI of the brain showing a bright signal from the medial temporal lobe on the left (A) and right (B) sides (arrows) consistent with limbic encephalitis.
Source: *Fahim et al. A case of limbic encephalitis presenting as a paraneoplastic manifestation of limited stage small cell lung cancer: a case report. J Med Case Rep 2010; 4:408.*

BRIEF INTRODUCTION

The **limbic system**, also known as the **'emotional or visceral brain'**, governs **memory**, **emotions**, **learning** and **social interactions**, all of which contribute to the generation of the distinctive **human behaviour**. The limbic system is one of the most complex and least understood parts of the nervous system (Figs. 15.2 and 15.3).

The basic concept of the limbic system is based on its functional connections; its anatomical structures are vaguely defined.

- Thomas Willis first introduced the limbic system in 1664.
- In the 1930s, Jamez Papez described the Papez circuit of emotions, which is essentially mediated by the limbic system.
- Additional significant observations were reported when bilateral removal of large parts of the temporal lobe resulted in a constellation of symptoms collectively known as **Klüver–Bucy syndrome** *(see Clinical Insight later in this chapter, p. 384)*.

A phylogenetically old part of the telencephalon, the limbic system is widely connected to subcortical centres, and its structures are composed of a combination of grey and white matter. A brief introduction about the phylogenetic classification of the cerebral cortex will help elucidate the origin of limbic system structures. In general, cortical structures fall into one of the following classifications:

- **Neocortex (neopallium, isocortex)** is composed of **six cell layers**. Examples include primary sensory area, primary motor area and association cortices.

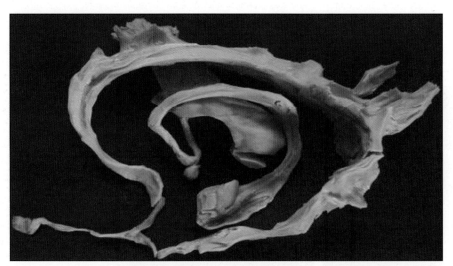

FIGURE 15.2 Photograph of a reconstructed model showing the various connections of the limbic system.
Source: *Shah, Abhidha. Analysis of the anatomy of the Papez circuit and adjoining limbic system by fiber dissection techniques. J Clin Neurosci 19(2): 289–298.*

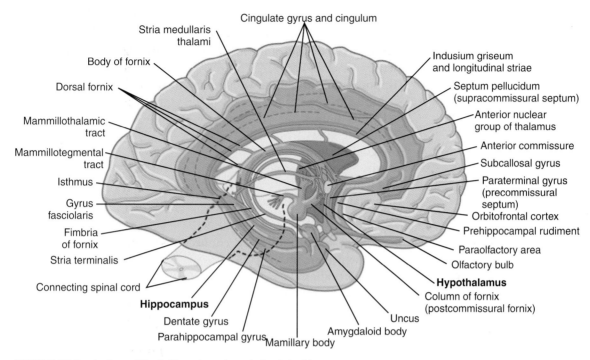

FIGURE 15.3 Anatomy of the limbic system, shown in the dark pink area.
Source: *Modified from Warwick R, Williams PL. Gray's anatomy, 35th ed. London: Longman Group Ltd; 1973.*

- **Allocortex** is composed of **less than six cell layers**. The allocortex is structurally and functionally associated with the limbic and olfactory systems and is further subclassified into:
  - **Paleocortex**, which includes areas composed of **3–5 cellular layers**, is represented by:
    - Entorhinal cortex comprising the **parahippocampal gyrus**.
    - Piriform cortex comprising the **uncus**.
    - **Lateral orbitofrontal gyrus (lateral olfactory gyrus)**, which overlies the lateral olfactory stria, a division of the olfactory tract.
  - **Archicortex**, which contains areas composed of **three cell layers**, is represented by:
    - **Dentate gyrus**.
    - **Hippocampus**.

LIMBIC SYSTEM COMPONENTS

The limbic system can be visualized as a group of cortical and subcortical structures forming an **inner** and an **outer arch**, with the hypothalamus located at the centre (Figs. 15.2 and 15.3):

- The **outer arch**, a C-shaped structure, is composed of:
  - **Orbitofrontal cortex**.
  - **Parahippocampal gyrus**.

- Cingulate (limbic) gyrus.
- Uncus (housing the primary olfactory cortex).
- The **inner arch** consists of the archicortical and paleocortical regions, namely:
  - **Hippocampal formation**, which is composed of:
    - Subiculum.
    - Hippocampus.
    - Dentate gyrus.
  - **Amygdaloid body.**
  - **Fornix.**
  - **Septal area.**
  - **Diagonal band of Broca.**
  - **Paraterminal gyrus.**

The limbic system establishes close connections with several subcortical nuclei, some of which are the (Fig. 15.4):

- **Mammillary bodies.**
- **Anterior nuclei of the thalamus.**

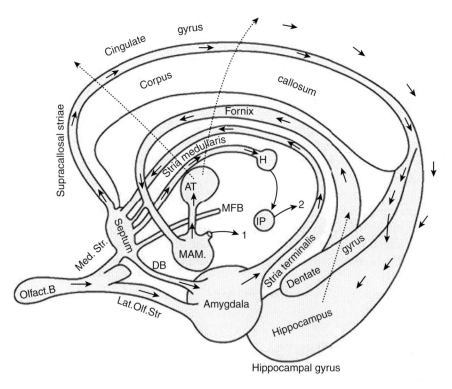

FIGURE 15.4 Internal connections within the limbic system: Olfact. B, olfactory bulb; Lat. Olf. Str, lateral olfactory stria; Med. Str, medial olfactory stria; AT, anterior nucleus of the thalamus; MFB, medial forebrain bundle; MAM, nucleus of the mammillary body; (1, connection to the midbrain reticular formation); DB, diagonal band of Broca; H, habenular nucleus; IP, interpeduncular nucleus; (2, connection to midbrain reticular formation).

Source: *(After McLean 1949.). Steele, J Douglas. Functional neuroanatomy. Companion to psychiatric studies. p. 17–43, Chapter 2.*

- **Habenular nuclei**, which lie medial to the thalamus and lateral to the ventricular wall and are connected to the pineal gland *(see chapter 10)*.
- **Midbrain nuclei**, including the:
  - **Interpeduncular nucleus.**
  - **Anterior tegmental nucleus.**
  - **Posterior tegmental nucleus.**

Hippocampal Formation [Figs. 15.5 and 15.6]

As mentioned earlier, the **hippocampal formation** is composed of the **subiculum**, **hippocampus** and **dentate gyrus**.

- Embryologically, the hippocampal formation originates dorsally and migrates ventrally and medially in the temporal lobe leaving remnant tissues behind (Fig. 15.7).
- The **subiculum** is a **transitional area** between the **hippocampus** and the **entorhinal cortex**; it plays an important role in the flow of information into the hippocampal formation.
- The **dentate gyrus** is a **continuation of the hippocampal pyramidal cells** and is made up of **dense granule cells.**
  - Medial to it lies the fimbria of the hippocampus and the sulcus that separates them, i.e., the fimbriodentate sulcus.
  - Lateral to it lies the subiculum and the sulcus that separates them, i.e., the hippocampal sulcus.

Hippocampus [Figs. 15.5 and 15.6]

The **hippocampus**, a term originating from the Greek word 'seahorse', is the main component of the archicortex.

- It lies on the **medial aspect** of the temporal lobe.
- Lateral to it, is the inferior (temporal) horn of the lateral ventricle.

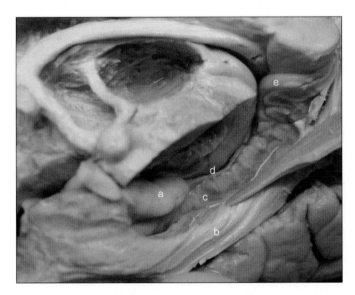

FIGURE 15.5 Photograph of the dissection of the mesial temporal structures: a, hippocampus; b, radiation of the cingulum; c, dentate gyrus; d, fimbria; e, fasciolar/subsplenial gyrus.
Source: *Shah, Abhidha. Analysis of the anatomy of the Papez circuit and adjoining limbic system by fiber dissection techniques. J Clin Neurosci 19(2): 289–298.*

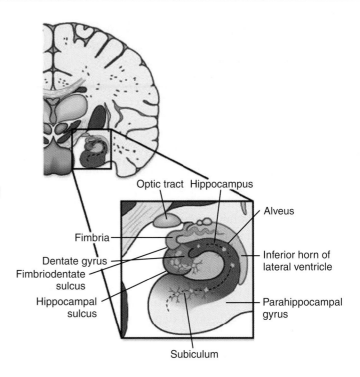

FIGURE 15.6 The hippocampal formation is found on the medial aspect of the temporal lobe, and it protrudes into the inferior horn of the lateral ventricle. Its major components are the hippocampus, the dentate gyrus and the subiculum, all of which are three-layered archicortex. The fimbria is the major output pathway from the hippocampal region to the mammillary body and the septal nuclei.
Source: *Koeppen, Bruce M., MD, PhD. Higher functions of the nervous system. Berne & Levy physiology. p. 201–217, Chapter 10.*

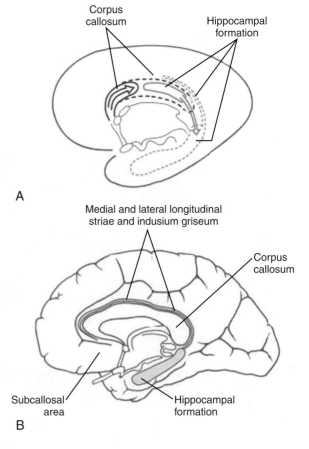

FIGURE 15.7 Developmental relationships between the corpus callosum (in red) and the hippocampal formation (in green). As the corpus callosum expands caudally from the general area of the anterior commissure (A), the hippocampal primordium migrates into the temporal lobe. In the adult brain, remnants of the hippocampal formation left behind during development are located dorsal to the corpus callosum (B).
Source: *Willis, M.A. The limbic system. Fundamental neuroscience for basic and clinical applications. p. 431–441.e1, Chapter 31.*

- From medial to lateral, the following structures are closely related to the hippocampus:
  - Fimbria of the hippocampus
  - Fimbriodentate sulcus
  - Dentate gyrus
  - Hippocampal sulcus
  - Subiculum and parahippocampal gyrus
- The hippocampal cortex forms a curled band, **Ammon's horn (hippocampus proper, cornu ammonis)**, which protrudes against the ventricle and is covered by a layer of fibres known as the **alveus** (Figs. 15.6 and 15.8).
- The **fimbria** lies on top of the hippocampus and continues as the **fornix** and **mammillary body** anteriorly (Fig. 15.9).
- The fimbria and the dentate gyrus run together posteriorly till the splenium of the corpus callosum, where the **dentate gyrus** becomes the **fasciolar gyrus** and continues as a band of grey matter along the superior aspect of the corpus callosum, in the anterior commissure region; this band is known as the **indusium griseum (supracallosal gyrus, gyrus epicallosus)** (Fig. 15.10).
  - In addition to the indusium griseum, there are two narrow fibre bundles that run lateral to the indusium griseum along the superior aspect of the corpus callosum, which are
    - Medial longitudinal stria of Lancini.
    - Lateral longitudinal stria of Lancini.

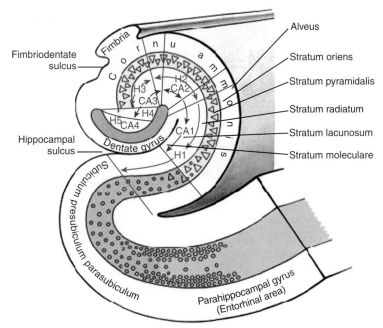

FIGURE 15.8 Hippocampal formation, showing the disposition of the various cell fields. Dentate gyrus, pink; hippocampus proper (cornu ammonis), yellow; areas of the subicular complex (subiculum), green; entorhinal cortex, blue. CA1–CA3, hippocampal cell fields. H1-H5, hippocampal sectors; H1 corresponds to CA1, H2 to CA2, H3 to CA3, and H4 and H5 to CA4.

Source: *Mancall, Elliott L., MD. Cerebral hemispheres. Gray's cinical neuroanatomy: the anatomic basis for clinical neuroscience. p. 279–312, Chapter 16.*

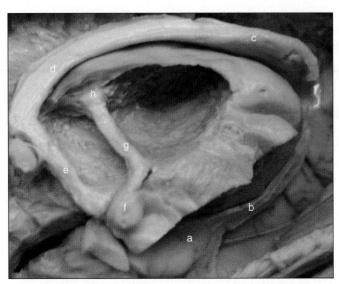

FIGURE 15.9 Photograph showing the mammillary body and surrounding structures after the removal of the dentate gyrus: a, hippocampus; b, fimbria; c, crus of the fornix; d, body of the fornix; e, column of the fornix; f, mammillary body; g, mammillothalamic tract; h, anterior nucleus of the thalamus.
Source: *Shah, Abhidha. Analysis of the anatomy of the Papez circuit and adjoining limbic system by fiber dissection techniques. J Clin Neurosci 19(2): 289–298.*

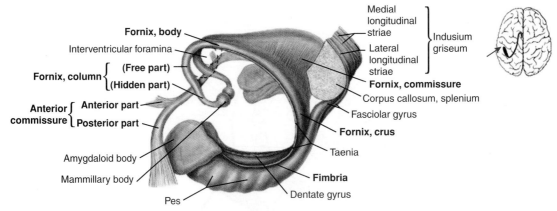

FIGURE 15.10 Anterior commissure, fornix and hippocampus formation, indusium griseum; view from the left side. All structures shown here are part of the limbic system, a functional concept with input from the telencephalon, diencephalon and mesencephalon. Relevant structures are the hippocampi, the amygdaloid bodies, the cingulate gyri and the septal nuclei. The limbic system regulates numerous functions, such as impulse, learning, memory, emotions, but also the regulation of food intake, digestion and reproduction by the autonomic nervous system. The anterior commissure is a fibre system (commissural fibres) composed of an anterior and posterior part. The anterior part connects the olfactory tracts and the olfactory cortices of both sides. The posterior part connects the rostral parts of the temporal lobes (particularly cortex and amygdaloid bodies). The amygdaloid body connects with the hippocampus. The hippocampus displays the hippocampal digitations of the pes and the fimbria which transition into the crus of fornix. An exchange of fibres occurs in the region of the column. In its rostral part, the columns of the fornix continue as free and hidden parts and the hidden part connects to the mammillary bodies.
Source: *Paulsen, F. Brain and spinal cord. Sobotta atlas of human anatomy, vol. 3. p. 211–342, Chapter 12.*

■ Both the **indusium griseum** and the **longitudinal striae**, which are **remnants of the hippocampal formation** during embryological migration, terminate in the **paraterminal gyrus**, forming the anterior end of the inner arch.

CLINICAL INSIGHT

■ **Rabies**
  ■ Patients who have **rabies disease**, the virus of which has a predilection for the **hippocampus** and **cerebellum**, are subject to anxiety, apprehensiveness and paroxysms of rage or terror.

Ammon's Horn (Fig. 15.8)

Ammon's horn is described either according to its four distinct regions or according to its six different layers. The four regions are classified based on size, cell count and width:

■ **CA1**, which contains **small pyramidal** cells.
■ **CA2**, which is a **narrow, dense band** of **large pyramidal** cells.
■ **CA3**, which is a **wide, loose band** of **large pyramidal** cells.
  ■ Dentate gyrus contains granule cells; these cells send mossy fibres that synapse on the large pyramidal cells of CA3.
■ **CA4**, which is a **loosely structured inner zone**.

CLINICAL INSIGHT

■ **Ammon's horn and hypoxia**
  ■ In ischaemic stroke, regions **CA1** and **CA4** are particularly **sensitive to hypoxia**, whereas **CA2** is **resistant to hypoxia**.

As mentioned earlier, Ammon's horn is composed of **six** different layers.

■ Alveus, which contains the efferent fibres.
■ Stratum oriens, which contains interneurons known as basket cells. Basket cells form a dense fibre network around pyramidal cells and are stimulated through collaterals of pyramidal cells
■ Stratum pyramidale.
■ Stratum radiatum.
■ Stratum lacunosum.
■ Stratum moleculare.

Afferent fibres to the hippocampus not only synapse on principal cells such as pyramidal and granule cells, but also synapse with **inhibitory neurons** such as **basket cells**.

Fibre Connections (Figs. 15.10 and 15.11)

■ **Afferent pathways to the hippocampal formation**
  ■ From the **entorhinal cortex**
    - Fibres from several areas terminate at the entorhinal cortex such

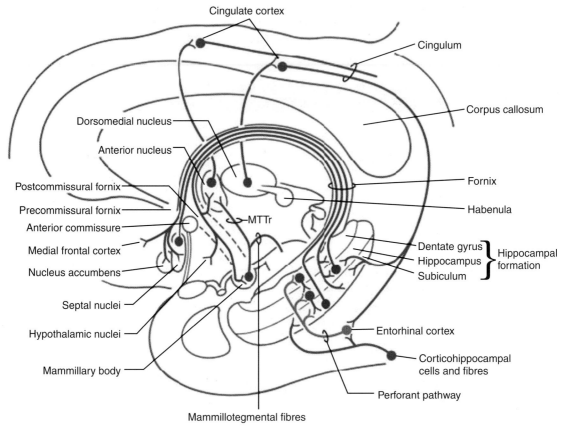

FIGURE 15.11 Diagrammatic representation of afferent and efferent connections of the hippocampal formation. MTTr, mammillo-thalamic tract.

Source: *Willis, M.A. The limbic system. Fundamental neuroscience for basic and clinical applications. p. 431–441.e1, Chapter 31.*

as the olfactory centre, amygdaloid body and various regions of the cerebrum. The entorhinal cortex integrates the information received from all these areas and sends it along afferent fibres to the hippocampal formation.

- These afferent fibres are the major input to the hippocampal formation and project mainly onto Ammon's horn by means of two pathways:
    - **Perforant pathway**, a major pathway that originates from the **lateral** part of the entorhinal cortex.
    - **Alvear pathway**, which originates from the **medial** part of the entorhinal cortex.
- The afferent pathways terminate on the **pyramidal dendrites**, which send fibres to the granule cells of the dentate gyrus. In return, the dentate gyrus sends **mossy fibres** to the pyramidal cells of the **hippocampus**.

- From the **cingulate gyrus**, whose fibres are condensed in the **cingulum** and project onto the subiculum (mainly) and hippocampus.
- The **fornix** contains fibre bundles from the septal nuclei but most importantly from the hippocampus and entorhinal cortex of the contralateral hemisphere. These fibres cross the **commissure of the fornix** to reach their targets in the **ipsilateral hippocampal formation**.
- **Efferent pathways of the hippocampal formation**
  - Originate primarily from cells of the **subiculum** and, to a lesser extent, from **pyramidal cells of the hippocampus.**
  - Axons leaving the subiculum and the hippocampus enter the **alveus** and merge to form the **fimbria** of the hippocampus, which continues as the **fornix**. Only a small number of fibres exit via the **longitudinal striae of Lancini**.
  - Axons of CA3 (large pyramidal cells) send collaterals, known as Schaffer collaterals, to CA1 cells (small pyramidal cells).

CLINICAL INSIGHT

- **Retrieval of information**
  - Stimuli from CA3 to CA1 assist in **retrieval of information** and project it to the neocortex. For example, object information are relayed to the inferior temporal visual cortex, spatial information are relayed to parietal allocentric spatial areas and reward and emotional information are relayed to the hippocampus, orbitofrontal cortex, amygdala and anterior cingulate gyrus.

Functional Correlations

The hippocampus is able to associate **object representations**, obtained from the **visual** and **auditory cortical areas** via the **entorhinal** and **perirhinal cortices**, with **spatial representations**, obtained from the **parietal cortical areas** (including posterior cingulate cortex) via the **parahippocampal area** *(see section on Parahippocampal Gyrus)*. It also helps to **consolidate long-term memories** from immediate and short-term memories.

CLINICAL INSIGHTS

- **Mesial temporal lobe sclerosis** [Fig. 15.12]
  - The most common type of **epilepsy** in adults occurs due to **sclerosis** involving the **hippocampus**, **amygdala** and **parahippocampal gyrus.**
- **Thiamine deficiency**
  - **Vitamin B1 (thiamine) deficiency** is seen in alcoholics, cancer patients and prolonged malnutrition states.
  - Thiamine deficiency can lead to **memory impairment** in addition to other symptoms that are grouped into one of two conditions: **Korsakoff psychosis** or **Wernicke encephalopathy**.
    - Mammillary bodies, dorsomedial nuclei of the thalamus and columns of the fornix are involved in both conditions.

- Wernicke encephalopathy is an **acute, reversible** condition characterized by **ophthalmoplegia**, **ataxia** and **confusion**, whereas Korsakoff psychosis is a **chronic, irreversible** condition characterized by **confabulations** as well as **anterograde** and **retrograde** amnesia.

■ **Hippocampal formation atrophy**

■ **Hippocampal** and **dentate gyrus atrophy** is seen in advanced dementia patients, especially in those with **Alzheimer disease** and **Pick disease**.

Fornix (Figs. 15.3, 15.4 and 15.9–15.11)

The **fornix** is composed of **two limbs** that converge to form the **fornix body** and **commissure**, the latter of which diverges into **two columns** anteriorly. The fornix carries the **major efferent pathways** from the hippocampus as well some afferent fibres.

- ■ The **efferent fibres** originate from the (Fig. 15.11):
  - ■ **Pyramidal cells of the hippocampus.**
  - ■ **Subiculum.**
- ■ The fimbria forms the **crura (s. crus) of fornix**, which curve superolaterally over the **pulvinar (posterior end) of the thalamus.**
- ■ The two crura meet anteriorly to form the body of the fornix; they are connected to each other by an interhemispheric commissure known as the **hippocampal commissure** (Fig. 15.10).
- ■ The body continues towards the anterior end of the thalamus where it arches downwards in front of the **foramina of Monro** as the columns of the fornix (Fig. 15.10).

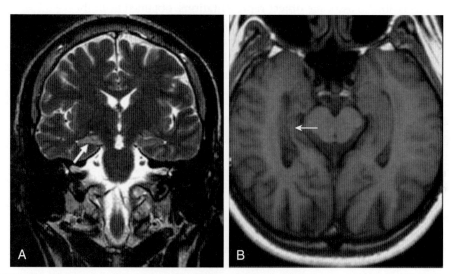

FIGURE 15.12 Right hippocampal sclerosis. Coronal T2-weighted image (A) shows hippocampal high signal intensity and volume loss (arrow). Axial T1-weighted image (B) shows atrophy in the hippocampal head, body and tail (arrow).
Source: *Ochoa-Escudero, Martin, MD. Congenital and acquired conditions of the mesial temporal lobe: a pictorial essay. Can Assoc Radiol J 66(3): 238–251.*

- Fibres of the fornix that approach the anterior commissure (not the same as the hippocampal commissure) are divided into (Fig. 15.11):
  - **Precommissural fibres**
    - Originate from the **pyramidal cells of the hippocampus**.
    - Relay input to:
      - Septal nuclei.
      - Lateral preoptic area.
      - Anterior part of the hypothalamus.
      - Nucleus of the diagonal band of Broca.
  - **Postcommissural fibres**
    - Originate from the **subiculum**.
    - Terminate in the.
      - Medial mammillary nucleus.
      - Anterior thalamic body.
      - Hypothalamus.
    - On their way, some of these fibres project onto the
      - Anterior nucleus of the thalamus, from which fibres radiate upwards and combine with fibres of the internal capsule reaching the cingulum and cingulate gyrus.
      - Lateral nucleus of the thalamus.
      - Lateral septal nuclei.

The efferent pathway may be summarized as follows (Fig. 15.11):
- Alveus and fimbria (hippocampal pyramidal cells) → Body of fornix → Precommissural fibres → Septal nuclei + Lateral preoptic area + Anterior part of the hypothalamus + Nucleus of the diagonal band of Broca
- Subiculum → Body of fornix → Postcommissural fibres
  → Medial mammillary nucleus + Anterior thalamic body + Hypothalamus
  In addition, some postcommissural fibres project onto:
  → Anterior nucleus of the thalamus, then to cingulum and cingulate gyrus + Lateral nucleus of the thalamus + Lateral septal nuclei

Moreover, postcommissural fibres reach the medial mammillary nucleus then ascend to the anterior nucleus of the thalamus forming the **mammillothalamic tract of Vicq d'Azyr**. The medial mammillary nucleus also gives rise to a smaller bundle, known as the **mammillotegmental tract of Gudden**, which terminates in the anterior tegmental nucleus, one of the nuclei of the midbrain reticular formation (Figs. 15.9 and 15.11).

Septal Area (Fig. 15.11)

The **septal area** is strongly connected to the hippocampus.
- Cholinergic and GABAergic neurons of the medial septal nucleus project to the hippocampus and dentate gyrus, which project back to the lateral septal nuclei.
- As with stimulation of the amygdaloid body, stimulation of the septal area triggers **oral**, **excretory** and **sexual reactions**.

Diagonal Band of Broca (Figs. 15.4 and 15.13)

The **diagonal band of Broca** contains **afferent fibres** from the **olfactory bulb** and forms the caudal limit of the olfactory cortex.

Parahippocampal Gyrus (Figs. 15.6 and 15.14)

The **parahippocampal gyrus** lies on the **medial aspect** of the temporal lobe.

- Anteriorly and medially, it extends to form the **uncus.**
- Anteriorly and laterally, it is limited by the rhinal sulcus, which marks the lateral extent of the entorhinal area.
- Posteriorly, it is divided by the **anterior calcarine sulcus** into
  - A **superior portion**, the **isthmus of the cingulate gyrus** that continues as the cingulate gyrus (Fig. 15.14-m).
  - An **inferior portion**, the **lingual gyrus** (Fig. 15.14-n).

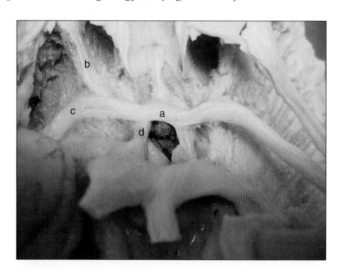

FIGURE 15.13 Photograph showing the inferior surface of the basal forebrain after deeper dissection: a, anterior commissure; b, anterior portion of anterior commissure; c, posterior portion of anterior commissure; d, diagonal band of Broca.
Source: *Shah, Abhidha. Analysis of the anatomy of the Papez circuit and adjoining limbic system by fiber dissection techniques. J Clin Neurosci 19(2): 289–298.*

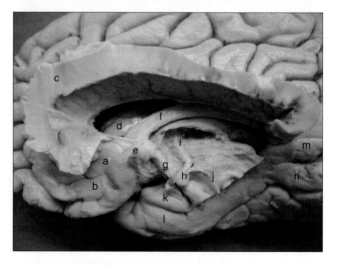

FIGURE 15.14 Photograph of the dissection of the medial aspect of the hemisphere: a, paraterminal gyrus; b, subcallosal gyrus; c, corpus callosum; d, caudate head in frontal horn of lateral ventricle; e, anterior commissure; f, body of fornix; g, columns of fornix; h, mammillary body; i, mammillothalamic tract; j, mammillotegmental tract; k, uncus; l, parahippocampal gyrus; m, parahippocampal gyrus continuing as cingulate gyrus superiorly; and as n, lingual gyrus inferiorly.
Source: *Shah, Abhidha. Analysis of the anatomy of the Papez circuit and adjoining limbic system by fiber dissection techniques. J Clin Neurosci 19(2): 289–298.*

- Medially, it curls inward towards the hippocampal fissure to form the **hippocampus**, which in turn curls inward to form the **dentate gyrus.**

Cingulate Gyrus (Fig. 15.3)

The **cingulate gyrus** extends above and around the corpus callosum.

- The cingulate gyrus is separated from the dentate gyrus by the **hippocampal sulcus.**
- Caudally, the isthmus of the cingulate gyrus is considered as a transition point.
- **Rostrally,** the cingulate gyrus tapers into the **paraterminal gyrus** and the **subcallosal (parolfactory area of Broca) area** (Fig. 15.15).
- The cingulate gyrus establishes connections with the (Fig. 15.16):
  - Olfactory cortex.
  - Hypothalamus.
  - Frontal cortex.
  - Caudal portion of the orbital cortex.
  - Rostral potion of the insular cortex.

The cortex of the cingulate gyrus has a strong influence on the **hypothalamus** and the **autonomic nervous system**; **rostral stimulation** of the cingulate gyrus leads to **changes in blood pressure, respiration** and **pulse rate.**

The **midcingulate gyrus,** as well as the orbitofrontal cortex, contains a representation area for **reward and punishment,** which are essential for learning the association between actions and their outcomes.

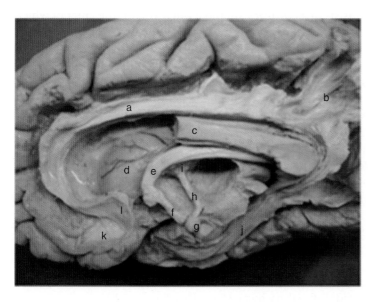

FIGURE 15.15 Photograph of the cingulum and surrounding structures after the anterior half of the corpus callosum had been cut and removed: a, cingulum; b, fibres of the cingulum entering into the parietal cortex; c, corpus callosum; d, head of caudate nucleus; e, body of the fornix; f, columns of the fornix; g, mammillary body; h, mammillothalamic tract; i, anterior nucleus of the thalamus; j, radiation of the cingulum; k, paraolfactory gyrus; l, paraterminal gyrus. Source: *Shah, Abhidha. Analysis of the anatomy of the Papez circuit and adjoining limbic system by fiber dissection techniques. J Clin Neurosci 19(2): 289–298.*

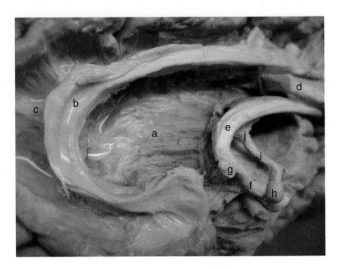

FIGURE 15.16 Photograph of the anterior thalamic radiation projecting to the cingulum after the caudate head had been removed in one piece. Fibres forming the cingulum can also be seen radiating to the frontal cortex: a, anterior thalamic radiation; b, cingulum; c, fibres from the cingulum entering the frontal cortex; d, cut end of the corpus callosum; e, body of fornix; f, column of fornix; g, anterior commissure; h, mammillary body; i, mammillothalamic tract; j, anterior nucleus of thalamus.

Source: *Shah, Abhidha. Analysis of the anatomy of the Papez circuit and adjoining limbic system by fiber dissection techniques. J Clin Neurosci 19(2): 289–298.*

CLINICAL INSIGHT

■ **Anterior cingulate gyrus**
  ▪ The **anterior cingulate gyrus**, **amygdala** and **orbitofrontal cortex** are sensitive to **social feedback**, which is important to change the human behaviour. Damage to the anterior cingulate gyrus leads to **emotional instability** and **apathy**.

Amygdaloid Body (Figs. 15.3 and 15.10)

Part of the **paleocortex**, the **amygdaloid body** or **amygdala**, is an **almond-shaped** group of cells that lie in the **medial part of the temporal lobe**.

The amygdala consists of a **cortical** part and a **nuclear** part, the latter of which is covered by the periamygdalar cortex that lies in the semilunar gyrus.

■ It has peptidergic neurons that secrete enkephalins and corticoliberin.
■ It is made of two different types of nuclear groups (Figs. 15.17 and 15.18):
  ▪ Phylogenetically old **corticomedial** group:
    - Consists of **superficial cortical** and **central nuclei**.
    - Receives afferent neurons from the olfactory bulb, hypothalamus, septal nuclei and brainstem nuclei.
    - Is the origin of **stria terminalis**.
  ▪ Phylogenetically new **basolateral** group:
    - Consists of **basal nuclei**, which has medial parvocellular and lateral magnocellular parts, and **lateral nuclei**, which establish fibre connections with the prepiriform (ambient gyrus) and entorhinal areas.
    - Receives input from the dorsal thalamus, prefrontal cortex, cingulate and parahippocampal gyrus, temporal and insular cortices and subiculum.
■ The **two major efferent** pathways are the **stria terminalis** and the **ventral amygdalofugal pathway** (Figs. 15.17 and 15.18).

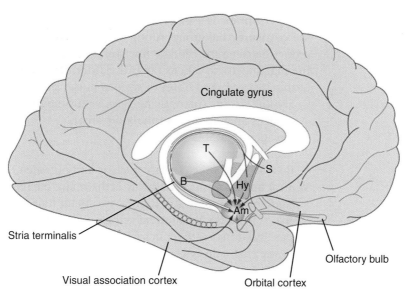

FIGURE 15.17 Major inputs to the basolateral (blue), central (red) and medial (green) nuclei of the amygdala (Am). Only inputs from visual association cortex to the basolateral nuclei are shown, although there are similar projections from most or all unimodal sensory areas. The inputs from the limbic cortex to the basolateral nuclei also include a major projection from the insula, which is not present in this view. B, brainstem (periaqueductal grey, parabrachial nuclei, other nuclei); Hy, hypothalamus; S, septal nuclei; T, thalamus (multiple nuclei). Source: *Modified from Warwick R, Williams PL. Gray's anatomy, Br ed 35. Philadelphia: WB Saunders; 1973.*

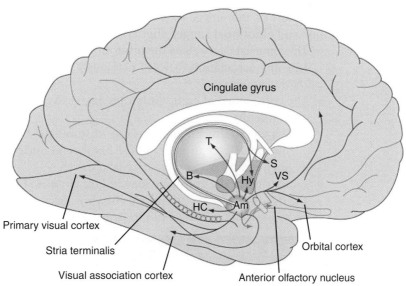

FIGURE 15.18 Major outputs from the basolateral (blue), central (red) and medial (green) nuclei of the amygdala (Am). These take three routes: (1) the stria terminalis, which reaches the septal nuclei (S) and hypothalamus (Hy); (2) the ventral amygdalofugal pathway to the hypothalamus (Hy), thalamus (T; mainly the dorsomedial nucleus), widespread areas of ventromedial prefrontal and insular cortex, ventral striatum (VS), olfactory structures and various brainstem sites (B); and (3) direct projections to the hippocampus (HC) and temporal and other neocortical areas.
Source: *Modified from Warwick R, Williams PL. Gray's anatomy, Br ed 35. Philadelphia: WB Saunders; 1973.*

- **Stria terminalis** is a small fibre bundle that originates from cells of the **corticomedial** group. Along most of its trajectory, it lies in the groove between the caudate nucleus and thalamus and passes below the thalamostriate vein as far as the **anterior commissure**. This tract terminates and send fibres to various nuclei such as:
  - Hypothalamus (preoptic nucleus, ventromedial nucleus, anterior nucleus and lateral hypothalamic area).
  - Nucleus accumbens.
  - Septal nuclei.
  - Rostral area of the caudate nucleus and putamen.
- **Ventral amygdalofugal pathway** is the major efferent pathway of the **amygdaloid complex** and follows two main trajectories.
  - Axons from the **basolateral** cell group synapse in the hippocampus and dorsomedial nucleus of the thalamus. They also project to the cingulate gyrus, ventral striatum, and orbital, primary visual and visual association cortices.
  - Fibres from the **central nucleus** project to the hypothalamus, septal nuclei and brainstem, specifically to the dorsal motor nucleus of the vagus, raphe nucleus, locus ceruleus and periaqueductal grey matter.
  - Fibres from the **medial nucleus** project to the olfactory nuclei.
- Another tract by which the amygdala and the hippocampus influence the brainstem is the **stria medullaris thalami**, which is a connection between the **septal nuclei** and the **habenular nucleus**.

Stimulation of the amygdala, as well as the stria terminalis, induces **autonomic** and **emotional (anger, flight) responses**.

- The amygdala, as well as the orbitofrontal cortex, is involved in the **learning association** between previously neutral stimuli and primary reinforcements.
- The **corticomedial** group promotes **aggressive behaviour**, **sexual drive** and **appetite**.
  - **Hypersexuality** might occur due to stimulation of this group, but also occurs due to injury of the basolateral nuclei, which have inhibitory control over other amygdalar nuclei.
- Other sites of the amygdala may induce alertness (along with turning the head towards the stimulus), chewing, licking, salivation, gastric secretions and motility, bulimia, urination and defecation.

CLINICAL INSIGHT

- **Klüver–Bucy syndrome**
  - Occurs secondary to **bilateral amygdaloid injury**.
  - Bilateral removal of the amygdala in monkeys produces behavioural changes such as **tameness, lack of emotional responsiveness, decreased fear responses, increased and disinhibited sexual behaviour and increased oral exploration**.
  - Cerebral oedema, herpes encephalitis, Alzheimer disease and Pick disease may cause bilateral amygdaloid injury.

OLFACTORY SYSTEM: CONNECTIONS TO THE LIMBIC SYSTEM

The limbic system is connected to the **olfactory system** through the **lateral olfactory striae**, which terminate in the **cortical part of the amygdaloid body** (Fig. 15.19).

- The **olfactory receptors** are specialized, ciliated nerve cells that reside in the olfactory epithelium of the nasal cavity. Their axons form the **olfactory nerve** that enters the cranial cavity through the **cribriform plate of the ethmoid bone**.
- The olfactory nerve projects to the **olfactory bulb**, where preliminary processing of olfactory information is mediated by **large mitral cells**. The olfactory bulb is connected to the olfactory cortex by the **olfactory tract**, which is divided at the **olfactory trigone** into the **medial** and **lateral olfactory striae** (Figs. 15.4, 15.19 and 15.20).

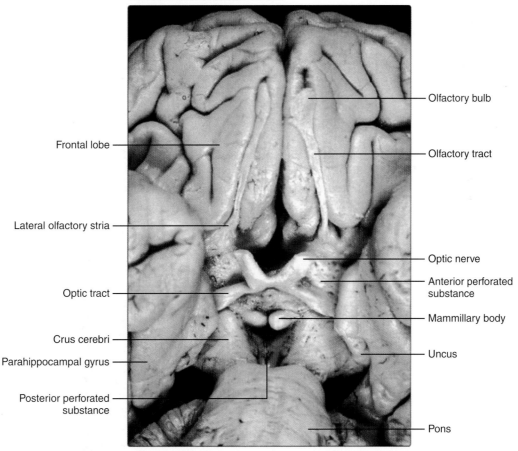

FIGURE 15.19   Ventral surface of the brain. The illustration shows the olfactory bulb and tract, the lateral olfactory stria and the primary olfactory area of the cerebral cortex (uncus).

Source: *Crossman, Alan R, PhD DSc. Hypothalamus, limbic system and olfactory system. Neuroanatomy: an ilustrated colour text. p. 160–170, Chapter 16.*

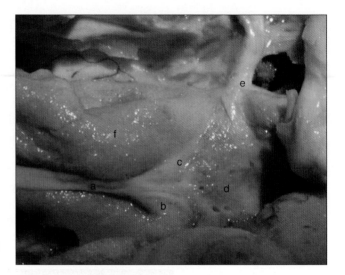

FIGURE 15.20 Photograph of the inferior surface of the brain showing the basal forebrain region: a, olfactory tract; b, lateral olfactory stria; c, medial olfactory stria; d, anterior perforated substance; e, anterior commissure; f, gyrus rectus.
Source: *Shah, Abhidha. Analysis of the anatomy of the Papez circuit and adjoining limbic system by fiber dissection techniques. J Clin Neurosci 19(2): 289–298.*

- From the olfactory bulb, all mitral cell fibres extend through the **lateral olfactory stria** to the **primary olfactory cortex in the uncus**, which is located at the inferomedial aspect of the temporal lobe. The components of the primary olfactory cortex are (Fig. 15.21):
  - Anterior perforated substance.
  - Prepiriform cortex, which is located within the ambient gyrus.
  - Periamygdalar cortex, which is located within the semilunar gyrus.
  - Superficial cortical nucleus of the amygdaloid body.
- The **prepiriform** and **periamygdalar cortices** are responsible for **conscious olfactory stimuli**.
- Fibre systems extend from the olfactory cortex to:
  - Entorhinal area.
  - Basolateral nuclei of the amygdaloid body.
  - Anterior and lateral portions of the hypothalamus.
  - Magnocellular part of the medial thalamic nuclei.

CLINICAL INSIGHT

- **Orbitofrontal cortex function and dysfunction**
  - The **orbitofrontal cortex** has representation of the reward/punishment value of many primary (unlearned) reinforcers such as taste, touch and pain, face expression, face beauty and auditory consonance.
  - **Pleasant stimuli** are represented **medially** in the orbitofrontal cortex, whereas **unpleasant stimuli** are represented **laterally**
  - Damage to the orbitofrontal cortex results in euphoria, irresponsibility, lack of affect, impulsiveness and inability to learn which stimuli are rewarding and which are not.
  - In **attention deficit hyperactivity disorder (ADHD)**, the connection between the amygdala and orbitofrontal cortex is damaged, leading to **disturbance in the perception of time** and contributing to the **behavioural disinhibition**. To compensate for this damage, the **hippocampus undergoes hypertrophy**

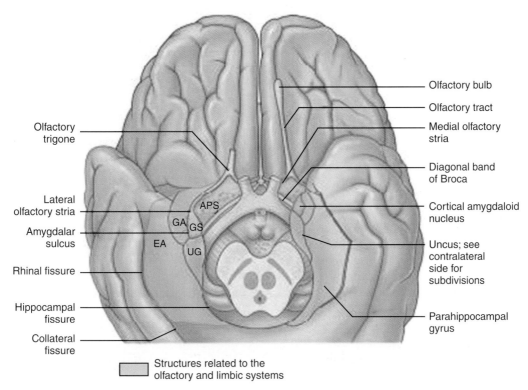

FIGURE 15.21   The inferior aspect of the brain. The brainstem has been removed and the right temporal pole has been displaced laterally to expose underlying structures. APS, anterior perforated substance; EA, entorhinal area; GA, ambient gyrus; GS, semilunar gyrus; UG, uncinate gyrus.

Source: *Standring, Susan, MBE, PhD, DSc, FKC, Hon FAS, Hon FRCS. Cerebral hemispheres. Gray's anatomy. p. 373–398.e2, Chapter 25.*

PAPEZ (MEDIAL LIMBIC) CIRCUIT (Fig. 15.22)

In 1937, James Papez proposed the **Papez circuit** in an attempt to explain the basis of **emotional experiences**. The circuit starts at the hippocampus and loops back to end where it started.

- Efferent fibres from the **hippocampus** reach the **mammillary body** through the **fornix**, which relays them to the **anterior thalamic nuclei** via the **mammillothalamic tract of Vicq d'Azyr**.
- The anterior thalamic nuclei project their fibres to the **posterior cortex of the cingulate gyrus**, which relays them to the **parahippocampal gyrus** and the **hippocampus via the cingulum**.

CLINICAL INSIGHT

- **Transient global amnesia**
  - This is a rare episodic disorder in which patients **lose memory** for a period ranging from a few to 48 hours and are **unable to learn new memories** during the episode. Although not much is known about this disorder, it is thought to be due to injuries to the **hippocampus** and **other structures of the Papez circuit.**

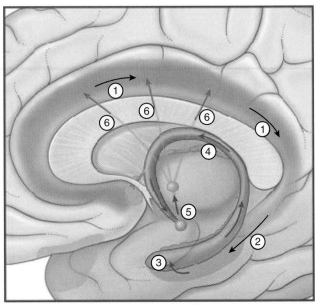

FIGURE 15.22 The Papez circuit. 1. Backward-projecting neurons in the cingulate gyrus. 2. Projection into the entorhinal cortex. 3. Projection into the hippocampus. 4. Fornix. 5. Mammillothalamic tract. 6. Projections from the anterior nucleus of the thalamus to the cingulate cortex. Source: *Mtui, Estomih, MD. Olfactory and limbic systems. Fitzgerald's clinical neuroanatomy and neuroscience.* p. 323–343, Chapter 34.

CASE STUDY DISCUSSION

Limbic encephalitis is a form of **autoimmune** encephalitis where autoantibodies attack limbic system structures. In many cases, it occurs as a **paraneoplastic syndrome**. Complete resection of the tumour is necessary to achieve cure.

Clinical Features

Symptoms develop over days to weeks and the hallmark is **short-term memory deficits**. Other symptoms include headache, irritability, sleep disturbance, seizures, delusions and hallucinations.

Investigations

CFS analysis may reveal leucocytosis, elevated protein level, elevated IgG and oligoclonal bands, but normal glucose levels.

    Brain MRI is the **cornerstone for diagnosis** and shows hyperintense signals involving the mesial temporal lobe on T2 images.

Diagnosis

The diagnosis is not straightforward and is usually delayed. The following four criteria are required to establish the diagnosis:

■ Subacute onset (<12 weeks) of seizures, short-term memory loss, confusion and psychiatric symptoms

■ Neuropathologic or radiologic evidence (MRI, single-photon emission computed tomography [SPECT], positron emission tomography [PET]) of involvement of the limbic system

■ Exclusion of other possible aetiologies of limbic dysfunction

■ Demonstration of cancer within 5 years of the diagnosis of neurologic symptoms, or the development of classic symptoms of limbic dysfunction in association with a well-characterized paraneoplastic antibody (Hu, Ma2, CV2, amphiphysin, Ri)

Treatment

The ultimate treatment is **complete resection of the tumour** if detected. Otherwise, IVIG, plasmapheresis and corticosteroid infusions may be tried.

CHAPTER 16

Autonomic Nervous System

Amanah Abraham, Mohammad Hassan A. Noureldine

CASE STUDY

Presentation and Physical Examination: A 72-year-old man presented to the neurology care unit with postural hypotension, leg stiffness and urinary incontinence. Upon interviewing the patient, he was most concerned about his urinary symptoms, which started many years ago as urinary urgencies but lately, he had become totally incontinent. Ten years earlier, he had developed impotence, which he attributed to the normal ageing process, followed by dizziness on standing with attacks of fainting similar to syncope. Few years later, he started suffering from progressive stiffness in both lower extremities, and shortly after that, he noticed respiratory abnormalities such as gasping on forced inspiration, occasional hiccupping and bursts of uncontrolled laughter. He had no family history of neurological diseases and no relevant medical history.

On examination, he had 'masked', parkinsonian facies. Cranial nerve (CN) examination was relevant for a hyperactive jaw jerk. Voluntary movements were slow and tone was increased in all four limbs causing a sustained resistance to passive movement and supportive of extrapyramidal rigidity. Cerebellar examination revealed upper extremities intentional tremor but no resting component. Deep tendon reflexes were brisk throughout with a left Babinski sign. Sensory and cognitive functions were normal.

Diagnosis, Management and Follow-Up: The approach to this unusual combination of neurological symptoms including autonomic symptoms (orthostatic hypotension, possibly impotence and urinary incontinence), extrapyramidal (parkinsonian facies, slow movements and rigidity) and pyramidal (brisk reflexes and Babinski) features, cerebellar symptoms (intention tremor) and respiratory abnormalities (stridor, hiccups) prompts us to think of a disease affecting multiple neurological systems.

Orthostatic hypotension was confirmed by asking the patient to stand up from a lying position, which was associated with a blood pressure drop from 160/100 to 80/50, with a heart rate increase from 75 to 90. Carotid massage did not lead to any significant change in heart rate. Electromyographic evaluation of the anal sphincter showed chronic denervation changes. Urodynamic testing of the bladder function displayed impaired detrusor contractility. Brain magnetic resonance imaging (MRI) revealed hyperintense T2 lesions, specifically in the pons ('hot-cross bun' sign), as well as putaminal T2 hypointensity, suggestive of a degenerative process (Fig. 16.1).

The patient was diagnosed with **multiple system atrophy (MSA)**, previously known as **Shy–Drager syndrome**, which was used to describe MSA patients with **predominant autonomic symptoms**. This term, however, is not used anymore since almost every MSA patient is affected by autonomic dysfunction.

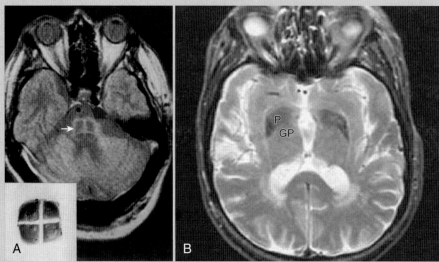

FIGURE 16.1 (A) Axial T2 magnetic resonance imaging (MRI) showing the 'hot-cross bun' sign (white arrow) in the basis pontis, suggesting pontocerebellar atrophy; compared to the actual hot cross bun in the left-hand corner. (B) Axial T2 image showing moderate putaminal (P) hypointensity relative to the globus pallidus (GP), suggesting degenerative changes.

Source: *(A) From Sitburana, Oraporn. Brain magnetic resonance imaging (MRI) in parkinsonian disorders. Parkinsonism Relat Disord 15(3): 165–174. (B) From Romero-Ortuno, Roman. Disorders of the autonomic nervous system. Brocklehurst's textbook of geriatric medicine and gerontology. p. 496–509.e4, Chapter 63.*

BRIEF INTRODUCTION

The peripheral nervous system (PNS) is functionally subdivided into somatic and autonomic systems. The autonomic nervous system (ANS) controls **autonomic** and **visceral** functions of the body and maintains its normal balance. Visceral organs such as cardiac muscle, smooth muscle (as in the gut and blood vessels) and glands function in response to **involuntary** stimuli. The **somatic system**, however, controls **voluntary** and most of the **conscious** functions such as skeletal muscle actions. In contrast to somatic motor efferent fibres that project directly onto end organs, autonomic projections from the spinal cord initially relay to autonomic ganglia located somewhere between the central nervous system (CNS) and visceral organs.

- The ANS is mainly controlled by higher centres such as the hypothalamus, brainstem nuclei, amygdala and several other regions of the limbic system.
- Autonomic responses are regulated by sensory afferent information corresponding to signals from internal receptors such as baroreceptors, chemoreceptors and osmoreceptors.
- The ANS is divided into two divisions of opposite functions: **sympathetic** and **parasympathetic**. Both innervate the same organs and function

simultaneously, but depending on the desired response, one or the other predominates and determines the final output (Fig. 16.2).

- The sympathetic nervous system (SNS) is a network of nerves that prepares the organs for **'fight or flight'** responses, i.e., **mobilization of energy**.

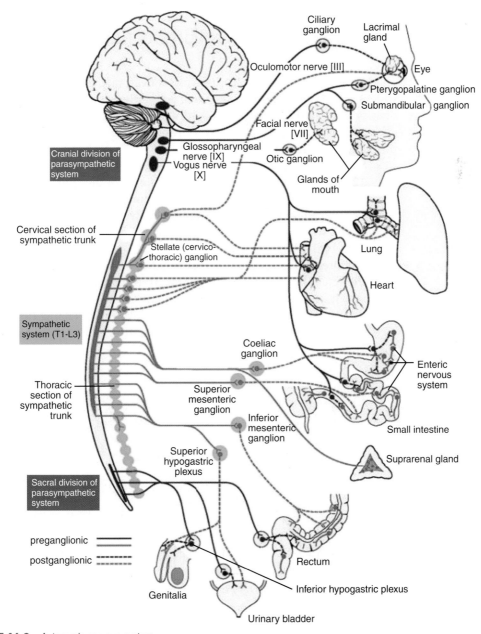

FIGURE 16.2 Autonomic nervous system.

Source: *Paulsen, F. General anatomy. Sobotta atlas of human anatomy, vol. p. 1, 1–38, Chapter 1.*

■ The parasympathetic nervous system orchestrates the vegetative **'rest and digest'** responses, i.e., **preservation of energy**.

This chapter describes the anatomy of the ANS and discusses the functions of its sympathetic and parasympathetic divisions, i.e., response of bodily organs to the activation of these divisions. Some of the relevant clinical correlations are described as well.

SYMPATHETIC/THORACOLUMBAR NERVOUS SYSTEM
(Fig. 16.2)

The **SNS** is generally **catabolic**. It increases heart rate, elevates blood pressure, widens the pupils and promotes adrenal medulla secretions. Both autonomic divisions have a distinctive **two-neuron system**, with one neuron in the CNS, giving rise to **preganglionic nerve fibres**, and one in the PNS, giving rise to **postganglionic nerve fibres**.

■ Structurally, the SNS is characterized by **preganglia** that reside in the **12 thoracic** and **upper 3 lumbar segments** of the spinal cord. Thus, the SNS is also known as the **thoracolumbar** nervous system.

■ The preganglionic neurons form distinctive lateral protrusions of grey matter within the spinal cord; these are known as the **lateral horns** (Fig. 16.3).

■ The preganglia send fibres that synapse on the ganglia of the **sympathetic chain** (also known as **paravertebral ganglia/trunk ganglia**), which lie parallel to the spinal cord and run from the upper neck down to the coccyx, where the two paravertebral chains fuse to form the **unpaired coccygeal ganglion** (ganglion of impar, ganglion of Walther).

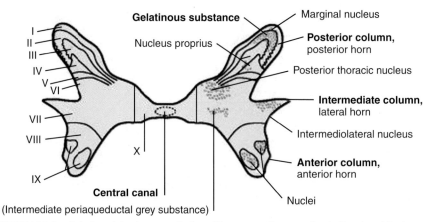

FIGURE 16.3 Spinal cord; laminar organization of the grey matter according to its cytoarchitecture [according to REXED, 1952], exemplified by the tenth thoracic segment (T10). The two lateral horns (spinal lamina VII) harbour neurons (intermediolateral nucleus) for autonomic efferents.

Source: *Paulsen, F. Brain and spinal cord. Sobotta atlas of human anatomy, vol. 3. p. 211–342, Chapter 12.*

Efferent (Motor) Pathway

- **Preganglionic sympathetic efferent pathway**
  - Preganglionic neurons reside in the grey matter of the lateral horns (T1–L3), specifically in the **intermediolateral column** that is situated in lamina VII (Fig. 16.3; *see chapter 6*), and send their fibres through the **ventral root** of the spinal cord.
  - Preganglionic fibres are mainly **myelinated** fibres; they form the **white communication rami** of thoracic and lumbar nerves (Fig. 16.4).
  - Preganglionic fibres follow one of three possible routes (Fig. 16.2):
    - Synapse on a postganglion situated at the same vertebral level.
    - Ascend or descend to synapse on another ganglion within the sympathetic chain, e.g., superior cervical, middle cervical and stellate sympathetic ganglia.
    - Pass through the ganglion chain without synapsing, form the splanchnic nerve and synapse on **prevertebral (collateral/intermediary/preaortic) ganglia**; these are the **coeliac, superior mesenteric** and **inferior mesenteric ganglia**.

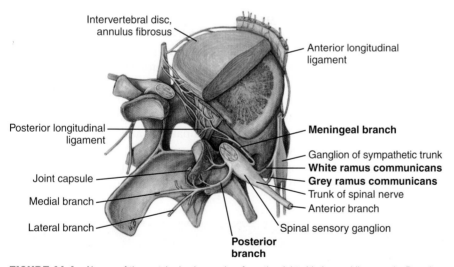

FIGURE 16.4 Nerves of the vertebral column; view from the right side in an oblique angle. Branches of the spinal nerve are shown which project to adjacent structures. These include the meningeal branch for the sensory innervation of the meningeal membranes of the spinal cord, smaller branches derived from the posterior branch for the joint capsule of the zygapophysial joints and the white and grey rami communicantes connecting with the sympathetic trunk. The white ramus communicans contains preganglionic sympathetic fibres from the lateral column of the spinal cord for the sympathetic trunk. The grey ramus communicans contains postganglionic sympathetic fibres of the sympathetic trunk, which project back to the spinal nerve. Autonomic nerve fibres from the sympathetic trunk innervate the intervertebral discs and ligaments of the vertebral column.

Source: *Paulsen, F. Trunk. Sobotta atlas of human anatomy, vol. 1. p. 39–126, Chapter 2.*

- Sympathetic fibres innervate almost every organ and tissue in the body, the segmental distribution of which proceeds as the following (Fig. 16.2):
  - T1–T4 fibres terminate in the **head**, **neck** and **thorax**.
  - T5–T12 fibres innervate the **abdomen**.
  - T10–L3 fibres supply the **legs**.
- Most preganglionic neurons utilize **acetylcholine** as their neurotransmitter but some exceptions exist.
- **Postganglionic sympathetic efferent pathway**
  - Postganglia within the paravertebral sympathetic chain extend to form the **grey communicans of rami** (Fig. 16.4).
  - The grey communicans of rami are generally **unmyelinated** fibres that join spinal nerves along their way to target organs; these fibres supply blood vessels, sweat glands and arrector pili muscles.
  - Postganglionic nerve fibres from **prevertebral ganglia** form nerves or **perivascular plexuses** that innervate the abdominal and pelvic regions.
  - An exception to the two-neuron relay system within the SNS is the adrenal gland (Fig. 16.2):
    - The preganglionic fibres pass from the intermediolateral horn cells of the spinal cord **without synapsing** on a ganglion.
    - They **synapse directly** in the **adrenal medulla/suprarenal glands** onto modified neuronal cells, which secrete epinephrine and nor-epinephrine into the bloodstream in response to stress.
  - Most sympathetic postganglionic neurons utilize **noradrenaline** as their neurotransmitter, but there are some exceptions; e.g., those innervating **sweat glands** and some **blood vessels** use **acetylcholine**.
  - It is worth mentioning that unlike most organs, **arteries** and **veins** do not have dual innervation by sympathetic and parasympathetic fibres; they **only receive sympathetic supply**.
  - The ratio of preganglionic to postganglionic sympathetic fibres is around **1:10**, which allows a **wide general sympathetic control** over the body.

CLINICAL INSIGHT

- **Pure autonomic failure (PAF)**
  - PAF is a **neurodegenerative** disease **purely** affecting the ANS.
  - While neurodegeneration in other conditions with autonomic dysfunction (such as MSA and Parkinson disease) occurs due to accumulation of alpha-synuclein in the CNS, pathologic examination shows involvement of the **intermediolateral cell column** with loss of small sympathetic neurons in PAF patients and sparing of the CNS.
  - Patients usually present with **idiopathic orthostatic hypotension**; other symptoms include **impotence** (very common in men), urinary retention, gastroparesis, angina pectoris (chest pain not related to atherosclerotic disease), decreased sweating, neck pain, fatigue and ophthalmologic disturbances.

- PAF is a diagnosis of exclusion; in the absence of other neurological conditions, these features are highly suggestive of PAF: **pronounced decrease** in blood pressure (systolic mainly) upon standing; **marked decrease** in **plasma** and **urinary catecholamine** (norepinephrine mainly, epinephrine, dopamine) levels.
- Treatment: vasopressor agents; manoeuvres to be able to keep upright position without fainting such as squatting, bending forward and crossing legs; compression stockings; increasing water intake.
- **Familial dysautonomia (Riley–Day syndrome)**
  - Is a hereditary **autosomal recessive** disorder mostly affecting Ashkenazi Jews.
  - Characterized by disruption of neurons in the **sensory**, **sympathetic** and **parasympathetic** systems.
  - Peripheral nerves have **decreased myelination** or **no myelin.**
  - Affected individuals also have **no catecholamines** (including epinephrine and norepinephrine) in their peripheral nerves.
  - Symptoms appear during infancy and include weak or absent suck reflex, hypotonia, lack of tears, delayed walking and speech, irregular body temperature, lung infections and irregular blood pressure. More symptoms appear with age; these include damage to optic nerves and loss of corneal reflex, indifference to pain and scoliosis, among others.
  - Survival rate is **low**; most patients die at infancy or early childhood.

PARASYMPATHETIC NERVOUS SYSTEM (Fig. 16.2)

Parasympathetic is derived from 'para' (meaning 'alongside') and 'sympathetic' as many of these nerves travel with sympathetic nerves.

- The ratio of preganglionic to postganglionic parasympathetic fibres is 1:4, which explains the **focused parasympathetic control** over the body, compared to the more generalized and widespread control of the sympathetic system.
- The parasympathetic activity of **'rest and digest'** involves salivation, lacrimation (tears), urination, digestion, defecation and sexual arousal. It lowers the blood pressure and heart rate, thus **preserving and restoring energy**.

Efferent (Motor) Pathway

- **Parasympathetic efferent pathway**
  - **Preganglionic** neurons reside in **brainstem nuclei** of CNs III, VII, IX, and X and **grey matter of sacral spinal segments (S2–S4)**; thus, the parasympathetic system is also known as the **craniosacral system** (Fig. 16.2).
  - **CN X (vagus nerve)** is the most prominent parasympathetic supply, giving rise to **75% of parasympathetic neurons**; these innervate numerous organs, including the heart, lungs, stomach, liver, pancreas, large intestine and small intestine, among others.
  - Preganglionic parasympathetic fibres are considerably **longer** than their sympathetic counterparts, because the **postganglia** of the parasympathetic system **lie closer to** or **within** the target organs (Fig. 16.2).

- Preganglionic as well as postganglionic neurons utilize **acetylcholine** as their neurotransmitter.
- **Cranial parasympathetic system**
  - **Oculomotor nerve (CN III)** (Fig. 16.2)
    - Fibres originate from the **accessory oculomotor (Edinger–Westphal) nucleus** and project onto the **ciliary ganglion,** which in turn extends its postganglionic fibres to the ciliary muscle and sphincter of the pupil, producing the accommodation reflex.
  - **Facial nerve (CN VII)** (Fig. 16.2)
    - Preganglionic fibres originate from the **superior salivatory nucleus** and project onto the **pterygopalatine** and **submandibular ganglia.**
    - Postganglionic fibres from the pterygopalatine ganglion extend to the lacrimal gland and mucosa of the nasal cavity, whereas those from the submandibular ganglion supply the submandibular and sublingual glands.
  - **Glossopharyngeal nerve (CN IX)** (Fig. 16.2)
    - Preganglionic fibres originate from the **inferior salivatory nucleus** and project onto the **otic ganglion,** which innervates the parotid gland.
  - **Vagus nerve (CN X)** (Fig. 16.2)
    - Preganglionic fibres originate from the **dorsal motor nucleus** and project onto the **intramural ganglia,** which innervate the viscera of the thorax and abdomen.
    - Another set of preganglionic fibres originate from the **nucleus ambiguus,** which projects onto the **intramural ganglia** of the heart and other organs. Within the heart, preganglionic fibres synapse onto the **sinoatrial (SA)** and **atrioventricular (AV) nodes.**
    - Effects of vagal stimulation include:
      - Heart: decreases heart rate.
      - Lungs: constricts bronchioles.
      - Gall bladder: excretes bile.
      - Stomach: secretes digestive enzymes.
      - Intestines: increases peristaltic movements and relaxes sphincters, allowing defecation.
- **Sacral parasympathetic system**
  - Preganglionic neurons reside in the spinal cord at **S2–S4 spinal segments** (Fig. 16.2).
  - Preganglionic fibres extend to S2–S4 spinal nerves through the sacral foramina, and then synapse onto autonomic ganglia situated near or within the target organ; these postganglia are known as **intramural ganglia/terminal ganglia.**
  - Sacral parasympathetic activity
    - Large intestines: relaxes sphincters.
    - Bladder: relaxes urethral sphincter and facilitates smooth muscle contraction of bladder wall (urine excretion).
    - Genitalia: penile and clitoral erection.

> **CLINICAL INSIGHT**
>
> ■ **SLUDGE syndrome**
>   - ■ SLUDGE stands for **S**alivation, **L**acrimation, **U**rination, **D**efecation, **G**astrointestinal motility and **E**mesis.
>   - ■ **Phosphorylation of acetylcholinesterase** by nerve gas, pesticides, some poisonous mushrooms or an overdose of cholinergic medications causes excessive stimulation of the parasympathetic system, the result of which is **SLUDGE syndrome.**

Table 16.1 summarizes the key characteristics of the sympathetic and parasympathetic systems.

ORGAN-SPECIFIC AUTONOMIC PATHWAYS AND EFFECTS (Fig. 16.2)

Eyes

- ■ Sympathetic:
  - ■ The **hypothalamic paraventricular nucleus** relays information to the **ciliospinal centre of Budge** in the intermediolateral cell column at **T1–T2 spinal segments**.
  - ■ Preganglionic fibres of the ciliospinal centre of Budge cross through the sympathetic chain and synapse onto the **superior cervical ganglion (SCG)**, which is part of the cervical plexus.
  - ■ The SCG extends postganglionic fibres around the internal carotid artery to form the internal carotid plexus.
  - ■ The internal carotid plexus carries **postganglionic** axons to the eye, lacrimal gland, mucous membranes of the mouth, nose and pharynx and numerous blood vessels in the head (Fig. 16.5).
  - ■ The ultimate effect is **vasoconstriction, pupillary dilation and decreased production of tears.**

Table 16.1 Summary of the key characteristics of the sympathetic and parasympathetic systems

	Sympathetic System	**Parasympathetic System**
Function	'Fight or flight' response	'Rest and digest' response
Origin/Location	Thoracolumbar (T1–L3 spinal segments)	Craniosacral (CNs III, VII, IX and X nuclei; S2–S4 spinal segments)
Location of ganglia	Closer to CNS	Closer to effector organs
Preganglionic fibres	Short	Long
Postganglionic fibres	Long	Short
Preganglionic neurotransmitter	Acetylcholine	Acetylcholine
Postganglionic neurotransmitter	Noradrenaline	Acetylcholine

Notes: *CNs, cranial nerves; CNS, central nervous system.*

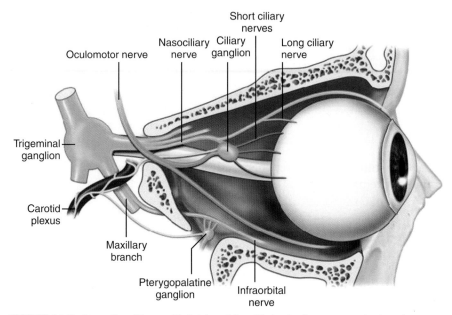

FIGURE 16.5   Innervation of the eye. Medial view of the orbit showing the sensory and autonomic nerves directed to the eye. The ophthalmic branch of the trigeminal ganglion gives the nasociliary nerve that sends long and short ciliary nerves to the eyeball, the last through the ciliary ganglion. Frontal and lacrimal nerves are not shown in this picture. The trigeminal maxillary branch gives the infraorbital nerve that innervates part of the eye and the lower lid. Sympathetic fibres from the superior cervical ganglion, travelling within the carotid plexus and parasympathetic branches of the ciliary and the pterygopalatine ganglia join short ciliary nerves. Source: *Adapted from Rubin M, Safdieh JE. Netter's concise neuroanatomy. Elsevier; 2007.*

- **Parasympathetic:**
  - The preganglionic **accessory oculomotor (Edinger–Westphal) nucleus** in the midbrain sends fibres along the **oculomotor nerve (CN III).**
  - Preganglionic fibres project onto the **ciliary ganglion**, which is located behind the eye.
  - The ciliary ganglion projects its postganglionic fibres via the **short ciliary nerve** to the sphincter muscle/pupillary sphincter of the iris, which **constricts the pupil,** and to the ciliary muscles/ciliaris, which **changes the shape of the lens** during accommodation (Fig. 16.5).

Heart

- **Sympathetic** (Fig. 16.6):
  - Preganglionic neurons in the **intermediolateral cell column (T1–T4)** relay to the **upper thoracic** and **cervical ganglia** within the sympathetic chain.
  - Postganglionic information is carried through the **cardiac nerve.**
  - The cardiac nerve synapses onto the atrial and ventricular walls as well as to the **SA** and **AV nodes**, leading to an **increase in heart rate** and **stronger myocardial contractions.**

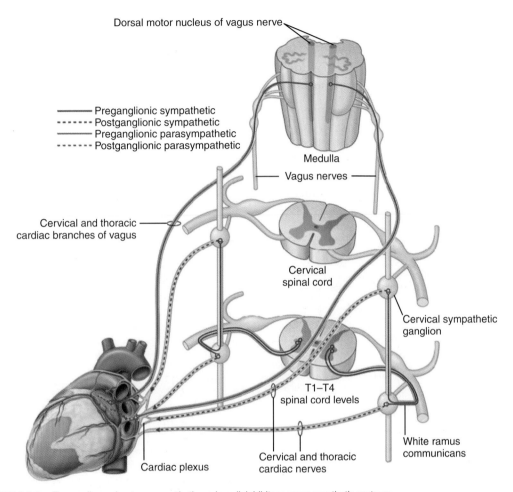

Dorsal motor nucleus of vagus nerve

—— Preganglionic sympathetic
······ Postganglionic sympathetic
—— Preganglionic parasympathetic
------ Postganglionic parasympathetic

Medulla

Vagus nerves

Cervical and thoracic
cardiac branches of vagus

Cervical
spinal cord

Cervical sympathetic
ganglion

T1–T4
spinal cord levels

White ramus
communicans

Cardiac plexus

Cervical and thoracic
cardiac nerves

FIGURE 16.6 The cardioacceleratory sympathetic and cardioinhibitory parasympathetic systems.
Source: *Reproduced with permission from Martini FH, Nath JL. Fundamentals of anatomy and physiology. 8th ed. San Francisco, CA: Pearson; 2008.*

- **Parasympathetic (**Fig. 16.6**):**
  - The preganglionic **nucleus ambiguus** sends its fibres through the **vagus nerve (CN X)** to the **intramural postganglia**, which in turn send fibres that synapse onto the **SA and AV nodes**.
  - Parasympathetic stimuli lead to **lower heart rate** and **weaker myocardial contractions**, promoting a restful state.

Lungs
- **Sympathetic:**
  - Preganglionic neurons synapse onto the **sympathetic trunk at T1–T4 vertebral levels**, are carried by the **pulmonary plexus** and then extend to the lungs, causing **bronchodilation** and **vasoconstriction**.

- **Parasympathetic:**
  - Preganglionic fibres arise from the **dorsal motor nucleus of the vagus** and project onto **postganglia in the pulmonary plexus,** which in turn send postganglionic fibres to the lungs, causing **bronchoconstriction, vasodilation** and **increased secretions.**

Bladder (Fig. 16.7)

- **Sympathetic:**
  - Fibres from **L1 to L3 spinal segments** extend to the **hypogastric** and **mesenteric plexuses,** which supply the internal sphincter and detrusor (bladder wall) muscles.

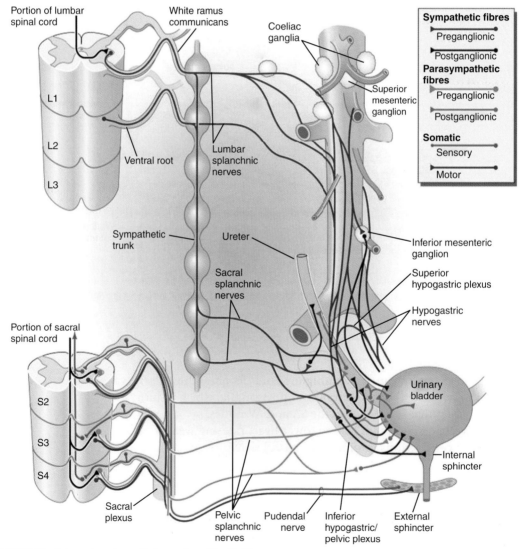

FIGURE 16.7 Autonomic and somatic innervation of the bladder.

Source: *Giebisch, Gerhard. Organization of the urinary system. Medical physiology. p. 722–738.e1, Chapter 33.*

- Distortion to the bladder's sympathetic system **does not cause a significant effect** because the bladder is **predominantly controlled by parasympathetic stimuli.**
- **Parasympathetic:**
  - **S2–S3 preganglia** extend their fibres through the **pelvic splanchnic nerve.**
  - The pelvic splanchnic nerve synapses onto the internal sphincter and detrusor (bladder wall) muscles, causing the **bladder to empty** by **contracting** the **detrusor and relaxing** the **internal sphincter muscles.**

CLINICAL INSIGHTS

- **Atonic bladder**
  - Injury to the **parasympathetic pathway** of the bladder leads to **atonic bladder.**
  - It is characterized by **overflow incontinence** (involuntary urination due to loss of urge to urinate).
  - It occurs **immediately after spinal injury** and may last from few days to several weeks.
- **Automatic reflex bladder**
  - It occurs **after the patient has recovered from a spinal cord shock** (due to any type of injury).
  - The area of injury **lies above the parasympathetic area (S2–S4).**
  - There is **no voluntary control** over the bladder; the bladder fills and empties due to **reflex**, similar to an infant's bladder.
  - Stretch receptors in the bladder wall relay messages to S2–S4 centres; these respond back and the bladder muscle contracts and the sphincter relaxes, leading to an **automatic reflex every 1–4 h.**
- **Autonomous bladder**
  - It is due to injury of the **sacral segments (S2–S4) of the spinal cord.**
  - It causes **loss of voluntary** and **reflex control** over the bladder.
  - The bladder becomes **flaccid** and its capacity increases.
  - The bladder is **manually emptied** (only partially) by manual compression over abdominal wall.

Genitalia (Fig. 16.2)

- **Sympathetic:**
  - **L1–L3 preganglionic** fibres pass through the sympathetic chain ganglia and synapse onto **pelvic ganglia** within the **superior hypogastric plexus,** which sends postganglionic fibres to the penis, leading to **vasoconstriction** and **loss of erection.**
  - **Postganglionic** fibres also synapse on the vas deferens, seminal vesicles and prostate, causing **smooth muscle contraction** and **ejaculation** in males.
- **Parasympathetic:**
  - **Preganglionic** fibres from **S2 to S4 spinal segments** synapse onto **ganglia of the inferior hypogastric plexuses.**
  - **Postganglionic** fibres synapse onto pudendal arteries within the erectile tissues of the penis and clitoris, causing **vasodilation** and **erection.**

> **CLINICAL INSIGHT**
>
> - **Erectile and ejaculation dysfunction**
>   - Injury to spinal segments **directly above S2** leads to loss of erection and ejaculation.
>   - Spontaneous or reflex erection and spontaneous ejaculation may occur after recovery if **S2–S4 spinal segments were not affected** by the injury.

Uterus

- Sympathetic:
  - **Lower lumbar preganglionic** fibres synapse onto the **sympathetic chain** and possibly onto the **inferior mesenteric/hypogastric series of plexuses**, from which **postganglionic** fibres arise and pass through the **uterovaginal plexus** to synapse onto the **uterus**, leading to uterine **contraction** and **vasoconstriction**.
- Parasympathetic:
  - **Preganglionic** fibres from **S2 to S4 spinal segments** extend through the pelvic splanchnic nerves and synapse onto the **pelvic ganglia**; **postganglionic** projections synapse onto the **uterus**, causing **relaxation** and **vasodilation**.

ENTERIC NERVOUS SYSTEM (Fig. 16.2)

The **enteric nervous system (ENS)** was historically considered as a third subdivision of the ANS. Today, it is recognized as a system that can function independent of the CNS, although it receives modulations from the CNS to a certain extent. Thus, it is known as the 'gut brain' or 'intrinsic nervous system of the gastrointestinal (GI) tract'.

- It contains an estimated **100 million neurons.**
- ENS neurons are surrounded by neuroglia-like cells that are comparable to astrocytes of the CNS.
- It regulates peristaltic movements, gland secretions, water and ion transfer, local blood flow to the GI tract, as well as some functions of the pancreas and gall bladder.
- It is modulated by the parasympathetic and sympathetic systems.
- **Parasympathetic** pathways regulate the upper GI tract through the **vagus nerve** and the **lower colon and rectum** through the **sacral nerves (S2–S4)** (Fig. 16.2).
- **Parasympathetic** inputs **relax sphincters** and **promote peristaltic movements** and **secretions.**
- **Sympathetic** pathways originate from **T5 to T12 spinal segments**, pass through the paravertebral ganglia without synapsing and terminate on the **prevertebral splanchnic ganglia** (coeliac, superior and inferior mesenteric ganglia) (Fig. 16.2).
- Coeliac, superior and inferior mesenteric **postganglionic** fibres terminate on smooth muscles of intestines and blood vessels.

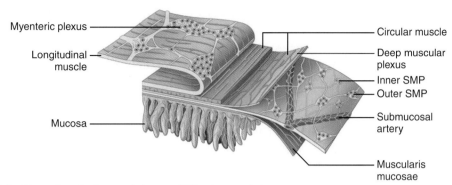

FIGURE 16.8 Myenteric and submucosal plexuses. SMP, submucosal plexus.

Source: *Redrawn with permission from Furness JB. The enteric nervous system and neurogastroenterology. Nat Rev Gastroenterol Hepatol 2012;9:286–294. Reprinted with permission from Nature Publishing Group.*

- **Sympathetic postganglionic** projections also terminate on parasympathetic nerves and are thought to **inhibit the parasympathetic activity**, thus:
  - **Inducing sphincter contractions**.
  - **Inhibiting peristaltic movements**.
  - **Inhibiting secretions**.
- Disruption of connections between the CNS and ENS leads to:
  - Little or no impairment in the functions of small and large intestines.
  - **Significant impairment** in the functions of **oesophagus and stomach**, which rely more on the ANS innervation; thus, an intact connection between the CNS and ENS is important for proper functioning of the upper digestive system.
- **Afferent** enteric fibres project to the CNS via the **vagus** and **splanchnic nerves**.

Enteric Plexuses (Fig. 16.8)

The ENS is made up of **two plexuses** that extend throughout the GI tract, **from the oesophagus to the rectum**. These plexuses are:
- **Myenteric (Auerbach's) plexus:**
  - That is located between the **outer longitudinal** and **inner circular muscle layers**.
  - Innervates nearly the **entire GI tract**.
  - Regulates **smooth muscle contractions** (movements of the gut walls).
- **Submucosal (Meissner's) plexus:**
  - Lies between the **mucosal** and **circular muscle layers**.
  - **Is absent** or **near absent** in the **oesophagus** and **stomach**.
  - Regulates **mucous membrane glandular secretions** and **blood flow**.

AUTONOMIC AFFERENT PATHWAY (Fig. 16.9)

Unlike the efferent autonomic pathways, **afferent** pathways **are not subdivided** into sympathetic and parasympathetic parts and relay information in the opposite direction: from organs and other parts of the body to the CNS.

- **Visceral pain** and other sensations such as hunger, nausea and smooth muscle stretch are transduced from the heart, upper GI tract, and kidneys through **thoracic** and **upper lumbar nerves** to the spinal cord, through which they are finally carried to the hypothalamus.
- **Sensory stimuli** from the pelvic organs, which help regulate sexual responses, micturition (voluntary urination) and defecation, pass through the **sacral nerves** to reach the spinal cord, through which they are carried to the hypothalamus.

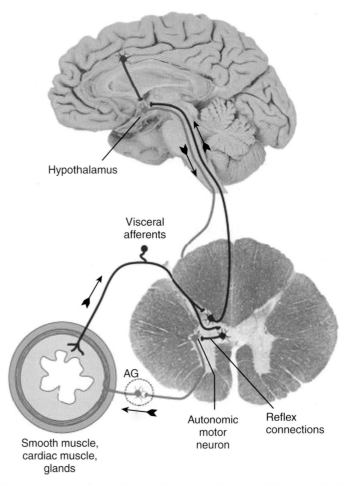

Hypothalamus

Visceral afferents

AG

Smooth muscle, cardiac muscle, glands

Autonomic motor neuron

Reflex connections

FIGURE 16.9 Autonomic afferents. The hypothalamus receives much of the ascending information and is a major source of descending pathways. Autonomic transmission to the periphery involves an intermediate synapse in an autonomic ganglion (AG).

Source: *Vanderah, Todd W., PhD. Spinal Cord. Nolte's the human brain. p. 233–271, Chapter 10.*

CLINICAL INSIGHT

- **Referred pain**
  - Somatic pain may merge with autonomic pain and cause **referred pain**. For example, myocardial ischaemia is accompanied with left arm pain or throat pain.
  - Referred pain occurs when pain fibres from a visceral organ and a specific dermatome enter the CNS at the **same spinal segment level**. The perception of pain is mistakenly attributed to a somatic area whose pain fibres enter the same spinal segment, whereas, in fact, the visceral organ is the source of pain.
- **Cardiovascular reflexes**
  - **Baroreceptors** in the aortic arch and carotid sinuses detect blood pressure changes and initiate the **baroreflex/baroreceptor reflex**. As blood pressure increases, baroreceptors in the carotid sinuses and aortic arch detect the changes and relay them to the CNS through afferent fibres in the glossopharyngeal nerve (CN IX) and vagus nerve (CN X), respectively.
  - Afferent fibres from both receptors project onto the **nucleus of the solitary tract (NTS)** in the brainstem
  - The NTS relays information to both the parasympathetic and sympathetic systems:
    - **Parasympathetic**: Fibres from the NTS synapse onto the **nucleus ambiguus** and dorsal nucleus of vagus nerve, **slowing** the heart rate.
    - **Sympathetic**: Fibres from the NTS synapse onto the **caudal ventrolateral medulla (CVLM)**, which inhibits the rostral ventrolateral medulla (RVLM), a central generator of sympathetic activity. Thus, the sympathetic outflow to the heart **is inhibited**, leading to a **decrease in blood pressure.**

CASE STUDY DISCUSSION

MSA is an **adult-onset, neurodegenerative disorder** that progresses insidiously over several years with **multiple neurological systems** involvement manifesting as a peculiar combination of signs/symptoms including, but not limited to, autonomic, pyramidal, extrapyramidal and cerebellar features.

Pathophysiology

The exact pathophysiological mechanism is not elucidated yet. However, histopathological studies demonstrated **accumulation of alpha-synuclein** inside glial cells, accompanied by loss of cells in different CNS sites such as the **nigrostriatal** and **olivopontocerebellar** structures, leading to the **parkinsonian** and **cerebellar** manifestations, as well as the progressive loss of **intermediolateral column** cells in the spinal cord, which is responsible for the **autonomic** symptoms. Thus, MSA is classified as a primary alpha-synucleinopathy.

Clinical Features

Given that MSA involves several neurological systems, the following list summarizes most of its clinical features according to the affected system:

- **Autonomic**: Erectile dysfunction, genitourinary dysfunction (incontinence or retention), severe orthostatic hypotension, postprandial hypotension, supine hypertension.
- **Extrapyramidal**: Akinesia, rigidity and stiffness, tremor (resting or 'pill-rolling'), decreased or absent response to levodopa.
- **Pyramidal**: Babinski sign, hyperreflexia, motor abnormalities.
- **Cerebellar**: Gait and limb ataxia, tremor (intention), dysarthria, nystagmus.

Prognosis

Prognosis of MSA is **very poor** as the disease **progresses rapidly** and current treatment is only **symptomatic**.

- Treatment to reverse or stop the progression of the disease is not available yet.
- Median age of survival **6–10 years.**
- Shorter duration of survival is associated with older age of onset.